Atypical Breast Proliferative Lesions and Benign Breast Disease

Farin Amersi • Kristine Calhoun
Editors

Atypical Breast Proliferative Lesions and Benign Breast Disease

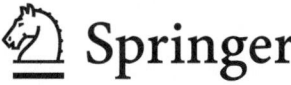

Editors
Farin Amersi
Samuel Oschin Comprehensive Cancer Inst
Cedars-Sinai Medical Center
Los Angeles, CA
USA

Kristine Calhoun
School of Medicine
University of Washington School
of Medicine
Seattle, WA
USA

ISBN 978-3-030-06482-2   ISBN 978-3-319-92657-5 (eBook)
https://doi.org/10.1007/978-3-319-92657-5

© Springer International Publishing AG, part of Springer Nature 2018
Softcover re-print of the Hardcover 1st edition 2018
This work is subject to copyright. All rights are reserved by the Publisher, whether the whole or part of the material is concerned, specifically the rights of translation, reprinting, reuse of illustrations, recitation, broadcasting, reproduction on microfilms or in any other physical way, and transmission or information storage and retrieval, electronic adaptation, computer software, or by similar or dissimilar methodology now known or hereafter developed.
The use of general descriptive names, registered names, trademarks, service marks, etc. in this publication does not imply, even in the absence of a specific statement, that such names are exempt from the relevant protective laws and regulations and therefore free for general use.
The publisher, the authors, and the editors are safe to assume that the advice and information in this book are believed to be true and accurate at the date of publication. Neither the publisher nor the authors or the editors give a warranty, express or implied, with respect to the material contained herein or for any errors or omissions that may have been made. The publisher remains neutral with regard to jurisdictional claims in published maps and institutional affiliations.

This Springer imprint is published by the registered company Springer Nature Switzerland AG
The registered company address is: Gewerbestrasse 11, 6330 Cham, Switzerland

Preface

The management of atypical breast lesions continues to evolve and become more complex. The days of surgical excision for any atypical lesion have been replaced by more nuanced decision making and individualized patient management. There is considerable controversy as to whether entities such as papillomas, radial scars, fibroepithelial lesions, pseudoangiomatous stromal hyperplasia (PASH), flat epithelial atypia (FEA), atypical ductal and lobular hyperplasia (ADH and ALH), lobular carcinoma in situ (LCIS), and ductal carcinoma in situ (DCIS) represent risk factors for future breast cancer or whether they are instead obligate precursor lesions that will themselves transform into malignancy. A better understanding of the prognostic and therapeutic implications of each of these lesions once diagnosed is important for assessing subsequent individual breast cancer risk. Risk assessment tools are available for screening high risk patients, and understanding the utility and limitations of these tools is important for all clinicians involved in the care of breast patients.

There have been significant advances in breast cancer screening in the last several years, including the addition of breast tomosynthesis to 2D mammogram, automated breast ultrasound, molecular imaging, as well as accelerated breast MRI protocols. This has led us to question whether women at risk for breast cancer need additional breast cancer screening using these newer imaging modalities or if standard mammography plus or minus MRI is sufficient. In addition, with these advances in imaging, many wonder if women with atypical proliferative lesions once diagnosed on pathologic analysis can be observed rather than proceed on to surgical excision. The role of observation, surgical excision, and even prophylactic mastectomy in women with atypical proliferative lesions continues to be debated; however, there is data that can guide physicians in the management of these complex patients.

Although sharing the terminology of in situ lesions, LCIS and DCIS are currently managed quite differently. LCIS in general is deemed a risk lesion, although a variant, pleomorphic lobular carcinoma in situ (PLCIS) is a distinct pathological entity within LCIS often managed much more like DCIS, despite limited natural history data and no clear consensus regarding surgical margins or the need for adjuvant treatment to prevent recurrence. Recently, ductal carcinoma in situ (DCIS) has been the subject of much controversy regarding whether it is truly a cancer or is instead best described as a precursor lesion. The traditional management of DCIS with surgery (lumpectomy and radiation versus mastectomy) is now being debated and recent data demonstrates that low-grade DCIS can be managed in nontraditional ways. Clinical trials are actively accruing patients with low- and intermediate-grade DCIS to observation and close surveillance instead of surgical excision. Finally, new guidelines for chemoprevention, as well as new agents in addition to traditional tamoxifen and raloxifen for women with atypical proliferative lesions, LCIS, PLCIS, and DCIS, are available and should be discussed as an option when guiding management of these patients.

The goal of this book is to provide a comprehensive review of atypical breast proliferative lesions and their management complexities. We hope it will serve as a valuable resource for nurse practitioners, physician assistants, breast and surgical oncology fellows, genetics counselors, geneticists, as well as other clinicians and surgeons who are referred and manage these complex breast patients. All chapters have been written by experts in the field who have research and clinical interest in each of these disease entities, and we the editors thank them for their willingness to contribute to an aspect of breast care that is less robustly discussed than malignancy. We hope that you learn much from their input and appreciate the opportunity to contribute to the growing information regarding atypical breast proliferative lesions. Thank you and enjoy.

Los Angeles, CA, USA Farin Amersi
Seattle, WA, USA Kristine Calhoun

Contents

1   **The Spectrum of Risk Lesions in Breast Pathology: Risk Factors or Cancer Precursors?** 1
Kimberly Allison and Kelly Mooney

2   **Lobular Carcinoma In Situ: Risk Factor or Cancer Precursor?** 21
Kevin M. Sullivan, Meghan R. Flanagan, Mark R. Kilgore, and Benjamin O. Anderson

3   **Ductal Carcinoma In Situ: Risk Factor or Cancer** 37
Nicci Owusu-Brackett and Funda Meric-Bernstam

4   **Diagnostic Management of Papillomas, Radial Scars, and Flat Epithelial Atypia: Core Biopsy Alone Versus Core Biopsy Plus Excision** 51
George Z. Li, Beth T. Harrison, and Faina Nakhlis

5   **Diagnostic Management of Fibroepithelial Lesions: When Is Excision Indicated?** 63
Nicholas Manguso and Catherine Dang

6   **Diagnostic Management of the Atypical Hyperplasias: Core Biopsy Alone Versus Excisional Biopsy** 79
Emily Siegel and Alice Chung

7   **Diagnostic Management of LCIS: Core Biopsy Alone Versus Core Biopsy plus Excision for Classic Versus Pleomorphic LCIS** 89
Batul Al-zubeidy and Nora Hansen

8   **Breast Cancer Risk Prediction in Women with Atypical Breast Lesions** 103
Suzanne B. Coopey and Kevin S. Hughes

9   **Advanced Screening Options and Surveillance in Women with Atypical Breast Lesions** 115
Erin Crane, Nicole Sondel Lewis, Erini Makariou, Janice Jeon, Judy Song, and Charlotte Dillis

10	**The Role of Chemoprevention in the Prevention of Breast Cancer** 129
	Jinny Gunn, E. Alexa Elder, and Sarah McLaughlin
11	**Prophylactic Mastectomy in Patients with Atypical Breast Lesions** 147
	Judy C. Boughey and Amy C. Degnim
12	**The Nonsurgical Management of Ductal Carcinoma In Situ (DCIS)** 159
	Alastair M. Thompson
13	**Surgical Treatment of Ductal Carcinoma In Situ** 171
	Meghan R. Flanagan and Kimberly J. Van Zee

Index 193

Contributors

E. Alexa Elder, MD Department of Surgery, Mayo Clinic, Jacksonville, FL, USA

Kimberly Allison, MD Department of Pathology, Stanford University, School of Medicine, Palo Alto, CA, USA

Batul Al-zubeidy, MD Lynn Sage Comprehensive Breast Center, Chicago, IL, USA

Benjamin O. Anderson, MD Department of Surgery, University of Washington, Seattle, WA, USA

Departments of Surgery and Global Health, University of Washington, Seattle, WA, USA

Surgery and Global Health Medicine, University of Washington, Seattle, WA, USA

Judy C. Boughey, MD Department of Surgery, Mayo Clinic, Rochester, MN, USA

Alice Chung, MD Cedars-Sinai Medical Center, Los Angeles, CA, USA

Suzanne B. Coopey, MD Division of Surgical Oncology, Massachusetts General Hospital, Boston, MA, USA

Erin Crane, MD Department of Radiology, Medstar Georgetown University Hospital, Washington, DC, USA

Catherine Dang, MD Cedars-Sinai Medical Center, Department of Surgery, Los Angeles, CA, USA

Amy C. Degnim, MD, FACS Department of Surgery, Mayo Clinic, Rochester, MN, USA

Charlotte Dillis, MD Department of Radiology, Medstar Georgetown University Hospital, Washington, DC, USA

Meghan R. Flanagan, MD, MPH Breast Service, Department of Surgery, Memorial Sloan Kettering Cancer Center, New York, NY, USA

Jinny Gunn, MD Department of Surgery, Mayo Clinic, Jacksonville, FL, USA

Nora Hansen, MD Lynn Sage Comprehensive Breast Center, Chicago, IL, USA

Beth T. Harrison, MD Department of Pathology, Brigham and Women's Hospital, Boston, MA, USA

Kevin S. Hughes, MD Division of Surgical Oncology, Massachusetts General Hospital, Boston, MA, USA

Janice Jeon, MD Department of Radiology, Medstar Georgetown University Hospital, Washington, DC, USA

Mark R. Kilgore, MD, FASCP, FCAP Department of Pathology, University of Washington, Seattle, WA, USA

Nicole Sondel Lewis, MD Department of Radiology, Medstar Georgetown University Hospital, Washington, DC, USA

George Z. Li, MD Department of Surgery, Brigham and Women's Hospital, Boston, MA, USA

Erini Makariou, MD Department of Radiology, Medstar Georgetown University Hospital, Washington, DC, USA

Nicholas Manguso, MD Cedars-Sinai Medical Center, Department of Surgery, Los Angeles, CA, USA

Sarah McLaughlin, MD Department of Surgery, Mayo Clinic, Jacksonville, FL, USA

Section of Surgical Oncology, Jacksonville, FL, USA

Funda Meric-Bernstam, MD Department of Surgical Oncology, The University of Texas MD Anderson Cancer Center, Houston, TX, USA

Department of Breast Surgical Oncology, The University of Texas MD Anderson Cancer Center, Houston, TX, USA

Department of Investigational Cancer Therapeutics (Phase I Clinical Trials Program), The University of Texas MD Anderson Cancer Center, Houston, TX, USA

Institute of Personalized Cancer Therapy, The University of Texas MD Anderson Cancer Center, Houston, TX, USA

Kelly Mooney, MD Department of Pathology, Stanford University, School of Medicine, Palo Alto, CA, USA

Faina Nakhlis Department of Surgery, Brigham and Women's Hospital, Boston, MA, USA

Nicci Owusu-Brackett, MD Department of Surgical Oncology, The University of Texas MD Anderson Cancer Center, Houston, TX, USA

Emily Siegel, MD Cedars-Sinai Medical Center, Los Angeles, CA, USA

Judy Song, MD Department of Radiology, Medstar Georgetown University Hospital, Washington, DC, USA

Kevin M. Sullivan, MD Department of Surgery, University of Washington, Seattle, WA, USA

Alastair M. Thompson, ALCM, BSc, MBChB, MD, FRCSEd Department of Breast Surgical Oncology, University of Texas MD Anderson Cancer Center, Houston, TX, USA

Kimberly J. Van Zee, MS, MD Breast Service, Department of Surgery, Memorial Sloan Kettering Cancer Center, New York, NY, USA

The Spectrum of Risk Lesions in Breast Pathology: Risk Factors or Cancer Precursors?

Kimberly Allison and Kelly Mooney

Abbreviations

ADH   Atypical ductal hyperplasia
ALH   Atypical lobular hyperplasia
DCIS Ductal carcinoma in situ
ER   Estrogen receptor
FEA   Flat epithelial atypia
FEL   Fibroepithelial lesion
RS   Radial scar

Terminology, Definitions, and Implications Relevant to Risk Lesions of the Breast

The category of "risk lesions" in breast pathology encompasses a wide variety of entities with incompletely characterized malignant potential, such as atypical ductal hyperplasia (ADH), atypical lobular hyperplasia (ALH), flat epithelial atypia (FEA), radial scar (RS), papillary lesions, and fibroepithelial lesions (FELs) [1, 2]. When identified as the worst lesion on a core needle biopsy sample, these entities each have a potential to "upgrade" to invasive carcinoma or carcinoma in situ on excision if an adjacent ductal carcinoma in situ (DCIS) or invasive carcinoma was not initially sampled [3, 4]. The upgrade rate of these lesions when identified on core biopsy is the focus of other chapters in this text (see Chaps. 4, 5, 6, and 7). This chapter focuses on the evidence regarding the overall lifetime risk of developing breast cancer associated with a diagnosis of ADH, ALH, FEA, RS, papillary lesions,

K. Allison (✉) · K. Mooney
Department of Pathology, Stanford University, School of Medicine, Palo Alto, CA, USA
e-mail: allisonk@stanford.edu; kelmoon@stanford.edu

and FELs, in addition to presenting knowledge regarding their role as possible precursor lesions for breast carcinoma.

A seminal review published in 1985, and updated in 1998, defined terms for nonmalignant breast lesions and presented their associated relative risks for future development of breast carcinoma, including a relative risk of 1.5–2.0-fold for complex fibroadenomas and papillomas, 4–5-fold for ADH and ALH, and 8–10-fold for ductal and lobular carcinoma in situ in either breast [5]. Numerous papers have published similar rates since, with a more recent retrospective review of over 14,000 cases showing that nearly 5% of women with atypia or LCIS were diagnosed with breast cancer in under 5 years compared to fewer than 1% of those with negative mammograms [6–8]. These reviews generally reported future risk of carcinoma developing in either breast. In contrast, other studies explored how these lesions could be clonal processes that could behave as non-obligate *precursors* with the potential to transform into cancers locally, with an ipsilateral risk of invasive cancer development (Fig. 1.1).

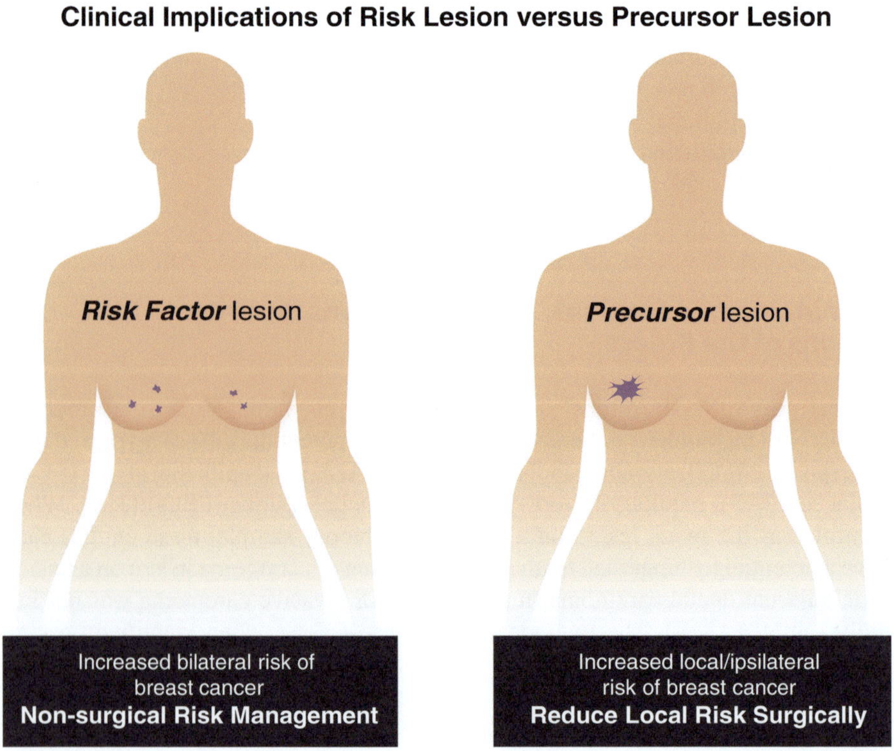

Fig. 1.1 Clinical implications of precursor versus risk factor lesions. This figure depicts the difference between a risk factor lesion and non-obligate precursor lesion, highlighting how risk factor lesions increase the risk of breast cancer developing in either breast (bilateral risk), while precursor lesions increase the risk of locoregional (ipsilateral) cancer and are amenable to surgical resection

The concept of precursor lesions of the breast was introduced as early as 1829, when Sir Astley Paston Cooper described a "nonmalignant category [of lesions]" and how "their extirpation may be rendered necessary; for malignancy may be lighted up in them" [9]. In 1975, Wellings published a morphologic description of the progression from the normal terminal duct lobular unit to invasive cancer, including "precancerous lesions" [10]. More recent advances in immunohistochemistry and genomics have refined our understanding of precursor lesions, particularly studies demonstrating shared genetic alterations in precursor alterations and breast carcinomas and supporting the concept of the non-obligate precursor [11, 12].

It is important to underscore that clonal neoplastic lesions may behave clinically either as a local (ipsilateral) risk factor for direct invasion ("non-obligate precursor") or as a generalized risk factor for the future development of invasive cancer in either breast ("risk lesion"). DCIS is the classic example of a lesion that is considered both a non-obligate precursor to invasion with an ipsilateral risk high enough that it is treated surgically to achieve negative margins and reduce this local risk of invasion. However, its presence also places the patient at an increased risk of cancer in either breast; thus it also behaves as a marker of future risk. Risk lesions of the breast as a general group have a much lower risk of local invasion, likely due to their smaller size in a given focus, but their scattered distribution pattern and likelihood of being present in the opposite breast creates a bilateral increased risk for future development of cancers. Since this risk is lower than DCIS and cannot as easily be managed surgically, it is more frequently managed by close imaging follow-up and/or medical risk reduction with hormonal therapies.

Precursors: A Primer on the Current Molecular Portrait of Breast Cancer Development

The original paradigm of breast carcinogenesis was based on morphology and lumped all ductal breast cancers into one broad pathway: ADH led to ductal carcinoma in situ (DCIS), which led to invasive ductal carcinomas [10, 13]. Subsequently, genetic information showed significant diversity within the ductal carcinomas, and it became clear that grade (degree of differentiation), hormone receptor and HER2 expression were powerful indicators of outcome within a particular histologic type [14–16].

Gene expression profiling studies allowed for segregation of breast cancers into "intrinsic subtypes" with similar gene expression signatures and significant prognostic relevance to survival. These primary intrinsic subtypes include the luminal subtypes (A and B), a HER2-enriched subtype, and a basal-like subtype [17–19]. The luminal subtypes express hormone receptor-related genes and are clinically estrogen receptor (ER) positive. The luminal subtypes (particularly luminal A cancers) have improved survival compared to the (typically) ER-negative, HER2-enriched, and commonly triple-negative basal-like subtypes [17–20].

The more recent breast carcinogenesis model builds on these findings and includes an "ER-positive neoplasia pathway" and an "ER-negative neoplasia pathway" (Fig. 1.2). "ER-positive neoplasia pathway" precursors include FEA, ADH, ALH, LCIS, and low-grade DCIS. In contrast, these lesions are not characteristic of the "ER-negative neoplasia pathway," which predominantly includes high-grade, ER-negative forms of DCIS or no precursor stage [11, 21, 22]. Lesions in the ER-positive neoplasia pathway have gains of 1q and losses of 16q, while lesions in the ER-negative neoplasia pathway are commonly characterized by complex karyotypes, high-level amplifications (including HER2), p53 mutations, BRCA1 dysfunction, high genomic instability, and very uncommonly gain of 1q and loss of 16q [23–28]. Of note, almost half of high-grade ER-positive cancers have the same 16q and 1q alterations as low-grade ER-positive cancers, suggesting that many evolve from lower-grade ER-positive cancers as additional mutations are acquired [24]. Complexities such as these, revealed by genetic analyses, will allow continued

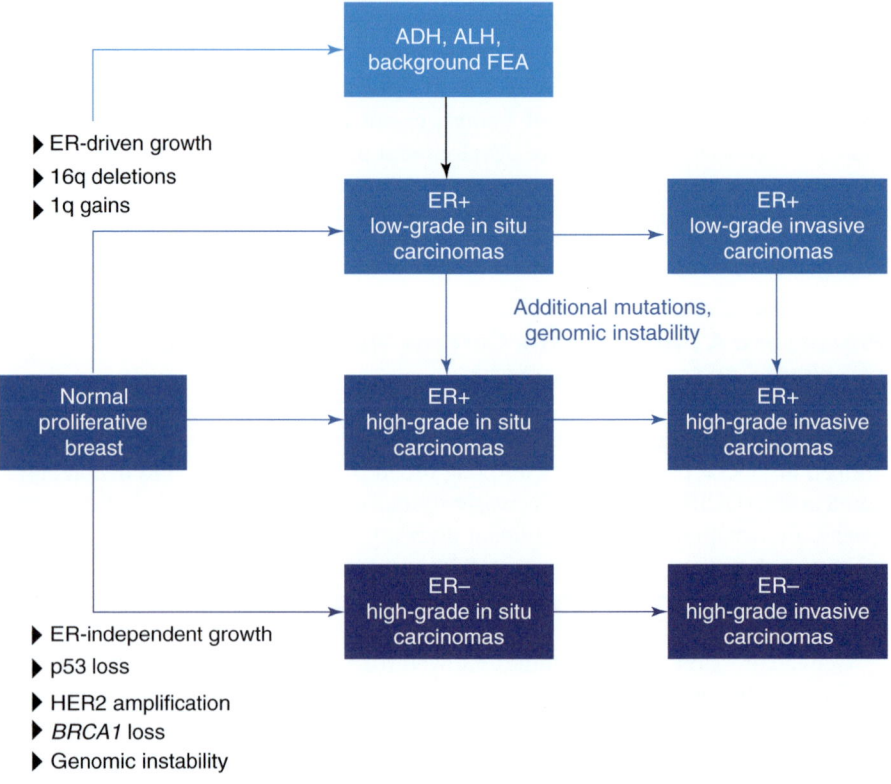

Fig. 1.2 A model of the molecular pathogenesis of breast cancers. This diagram summarizes the current concepts of ER-positive and ER-negative neoplasia pathways of breast carcinogenesis

refinement of our understanding of breast carcinogenesis and inform prognostication. In terms of outcomes, ER-negative DCIS and invasive cancers have a relatively shorter-term risk of recurrence/progression (highest within 5 years) when compared to the timeline for progression of lesions in the ER-positive pathway (extends far beyond 5 years).

Flat Epithelial Atypia and Breast Cancer Risk

Flat epithelial atypia (FEA) is considered to lie within the spectrum of columnar cell lesions and is histologically characterized by terminal duct lobular units with one to several layers of cuboidal to columnar epithelial cells possessing low-grade monomorphic cytologic atypia, including round nuclei and small nucleoli [29].

Rosen was among the first to describe how FEA is often seen in close association with LCIS, both with and without low-grade well-differentiated (tubular) carcinoma [30, 31]. In honor of this description, the "Rosen triad" refers to the common coexistence of FEA with LCIS and low-grade invasive carcinoma [32]. Rosen also noted that FEA and lobular neoplasia could be frequently seen in the setting of calcifications *without* carcinoma. This observation that FEA is frequently associated with neighboring lesions was later expanded to other members of the ER-positive neoplasia family including ADH, ALH, and ER-positive, low-grade DCIS [11, 30, 33–36]. The genetic similarities of FEA with these other ER-positive lesions [36, 37] clearly place FEA in the ER-positive neoplasia family of lesions and the molecular pathway to ER-positive breast cancer development. However, the future risk of developing breast cancer with a diagnosis of FEA alone appears to be significantly lower than that associated with a diagnosis of ADH or ALH. In one study, FEA alone was associated with a relative future bilateral risk of developing breast cancer of approximately 2.0 (95% CI: 1.23–3.19), which is nearly the same as that for women with a breast biopsy containing proliferative disease without atypia (relative risk 1.90, confidence interval 1.72–2.09) ($p = 0.76$) [38]. Since FEA is frequently found to be associated with ADH or ALH (which then implies a relative risk of cancer for these lesions), it is often a "red flag" for the potential presence of these additional risk-bearing atypical lesions. If FEA alone is identified on a core needle biopsy, pathologists frequently perform additional levels to rule out the presence of these other atypias because of the higher clinical impact of these lesions.

FEA may represent the earliest detectable clonal but non-obligate precursor lesion, as comparative genomic hybridization and other techniques have shown a morphologic and molecular continuum in columnar cell lesions, ranging from columnar cell change to flat epithelial atypia, including genetic alterations and recurrent 16q loss, features that are similar to those of low-grade in situ and invasive carcinoma [36, 39–41]. However, the cancer risk associated with FEA alone is so low that it is reasonable to assume that the vast majority of these lesions either regress, remain stable, or very slowly progress to other atypias.

Atypical Ductal Hyperplasia and Breast Cancer Risk

Atypical ductal hyperplasia (ADH) is defined as a lesion with "some but not all of the features of low grade DCIS" or a lesion that fulfills all criteria for a low-grade DCIS diagnosis but is very limited in extent (under 2–3 mm) [29]. Because the qualitative criteria are necessarily subjective, an ADH diagnosis may be associated with frequent diagnostic disagreement between pathologists, with UDH and low-grade DCIS frequently in the differential [42]. This factor should be considered when making clinical decisions on individual patients. However, in larger population-based studies where this may play less of a factor, it has become clear that ADH is a well-established risk marker for future development of breast cancer in either breast. Although the reported relative risk ranges from 2.4 to 13.0, the largest studies with long-term follow-up report relative risks ranging from 3.0 to 5.0 [43–52]. Although typically considered a risk factor for developing carcinoma in either breast, some studies have shown a higher likelihood of breast cancer developing in the same breast as a prior ADH diagnosis, raising the possibility that ADH can also act as a non-obligate precursor lesion [43, 45]. In loss of heterozygosity studies, ADH demonstrated chromosomal imbalances almost identical to those seen in low-grade DCIS, including recurrent 16q and 17p loss and 1q gains [53–56]. This genetic and morphologic similarity to ER-positive low-grade in situ and invasive carcinomas supports ADH's place in the low-grade pathway to invasion, although the relatively low annual risk of invasion with ADH and frequent multifocality/non-localized nature of the lesion support its current clinical management as a bilateral risk lesion.

Atypical Lobular Hyperplasia and Breast Cancer Risk

ALH is defined as a proliferation of small, monomorphic, discohesive cells within the terminal duct lobular unit. It is distinguished morphologically from LCIS on the basis of the degree of lobular distension present, with the threshold for an LCIS diagnosis defined as over half of the terminal duct lobular units "filled and distended" with the population. Given that these two entities are identical on a molecular level and are separated morphologically purely on this qualitative measure of extent/development, ALH and LCIS are frequently seen together and sometimes categorized together as "in situ lobular neoplasia" [29]. However, just like ADH and low-grade DCIS share many morphologic and genetic similarities but different relative risks, ALH and LCIS also have different relative risks of developing breast cancer.

Many studies also combine ALH and ADH under the heading "atypical hyperplasia," reporting similar relative risk values for both ALH and ADH (three- to five-fold) [44, 45, 57, 58]. There is some debate about whether the risk associated with ALH is bilateral or unilateral. In one retrospective study looking specifically at outcomes for ALH in 252 women over 35 years, invasive breast cancer was 3.1 times more likely to develop in the ipsilateral breast than the contralateral breast [59]. Another study showed a statistically insignificant greater risk of ipsilateral breast cancer in women with ALH compared to those with ADH (61.3% vs 55.9%) [46].

For many years, due to lesion rarity and long duration between lesion identification and carcinoma development, lobular neoplasia was believed to be solely a risk factor for breast cancer, but genetic data suggest that ALH can also act as a nonobligate precursor lesion. Comparative genomic hybridization analysis showed ALH and LCIS have loss of material from 16p, 16q, 17p, and 22q and gain of material from 6q at the same rates [60]. Losses at 1q, 16q, and 17p have also been seen in invasive lobular carcinomas [15, 61]. Genomics studies demonstrate similar molecular profiles between lobular neoplasia and concurrent adjacent invasive lobular carcinoma, including alteration characteristic of the low-grade pathway (gain of 1q and loss of 16q) and presence of the same truncating mutations and loss of heterozygosity of the wild-type E-cadherin in the LCIS component and in the adjacent invasive lobular carcinoma [62]. Similar to ADH and FEA, ALH confers a moderately increased overall risk of developing cancer over time but also clearly is a nonobligate precursor lesion with a very low local risk of invasion. Its scattered distribution pattern supports its clinical management as a nonsurgical, bilateral risk lesion.

Clinical and Histologic Risk Modifiers

Clinical and histologic factors have been explored as possible risk modifiers in the setting of high-risk breast lesions. For atypical hyperplasia, younger age at diagnosis increases the chances that a diagnosis of breast cancer will ensue [45, 49, 63]. A family history of breast cancer has been reported in some studies to increase the risk associated with a diagnosis of atypical hyperplasia [38]; however, most larger recent studies demonstrate similar risk of breast cancer in women with an atypical hyperplasia diagnosis regardless of whether or not a family history is reported [44–46].

On histology, greater numbers of atypical foci are associated with higher risk, and greater involution of background lobular units is associated with lower risk [45, 64]. More specifically, marked elevations in relative risk up to 10.35-fold (95% CI, 6.13–16.4) were seen with multiple foci of ADH (defined as three or more foci with calcifications), with the highest relative risk in women younger than 45 years old [44]. Extensive lobular in situ neoplasia, defined as over ten affected lobular units, has also been associated with an increased risk (from 8% to 24%) of subsequent development of invasive lobular carcinoma [65].

Radial Scar and Breast Cancer Risk

Atypias from the ER-positive neoplasia pathway can also be observed arising in other clinically identified lesions such as radial scar, papilloma, or fibroadenoma [66, 67]. Histologically, radial scars are characterized by ducts and lobules radiating out from a central nidus of fibroelastotic stroma to create an architectural pattern "reminiscent of a flower head," while "complex sclerosing lesion" denotes larger less organized lesions without an obvious central fibroelastotic nidus (although often these terms are used interchangably) [29, 68].

Most studies describing radial scars have identified this lesion as an independent, albeit low-risk, factor for breast cancer. Early autopsy studies compared the burden of radial scar lesions in the breasts with and without known carcinoma, with inconsistent findings [69, 70]. However, in a study with nearly entire mammary gland sampling, radial scars were significantly more common in the breasts containing carcinoma compared to breasts without carcinoma [69–71]. Radial scar cases from the Nurses' Health Study were reported to have an increased risk of breast cancer development when compared to women without radial scar (odds ratio 1.6, 95% confidence interval 1.1–2.3), particularly among women over 50 years old [72]. Another study involving the Nurses' Health Study cohort calculated that women with radial scars had twice the risk of developing ipsilateral or contralateral breast cancer compared to those without (RR 1.8, 95% CI 1.1–2.9), and that increased number or lesion size was associated with an increased risk [73]. A meta-analysis of a subgroup of larger studies (sample size over 2000) showed that the presence of radial scar was associated with a 1.6-fold breast cancer risk [74]. In a prospective cohort analysis of 149 women with only a radial scar/complex sclerosing lesion diagnosis, 5 (3.3%) developed breast cancer (mean follow-up 5.6 years), at a rate of 0.84% per year, higher than the 0.32% per year rate in the normal population (relative risk 2.6, 95% confidence interval 0.86–6.0) [75].

The pathophysiology behind the increased risk of breast cancer among women with radial scars is unclear. Some have postulated that a disturbance in the relationship between the breast stroma and epithelium exists [76]. One explanation may be that the ducts and lobules emanating from radial scars can serve as the milieu for atypia, DCIS, and invasive carcinoma in a minority of radial scars [68, 77–79]. In one retrospective study of 175 patients with radial scars, 15.7% of "symptomatic" radial scars compared to 7% of screening-detected radial scars were associated with in situ or invasive carcinoma [79]. Similarly, larger radial scars (mammographically detectable) in older patients (41–50 years old) were more likely to contain carcinoma [68].

One small study microdissected targeted benign proliferative lesions (i.e., usual hyperplasia, adenosis) within radial scars and detected allelic imbalances of chromosomes 16q and 8p, indicating that at least some areas of radial scars may be clonal and neoplastic [80]. However, there is a dearth of genetic information exploring the biological precursor nature of radial scar. Whether or not radial scar/complex sclerosing lesion is a definite precursor lesion remains unproven [81].

Papillary Lesions and Breast Cancer Risk

Papillary lesions of the breast are a heterogeneous group of lesions characterized by finger-like projections composed of central fibrovascular cores covered by epithelium [29]. Papillomas were considered malignant or precancerous and treated with mastectomy in the early 1900s before local excision became the preferred treatment [82–85]. Historical reports of cancer incidence following diagnosis of papilloma varied considerably (<1% to over 10%), likely due to varying morphologic criteria [83, 85–87]. More recent studies show that papillomas lacking cytologic atypia are associated with an approximately twofold risk of subsequent breast cancer, similar to that seen with usual ductal hyperplasia or proliferative fibrocystic disease [88–90].

Significantly, multiple papillomas have been associated with a particularly increased cancer risk [91, 92]. In a retrospective clinicopathologic study of 28 cases of multiple papillomas (defined as at least five in at least two nonconsecutive blocks), 12 (43%) were associated with atypical hyperplasia (ADH or ALH), and three (23%) developed invasive contralateral carcinoma.

The most comprehensive study evaluating breast cancer risk after papilloma diagnosis included 372 non-atypical papillomas, 54 atypical papillomas (with ADH or ALH), 41 multiple papillomas, and 13 multiple atypical papilloma cases. Cases were compared to cases of nonproliferative disease without papillomas ($n = 2308$) and atypical hyperplasia ADH/ALH cases ($n = 41$) [89]. The relative risk of breast cancer development was 2.04 for a benign papilloma (95% CI 1.43–2.81), 5.11 for a single atypical papilloma (95% CI 2.64–8.92), 3.01 for multiple papillomas (95% CI 1.10–6.55), and 7.01 for multiple papillomas with atypia (95% CI 1.91–17.97). The authors concluded that a single papilloma imparts cancer risk similar to fibrocystic change, that atypia in a papilloma does not modify the risk of atypical hyperplasia overall, and that multiple papillomas constitute breast disease with unique clinical and biological behavior.

While an association has been made between overall breast cancer overall risk and multiple papillomas, the relationship between papillary lesions and carcinogenesis is uncertain. Papillomas have been shown to be clonal in studies of X-inactivation patterns [93, 94]. Subsequent studies reported conflicting results regarding large-scale chromosomal alterations in benign papillary lesions [95–100]. A recent study detected mutations in PIK3CA and AKT1 in a majority of papillary lesions, with predominantly AKT1 mutations in papillomas, predominantly PIK3CA in atypical papillomas, and lower frequencies of mutations in papillary carcinoma cases, concluding that papillomas are driven by PI3CA/AKT pathway mutations and that some papillary carcinomas may arise from these lesions, with others having different molecular origins [101]. The shared mutations in papillary lesions and papillary carcinomas suggest a precursor role of papillomas, but additional research is needed to further define this risk.

Fibroepithelial Lesions and Malignancy Risk

Fibroepithelial lesions are defined by a biphasic proliferation of epithelium and stroma and include a spectrum of histologically and clinically diverse lesions, ranging from benign fibroadenoma to benign, borderline, and malignant phyllodes tumors [29].

A diagnosis of fibroadenoma is associated with an approximate relative risk of developing carcinoma of 1.5–2.0 times that of age-matched women in the general population [102–104]. A slightly increased relative risk of 2.3–3 has been reported for complex fibroadenomas, which are defined by the presence of associated cysts, sclerosing adenosis, epithelial calcifications, or papillary apocrine changes [102, 104]. Very rarely, ALH, ADH, LCIS, DCIS, and invasive carcinoma are seen associated with fibroadenomas [105–108]. One study showed no increased risk of invasive carcinoma in women with fibroadenomas containing ADH or ALH; however, the study was small (13 patients) [103]. Additional larger studies are warranted to further explore the clinical and biological behavior of fibroadenomas with epithelial atypia.

It is important to highlight that classification of fibroepithelial lesions can have diagnostic variablity, largely because of overlapping features in the various diagnostic WHO categories [109, 110].

Multiple attempts have been made to stratify fibroepithelial lesions into those at higher risk for recurrence/malignancy [74, 111–116]. Genome sequencing revealed mediator complex subunit 12 (MED12) somatic mutations in 59–67% of fibroadenomas and 45–67% of phyllodes tumors [117–120]. Studies have demonstrated recurrent chromosomal imbalances in phyllodes tumors, with1q gain and 13q loss in borderline and malignant phyllodes tumors, and benign phyllodes tumors showing few or no alterations [121, 122]. However, 1q gain did not correlate with phyllodes category, and 1q gains were reported in benign phyllodes tumors [116, 123].

By differential gene methylation analysis, most fibroadenomas demonstrated polyclonal epithelium and stroma, and fibroadenomas that later became phyllodes tumors demonstrated monoclonality on retrospective review [124, 125]. These studies pointed toward a stromal origin of phyllodes tumors; however, other studies found epithelial and stromal changes and sparked consideration of the significance of stromal and epithelial interactions in the pathogenesis of phyllodes tumors [126–129]. Whether some fibroadenomas represent a non-obligate phyllodes tumor precursor remains unclear.

Breast Risk Lesions: Putting Future Risk of Breast Cancer in Perspective

In this chapter, evidence from case reviews, genomics, and genetics studies have been used to define the long-term bilateral risk of breast malignancy and precursor role, respectively, for six categories of breast risk lesions (Table 1.1). Fairly compelling genetic data support the hypothesis that ADH, ALH, and FEA are non-obligate precursor lesions in breast carcinogenesis, while more research is needed to understand the biological relationship between radial scars and carcinoma, papillomas and carcinomas, and fibroadenomas/FELs and malignant phyllodes tumors.

The lesions described here are associated with a low absolute risk of future breast cancer diagnosis, and an even lower absolute risk of mortality, particularly since the carcinoma that develops in the setting of these lesions is often ER positive [1, 130]. For example, if the absolute risk of a 40-year-old woman developing breast cancer in the next 10 years is 1 in 67, then the chance of developing breast cancer if she gets a diagnosis of atypical ductal hyperplasia is 5 in 67, or 1 in 13 (8%), with overall survival in the setting of a DCIS or low-grade carcinoma diagnosis approaching 100% [5, 131] (Fig. 1.3).

While risk lesions of the breast are diagnosed in a small minority of breast biopsies, their rarity and incomplete characterization as risk factors occasionally cause confusion regarding management. Continued progress may help predict which lesions will transform into clinically relevant malignancies [132]. For now,

Table 1.1 Summary of risk lesions of the breast

	Approximate relative risk of developing carcinoma in either breast	Evidence of precursor role
ADH	4.0–5.0×	Yes (ER-positive neoplasia pathway)
	10.0× (with over two foci)	
ALH	4.0–5.0×	Yes (ER-positive neoplasia pathway)
FEA	2.0×	Yes (ER-positive neoplasia pathway)
Radial scar	2.0×	No definite; however, evidence of clonality
Papillary lesion	2.0× (without atypia)	No definite; however, evidence of shared genetic alterations with papillary carcinoma
	3.0× (over five foci)	
	4.0× (with atypia)	
Fibroepithelial lesion	1.5–2.0×	No definite; however, evidence of shared genetic alterations among fibroadenomas and phyllodes tumors
	2.0–3.0× (complex)	

Approximate relative risks of breast carcinoma, in addition to evidence of precursor role, are listed here for reference, for the six "risk" lesions discussed in this chapter

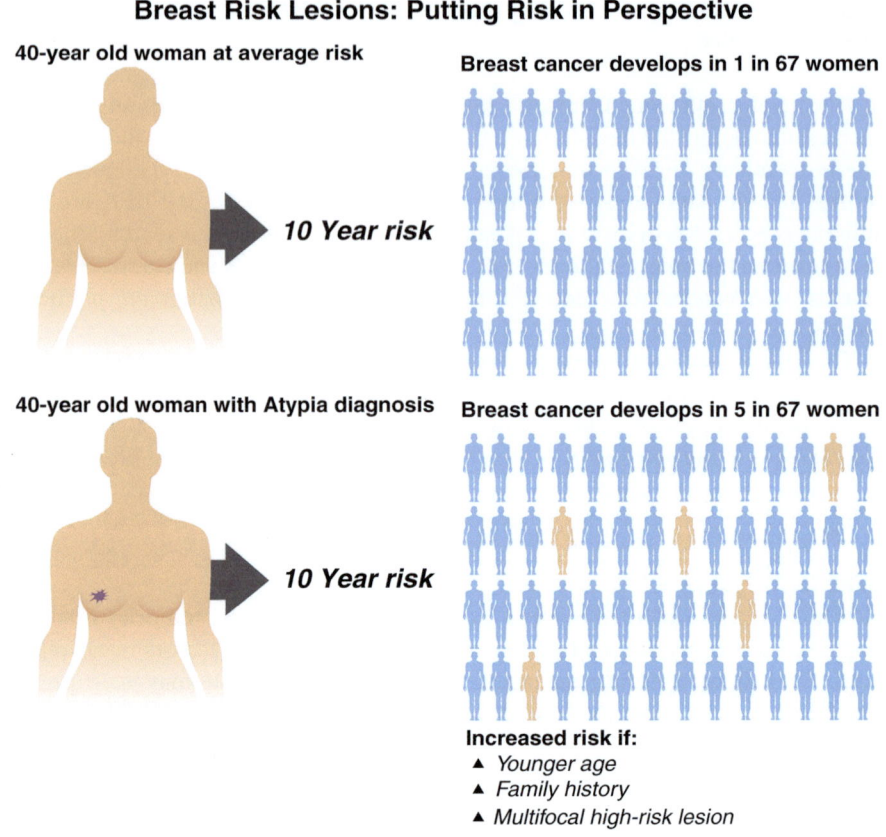

Fig. 1.3 Breast risk lesions: putting risk in perspective. Overall, the 10-year risk of developing breast cancer with a diagnosis of atypia on breast biopsy is low but increased relative to average risk

in the setting of increased public awareness and advances in imaging with more early breast cancer detection, an understanding of the risk associated with these lesions can be used to help counsel women found to have one of these lesions.

References

1. Mayer S, Kayser G, Rücker G, Bögner D, Hirschfeld M, Hug C, et al. Absence of epithelial atypia in B3-lesions of the breast is associated with decreased risk for malignancy. Breast. 2017;31(Supplement C):144–9.
2. Perry N, Broeders M, de Wolf C, Törnberg S, Holland R, von Karsa L. European guidelines for quality assurance in breast cancer screening and diagnosis. Fourth edition—summary document. Ann Oncol. 2008;19(4):614–22.
3. Houssami N, Ciatto S, Bilous M, Vezzosi V, Bianchi S. Borderline breast core needle histology: predictive values for malignancy in lesions of uncertain malignant potential (B3). Br J Cancer. 2007;96(8):1253–7.

4. Noske A, Pahl S, Fallenberg E. Flat epithelial atypia is a common subtype of B3 breast lesions and is associated with noninvasive cancer but not with invasive cancer in final excision histology. Hum Pathol. 2010;41:522–7.
5. Fitzgibbons PL, Henson DE, Hutter RV. Benign breast changes and the risk for subsequent breast cancer: an update of the 1985 consensus statement. Cancer Committee of the College of American Pathologists. Arch Pathol Lab Med. 1998;122(12):1053–5.
6. Ashbeck EL, Rosenberg RD, Stauber PM, Key CR. Benign breast biopsy diagnosis and subsequent risk of breast cancer. Cancer Epidemiol Prev Biomark. 2007;16(3):467–72.
7. Sauter ER, Daly MB, editors. Breast cancer risk reduction and early detection [Internet]. Boston: Springer; 2010. [cited 2017 Oct 2]. Available from: http://link.springer.com/10.1007/978-0-387-87583-5
8. Silvera SAN, Rohan TE. Benign proliferative epithelial disorders of the breast: a review of the epidemiologic evidence. Breast Cancer Res Treat. 2008;110(3):397–409.
9. Cooper A, Royal College of Physicians of Edinburgh. Illustrations of the diseases of the breast ... Part 1 [Internet]. London: Longman, Rees, Orme, Brown, Green, and Longman; 1829 [cited 2017 Oct 2]. p. 150. Available from: http://archive.org/details/b21913249
10. Wellings SR, Jensen HM, Marcum RG. An atlas of subgross pathology of the human breast with special reference to possible precancerous lesions. J Natl Cancer Inst. 1975;55(2):231–73.
11. Simpson PT, Reis-Filho JS, Gale T, Lakhani SR. Molecular evolution of breast cancer. J Pathol. 2005;205(2):248–54.
12. Begg CB, Ostrovnaya I, Carniello JVS, Sakr RA, Giri D, Towers R, et al. Clonal relationships between lobular carcinoma in situ and other breast malignancies. Breast Cancer Res BCR. 2016;18(1):66.
13. Wellings SR, Jensen HM. On the origin and progression of ductal carcinoma in the human breast. J Natl Cancer Inst. 1973;50(5):1111–8.
14. Reis-Filho JS, Simpson PT, Jones C, Steele D, Mackay A, Iravani M, et al. Pleomorphic lobular carcinoma of the breast: role of comprehensive molecular pathology in characterization of an entity. J Pathol. 2005;207(1):1–13.
15. Buerger H, Mommers EC, Littmann R, Simon R, Diallo R, Poremba C, et al. Ductal invasive G2 and G3 carcinomas of the breast are the end stages of at least two different lines of genetic evolution. J Pathol. 2001;194(2):165–70.
16. Roylance R, Gorman P, Harris W, Liebmann R, Barnes D, Hanby A, et al. Comparative genomic hybridization of breast tumors stratified by histological grade reveals new insights into the biological progression of breast cancer. Cancer Res. 1999;59(7):1433–6.
17. Perou CM, Sørlie T, Eisen MB, van de Rijn M, Jeffrey SS, Rees CA, et al. Molecular portraits of human breast tumours. Nature. 2000;406(6797):747–52.
18. Sørlie T, Tibshirani R, Parker J, Hastie T, Marron JS, Nobel A, et al. Repeated observation of breast tumor subtypes in independent gene expression data sets. Proc Natl Acad Sci. 2003;100(14):8418–23.
19. van't Veer LJ, Dai H, van de Vijver MJ, He YD, AAM H, Mao M, et al. Gene expression profiling predicts clinical outcome of breast cancer. Nature. 2002;415(6871):530–6.
20. Sørlie T, Perou CM, Tibshirani R, Aas T, Geisler S, Johnsen H, et al. Gene expression patterns of breast carcinomas distinguish tumor subclasses with clinical implications. Proc Natl Acad Sci. 2001;98(19):10869–74.
21. King TA, Sakr RA, Muhsen S, Andrade VP, Giri D, Zee KJV, et al. Is there a low-grade precursor pathway in breast Cancer? Ann Surg Oncol. 2012;19(4):1115–21.
22. Lopez-Garcia MA, Geyer FC, Lacroix-Triki M, Marchió C, Reis-Filho JS. Breast cancer precursors revisited: molecular features and progression pathways. Histopathology. 2010;57(2):171–92.
23. Natrajan R, Lambros MB, Rodríguez-Pinilla SM, Moreno-Bueno G, Tan DSP, Marchió C, et al. Tiling path genomic profiling of grade 3 invasive ductal breast cancers. Clin Cancer Res. 2009;15(8):2711–22.

24. Natrajan R, Weigelt B, Mackay A, Geyer FC, Grigoriadis A, Tan DSP, et al. An integrative genomic and transcriptomic analysis reveals molecular pathways and networks regulated by copy number aberrations in basal-like, HER2 and luminal cancers. Breast Cancer Res Treat. 2010;121(3):575–89.
25. Bombonati A, Sgroi DC. The molecular pathology of breast cancer progression. J Pathol. 2011;223(2):308–18.
26. Andre F, Job B, Dessen P, Tordai A, Michiels S, Liedtke C, et al. Molecular characterization of breast cancer with high-resolution oligonucleotide comparative genomic hybridization array. Clin Cancer Res Off J Am Assoc Cancer Res. 2009;15(2):441–51.
27. Chin SF, Teschendorff AE, Marioni JC, Wang Y, Barbosa-Morais NL, Thorne NP, et al. High-resolution aCGH and expression profiling identifies a novel genomic subtype of ER negative breast cancer. Genome Biol. 2007;8:R215.
28. Jönsson G, Staaf J, Vallon-Christersson J, Ringnér M, Holm K, Hegardt C, et al. Genomic subtypes of breast cancer identified by array-comparative genomic hybridization display distinct molecular and clinical characteristics. Breast Cancer Res. 2010;12:R42.
29. Schnitt SJ, Collins LC. Biopsy interpretation of the breast. 2nd ed. Philadelphia: LWW; 2012. p. 512.
30. Rosen PP. Columnar cell hyperplasia is associated with lobular carcinoma in situ and tubular carcinoma. Am J Surg Pathol. 1999;23(12):1561.
31. Azzopardi JG, Ahmed A, Millis RR. Problems in breast pathology. Major Probl Pathol. 1979;11:i–xvi, 1–466.
32. Brandt SM, Young GQ, Hoda SA. The "Rosen Triad": tubular carcinoma, lobular carcinoma in situ, and columnar cell lesions. Adv Anat Pathol. 2008;15(3):140–6.
33. Abdel-Fatah TMA, Powe DG, Hodi Z, Lee AHS, Reis-Filho JS, Ellis IO. High frequency of coexistence of columnar cell lesions, lobular neoplasia, and low grade ductal carcinoma in situ with invasive tubular carcinoma and invasive lobular carcinoma. Am J Surg Pathol. 2007;31(3):417–26.
34. Fraser JL, Raza S, Chorny K, Connolly JL, Schnitt SJ. Columnar alteration with prominent apical snouts and secretions: a spectrum of changes frequently present in breast biopsies performed for microcalcifications. Am J Surg Pathol. 1998;22(12):1521–7.
35. Goldstein NS, O'Malley BA. Cancerization of small ectatic ducts of the breast by ductal carcinoma in situ cells with apocrine snouts: a lesion associated with tubular carcinoma. Am J Clin Pathol. 1997;107(5):561–6.
36. Simpson PT, Gale T, Reis-Filho JS, Jones C, Parry S, Sloane JP, et al. Columnar cell lesions of the breast: the missing link in breast cancer progression? A morphological and molecular analysis. Am J Surg Pathol. 2005;29(6):734–46.
37. McLaren BK, Gobbi H, Schuyler PA, Olson SJ, Parl FF, Dupont WD, et al. Immunohistochemical expression of estrogen receptor in enlarged lobular units with columnar alteration in benign breast biopsies: a nested case-control study. Am J Surg Pathol. 2005;29(1):105–8.
38. Webb PM, Byrne C, Schnitt SJ, Connolly JL, Jacobs T, Peiro G, et al. Family history of breast cancer, age and benign breast disease. Int J Cancer. 2002;100(3):375–8.
39. Moinfar F, Man YG, Bratthauer GL. Genetic abnormalities in mammary ductal intraepithelial neoplasia-flat type ('clinging ductal carcinoma in situ'): a simulator of normal mammary epithelium. Cancer. 2000;88:2072–81.
40. Dabbs DJ, Carter G, Fudge M, Peng Y, Swalsky P, Finkelstein S. Molecular alterations in columnar cell lesions of the breast. Mod Pathol Off J U S Can Acad Pathol Inc. 2006;19(3):344–9.
41. Sinn H-P, Elsawaf Z, Helmchen B, Aulmann S. Early breast Cancer precursor lesions: lessons learned from molecular and clinical studies. Breast Care Basel Switz. 2010;5(4):218–26.
42. Elmore JG, Longton GM, Carney PA, Geller BM, Onega T, Tosteson ANA, et al. Diagnostic concordance among pathologists interpreting breast biopsy specimens. JAMA. 2015;313(11):1122–32.

43. Dupont WD, Page DL. Risk factors for breast cancer in women with proliferative breast disease. N Engl J Med. 1985;312(3):146–51.
44. Degnim AC, Visscher DW, Berman HK, Frost MH, Sellers TA, Vierkant RA, et al. Stratification of breast cancer risk in women with atypia: a mayo cohort study. J Clin Oncol. 2007;25(19):2671–7.
45. Hartmann LC, Radisky DC, Frost MH, Santen RJ, Vierkant RA, Benetti LL, et al. Understanding the premalignant potential of atypical hyperplasia through its natural history: a longitudinal cohort study. Cancer Prev Res Phila Pa. 2014;7(2):211–7.
46. Collins LC, Baer HJ, Tamimi RM, Connolly JL, Colditz GA, Schnitt SJ. Magnitude and laterality of breast cancer risk according to histologic type of atypical hyperplasia: results from the nurses' health study. Cancer. 2007;109(2):180–7.
47. Carter CL, Corle DK, Micozzi MS, Schatzkin A, Taylor PR. A prospective study of the development of breast cancer in 16,692 women with benign breast disease. Am J Epidemiol. 1988;128(3):467–77.
48. McDivitt RW, Stevens JA, Lee NC, Wingo PA, Rubin GL, Gersell D. Histologic types of benign breast disease and the risk for breast cancer. The cancer and steroid hormone study group. Cancer. 1992;69(6):1408–14.
49. London SJ, Connolly JL, Schnitt SJ, Colditz GA. A prospective study of benign breast disease and the risk of breast cancer. JAMA. 1992;267(7):941–4.
50. Gomes DS, Porto SS, Balabram D, Gobbi H. Inter-observer variability between general pathologists and a specialist in breast pathology in the diagnosis of lobular neoplasia, columnar cell lesions, atypical ductal hyperplasia and ductal carcinoma in situ of the breast. Diagn Pathol. 2014;9:121.
51. Tan PH, Ho BC-S, Selvarajan S, Yap WM, Hanby A. Pathological diagnosis of columnar cell lesions of the breast: are there issues of reproducibility? J Clin Pathol. 2005;58(7):705–9.
52. O'Malley FP, Mohsin SK, Badve S, Bose S, Collins LC, Ennis M, et al. Interobserver reproducibility in the diagnosis of flat epithelial atypia of the breast. Mod Pathol Off J U S Can Acad Pathol Inc. 2006;19(2):172–9.
53. Gong G, DeVries S, Chew KL, Cha I, Ljung BM, Waldman FM. Genetic changes in paired atypical and usual ductal hyperplasia of the breast by comparative genomic hybridization. Clin Cancer Res Off J Am Assoc Cancer Res. 2001;7(8):2410–4.
54. Amari M, Suzuki A, Moriya T, Yoshinaga K, Amano G, Sasano H, et al. LOH analyses of premalignant and malignant lesions of human breast: frequent LOH in 8p, 16q, and 17q in atypical ductal hyperplasia. Oncol Rep. 1999;6(6):1277–80.
55. Lakhani SR, Collins N, Stratton MR, Sloane JP. Atypical ductal hyperplasia of the breast: clonal proliferation with loss of heterozygosity on chromosomes 16q and 17p. J Clin Pathol. 1995;48(7):611–5.
56. Larson PS, de las Morenas A, Cerda SR, Bennett SR, Cupples LA, Rosenberg CL. Quantitative analysis of allele imbalance supports atypical ductal hyperplasia lesions as direct breast cancer precursors. J Pathol. 2006;209(3):307–16.
57. McDivitt RW, Hutter RV, Foote FW, Stewart FW. In situ lobular carcinoma. A prospective follow-up study indicating cumulative patient risks. JAMA. 1967;201(2):82–6.
58. Bodian CA, Perzin KH, Lattes R. Lobular neoplasia. Long term risk of breast cancer and relation to other factors. Cancer. 1996;78(5):1024–34.
59. Page DL, Schuyler PA, Dupont WD, Jensen RA, Plummer WD, Simpson JF. Atypical lobular hyperplasia as a unilateral predictor of breast cancer risk: a retrospective cohort study. Lancet Lond Engl. 2003;361(9352):125–9.
60. Lu YJ, Osin P, Lakhani SR, Di Palma S, Gusterson BA, Shipley JM. Comparative genomic hybridization analysis of lobular carcinoma in situ and atypical lobular hyperplasia and potential roles for gains and losses of genetic material in breast neoplasia. Cancer Res. 1998;58(20):4721–7.
61. Nishizaki T, Chew K, Chu L, Isola J, Kallioniemi A, Weidner N, et al. Genetic alterations in lobular breast cancer by comparative genomic hybridization. Int J Cancer. 1997;74(5):513–7.

62. Hwang ES, Nyante SJ, Yi Chen Y, Moore D, DeVries S, Korkola JE, et al. Clonality of lobular carcinoma in situ and synchronous invasive lobular carcinoma. Cancer. 2004;100(12):2562–72.
63. Hartmann LC, Sellers TA, Frost MH, Lingle WL, Degnim AC, Ghosh K, et al. Benign breast disease and the risk of breast cancer. N Engl J Med. 2005;353(3):229–37.
64. Baer HJ, Collins LC, Connolly JL, Colditz GA, Schnitt SJ, Tamimi RM. Lobule type and subsequent breast cancer risk: results from the nurses' health studies. Cancer. 2009;115(7):1404–11.
65. Ottesen GL, Graversen HP, Blichert-Toft M, Zedeler K, Andersen JA. Lobular carcinoma in situ of the female breast. Short-term results of a prospective nationwide study. The Danish breast cancer cooperative group. Am J Surg Pathol. 1993;17(1):14–21.
66. Sanders ME, Page DL, Simpson JF, Schuyler PA, Dale Plummer W, Dupont WD. Interdependence of radial scar and proliferative disease with respect to invasive breast carcinoma risk in patients with benign breast biopsies. Cancer. 2006;106(7):1453–61.
67. Page DL, Salhany KE, Jensen RA, Dupont WD. Subsequent breast carcinoma risk after biopsy with atypia in a breast papilloma. Cancer. 1996;78(2):258–66.
68. Sloane JP, Mayers MM. Carcinoma and atypical hyperplasia in radial scars and complex sclerosing lesions: importance of lesion size and patient age. Histopathology. 1993;23(3):225–31.
69. Anderson TJ, Battersby S. Radial scars of benign and malignant breasts: comparative features and significance. J Pathol. 1985;147(1):23–32.
70. Wellings SR, Alpers CE. Subgross pathologic features and incidence of radial scars in the breast. Hum Pathol. 1984;15(5):475–9.
71. Nielsen M, Jensen J, Andersen JA. An autopsy study of radial scar in the female breast. Histopathology. 1985;9(3):287–95.
72. Aroner SA, Collins LC, Connolly JL, Colditz GA, Schnitt SJ, Rosner BA, et al. Radial scars and subsequent breast cancer risk: results from the nurses' health studies. Breast Cancer Res Treat. 2013;139(1):277–85.
73. Jacobs TW, Byrne C, Colditz G, Connolly JL, Schnitt SJ. Radial scars in benign breast-biopsy specimens and the risk of breast cancer. N Engl J Med. 1999;340(6):430–6.
74. Lv M, Zhu X, Zhong S, Chen W, Hu Q, Ma T, et al. Radial scars and subsequent breast cancer risk: a meta-analysis. PLoS One. 2014;9(7):e102503.
75. Bunting DM, Steel JR, Holgate CS, Watkins RM. Long term follow-up and risk of breast cancer after a radial scar or complex sclerosing lesion has been identified in a benign open breast biopsy. Eur J Surg Oncol J Eur Soc Surg Oncol Br Assoc Surg Oncol. 2011;37(8):709–13.
76. Rønnov-Jessen L, Petersen OW, Bissell MJ. Cellular changes involved in conversion of normal to malignant breast: importance of the stromal reaction. Physiol Rev. 1996;76(1):69–125.
77. Mokbel K, Price RK, Mostafa A, Williams N, Wells CA, Perry N, et al. Radial scar and carcinoma of the breast: microscopic findings in 32 cases. Breast Edinb Scotl. 1999;8(6):339–42.
78. Alvarado-Cabrero I, Tavassoli FA. Neoplastic and malignant lesions involving or arising in a radial scar: a clinicopathologic analysis of 17 cases. Breast J. 2000;6(2):96–102.
79. Patterson JA, Scott M, Anderson N, Kirk SJ. Radial scar, complex sclerosing lesion and risk of breast cancer. Analysis of 175 cases in Northern Ireland. Eur J Surg Oncol J Eur Soc Surg Oncol Br Assoc Surg Oncol. 2004;30(10):1065–8.
80. Iqbal M, Shoker BS, Foster CS, Jarvis C, Sibson DR, Davies MPA. Molecular and genetic abnormalities in radial scar. Hum Pathol. 2002;33(7):715–22.
81. Fisher ER, Palekar AS, Kotwal N, Lipana N. A nonencapsulated sclerosing lesion of the breast. Am J Clin Pathol. 1979;71(3):240–6.
82. Adair FE. Sanguineous discharge from the nipple and its significance in relation to cancer of the breast: a study based on 108 cases. Ann Surg. 1930;91(2):197–209.
83. Carter D. Intraductal papillary tumors of the breast: a study of 78 cases. Cancer. 1977;39(4):1689–92.
84. Lewison EF, Lyons JG. Relationship between benign breast disease and cancer. AMA Arch Surg. 1953;66(1):94–114.

85. Haagensen CD, Stout AP, Phillips JS. The papillary neoplasms of the breast. I. Benign intraductal papilloma. Ann Surg. 1951;133(1):18–36.
86. Buhl-Jorgensen SE, Fischermann K, Johansen H, Petersen B. Cancer risk in intraductal papilloma and papillomatosis. Surg Gynecol Obstet. 1968;127(6):1307–12.
87. Kilgore AR, Fleming R, Ramos MM. The incidence of cancer with nipple discharge and the risk of cancer in the presence of papillary disease of the breast. Surg Gynecol Obstet. 1953;96(6):649–60.
88. Mulligan AM, O'malley FP. Papillary lesions of the breast: a review. Adv Anat Pathol. 2007;14(2):108–19.
89. Lewis JT, Hartmann LC, Vierkant RA, Maloney SD, Shane Pankratz V, Allers TM, et al. An analysis of breast cancer risk in women with single, multiple, and atypical papilloma. Am J Surg Pathol. 2006;30(6):665–72.
90. Ciatto S, Andreoli C, Cirillo A, Bonardi R, Bianchi S, Santoro G, et al. The risk of breast cancer subsequent to histologic diagnosis of benign intraductal papilloma follow-up study of 339 cases. Tumori. 1991;77(1):41–3.
91. Pellettiere EV. The clinical and pathologic aspects of papillomatous disease of the breast: a follow-up study of 97 patients treated by local excision. Am J Clin Pathol. 1971;55(6):740–8.
92. Ali-Fehmi R, Carolin K, Wallis T, Visscher DW. Clinicopathologic analysis of breast lesions associated with multiple papillomas. Hum Pathol. 2003;34(3):234–9.
93. Noguchi S, Motomura K, Inaji H, Imaoka S, Koyama H. Clonal analysis of solitary intraductal papilloma of the breast by means of polymerase chain reaction. Am J Pathol. 1994;144(6):1320–5.
94. Noguchi S, Aihara T, Koyama H, Motomura K, Inaji H, Imaoka S. Clonal analysis of benign and malignant human breast tumors by means of polymerase chain reaction. Cancer Lett. 1995;90(1):57–63.
95. Tsuda H, Takarabe T, Inazawa J, Hirohashi S. Detection of numerical alterations of chromosomes 3, 7, 17 and X in low-grade Intracystic papillary tumors of the breast by multi-color fluorescence in situ hybridization. Breast Cancer Tokyo Jpn. 1997;4(4):247–52.
96. Lininger RA, Park WS, Man YG, Pham T, MacGrogan G, Zhuang Z, et al. LOH at 16p13 is a novel chromosomal alteration detected in benign and malignant microdissected papillary neoplasms of the breast. Hum Pathol. 1998;29(10):1113–8.
97. Di Cristofano C, Mrad K, Zavaglia K, Bertacca G, Aretini P, Cipollini G, et al. Papillary lesions of the breast: a molecular progression? Breast Cancer Res Treat. 2005;90(1):71–6.
98. Boecker W, Buerger H, Schmitz K, Ellis IA, van Diest PJ, Sinn HP, et al. Ductal epithelial proliferations of the breast: a biological continuum? Comparative genomic hybridization and high-molecular-weight cytokeratin expression patterns. J Pathol. 2001;195(4):415–21.
99. Dietrich CU, Pandis N, Teixeira MR, Bardi G, Gerdes AM, Andersen JA, et al. Chromosome abnormalities in benign hyperproliferative disorders of epithelial and stromal breast tissue. Int J Cancer. 1995;60(1):49–53.
100. Komoike Y, Motomura K, Inaji H, Koyama H. Diagnosis of ductal carcinoma in situ (DCIS) and intraductal papilloma using fluorescence in situ hybridization (FISH) analysis. Breast Cancer Tokyo Jpn. 2000;7(4):332–6.
101. Troxell ML, Levine J, Beadling C, Warrick A, Dunlap J, Presnell A, et al. High prevalence of PIK3CA/AKT pathway mutations in papillary neoplasms of the breast. Mod Pathol. 2009;23(1):27–37.
102. Dupont WD, Page DL, Parl FF, Vnencak-Jones CL, Plummer WDJ, Rados MS, et al. Long-term risk of breast cancer in women with Fibroadenoma. N Engl J Med. 1994;331(1):10–5.
103. Carter BA, Page DL, Schuyler P, Parl FF, Simpson JF, Jensen RA, et al. No elevation in long-term breast carcinoma risk for women with fibroadenomas that contain atypical hyperplasia. Cancer. 2001;92(1):30–6.
104. Nassar A, Visscher DW, Degnim AC, Frank RD, Vierkant RA, Frost M, et al. Complex fibroadenoma and breast cancer risk: a mayo clinic benign breast disease cohort study. Breast Cancer Res Treat. 2015;153(2):397–405.

105. Hua B, Xu J-Y, Jiang L, Wang Z. Fibroadenoma with an unexpected lobular carcinoma in situ: a case report and review of the literature. Oncol Lett. 2015;10(3):1397–401.
106. Buzanowski-Konakry K, Harrison EG, Payne WS. Lobular carcinoma arising in fibroadenoma of the breast. Cancer. 1975;35(2):450–6.
107. Diaz NM, Palmer JO, McDivitt RW. Carcinoma arising within fibroadenomas of the breast. A clinicopathologic study of 105 patients. Am J Clin Pathol. 1991;95(5):614–22.
108. Fives C, O'Neill CJ, Murphy R, Corrigan MA, O'Sullivan MJ, Feeley L, et al. When pathological and radiological correlation is achieved, excision of fibroadenoma with lobular neoplasia on core biopsy is not warranted. Breast Edinb Scotl. 2016;30:125–9.
109. Lawton TJ, Acs G, Argani P, Farshid G, Gilcrease M, Goldstein N, et al. Interobserver variability by pathologists in the distinction between cellular fibroadenomas and phyllodes tumors. Int J Surg Pathol. 2014;22(8):695–8.
110. Krings G, Bean GR, Chen Y-Y. Fibroepithelial lesions; the WHO spectrum. Semin Diagn Pathol. 2017;34(5):438–52.
111. Tan PH, Thike AA, Tan WJ, Thu MMM, Busmanis I, Li H, et al. Predicting clinical behaviour of breast phyllodes tumours: a nomogram based on histological criteria and surgical margins. J Clin Pathol. 2012;65(1):69–76.
112. Tan WJ, Cima I, Choudhury Y, Wei X, Lim JCT, Thike AA, et al. A five-gene reverse transcription-PCR assay for pre-operative classification of breast fibroepithelial lesions. Breast Cancer Res BCR. 2016;18(1):31.
113. Yasir S, Gamez R, Jenkins S, Visscher DW, Nassar A. Significant histologic features differentiating cellular fibroadenoma from phyllodes tumor on core needle biopsy specimens. Am J Clin Pathol. 2014;142(3):362–9.
114. Tse GMK, Lee CS, Kung FYL, Scolyer RA, Law BKB, Lau T, et al. Hormonal receptors expression in epithelial cells of mammary phyllodes tumors correlates with pathologic grade of the tumor: a multicenter study of 143 cases. Am J Clin Pathol. 2002;118(4):522–6.
115. Jacobs TW, Chen Y-Y, Guinee DG, Holden JA, Cha I, Bauermeister DE, et al. Fibroepithelial lesions with cellular stroma on breast core needle biopsy: are there predictors of outcome on surgical excision? Am J Clin Pathol. 2005;124(3):342–54.
116. Lu YJ, Birdsall S, Osin P, Gusterson B, Shipley J. Phyllodes tumors of the breast analyzed by comparative genomic hybridization and association of increased 1q copy number with stromal overgrowth and recurrence. Genes Chromosomes Cancer. 1997;20(3):275–81.
117. Yoshida M, Sekine S, Ogawa R, Yoshida H, Maeshima A, Kanai Y, et al. Frequent MED12 mutations in phyllodes tumours of the breast. Br J Cancer. 2015;112(10):1703–8.
118. Piscuoglio S, Murray M, Fusco N, Marchiò C, Loo FL, Martelotto LG, et al. MED12 somatic mutations in fibroadenomas and phyllodes tumours of the breast. Histopathology. 2015;67(5):719–29.
119. Nagasawa S, Maeda I, Fukuda T, Wu W, Hayami R, Kojima Y, et al. MED12 exon 2 mutations in phyllodes tumors of the breast. Cancer Med. 2015;4(7):1117–21.
120. Cani AK, Hovelson DH, McDaniel AS, Sadis S, Haller MJ, Yadati V, et al. Next-gen sequencing exposes frequent MED12 mutations and actionable therapeutic targets in phyllodes tumors. Mol Cancer Res MCR. 2015;13(4):613–9.
121. Laé M, Vincent-Salomon A, Savignoni A, Huon I, Fréneaux P, Sigal-Zafrani B, et al. Phyllodes tumors of the breast segregate in two groups according to genetic criteria. Mod Pathol Off J U S Can Acad Pathol Inc. 2007;20(4):435–44.
122. Jones AM, Mitter R, Springall R, Graham T, Winter E, Gillett C, et al. A comprehensive genetic profile of phyllodes tumours of the breast detects important mutations, intra-tumoral genetic heterogeneity and new genetic changes on recurrence. J Pathol. 2008;214(5):533–44.
123. Lv S, Niu Y, Wei L, Liu Q, Wang X, Chen Y. Chromosomal aberrations and genetic relations in benign, borderline and malignant phyllodes tumors of the breast: a comparative genomic hybridization study. Breast Cancer Res Treat. 2008;112(3):411–8.
124. Noguchi S, Motomura K, Inaji H, Imaoka S, Koyama H. Clonal analysis of fibroadenoma and phyllodes tumor of the breast. Cancer Res. 1993;53(17):4071–4.

125. Noguchi S, Yokouchi H, Aihara T, Motomura K, Inaji H, Imaoka S, et al. Progression of fibroadenoma to phyllodes tumor demonstrated by clonal analysis. Cancer. 1995;76(10):1779–85.
126. Sawyer EJ, Hanby AM, Ellis P, Lakhani SR, Ellis IO, Boyle S, et al. Molecular analysis of phyllodes tumors reveals distinct changes in the epithelial and stromal components. Am J Pathol. 2000;156(3):1093–8.
127. Sawyer EJ, Hanby AM, Rowan AJ, Gillett CE, Thomas RE, Poulsom R, et al. The Wnt pathway, epithelial-stromal interactions, and malignant progression in phyllodes tumours. J Pathol. 2002;196(4):437–44.
128. Wang ZC, Buraimoh A, Iglehart JD, Richardson AL. Genome-wide analysis for loss of heterozygosity in primary and recurrent phyllodes tumor and fibroadenoma of breast using single nucleotide polymorphism arrays. Breast Cancer Res Treat. 2006;97(3):301–9.
129. Sawhney N, Garrahan N, Douglas-Jones AG, Williams ED. Epithelial – stromal interactions in tumors. A morphologic study of fibroepithelial tumors of the breast. Cancer. 1992;70(8):2115–20.
130. Mooney KL, Bassett LW, Apple SK. Upgrade rates of high-risk breast lesions diagnosed on core needle biopsy: a single-institution experience and literature review. Mod Pathol. 2016;29(12):1471–84.
131. Cancer of the breast (female) – SEER cancer stat facts [Internet]. [cited 2017 Oct 2]. Available from: https://seer.cancer.gov/statfacts/html/breast.html
132. Cheeney S, Rahbar H, Dontchos BN, Javid SH, Rendi MH, Partridge SC. Apparent diffusion coefficient values may help predict which MRI-detected high-risk breast lesions will upgrade at surgical excision. J Magn Reson Imaging JMRI. 2017;46(4):1028–36.

Lobular Carcinoma In Situ: Risk Factor or Cancer Precursor?

Kevin M. Sullivan, Meghan R. Flanagan, Mark R. Kilgore, and Benjamin O. Anderson

Abbreviations

ADH	Atypical ductal hyperplasia
AI	Aromatase inhibitor
ALH	Atypical lobular hyperplasia
CGH	Comparative genomic hybridization
CI	Confidence interval
DCIS	Ductal carcinoma in situ
ER	Estrogen receptor
H&E	Hematoxylin and eosin
HER2	Human epidermal growth factor receptor 2
HR	Hazard ratio
IDC	Invasive ductal carcinoma
IHC	Immunohistochemistry

K. M. Sullivan
Department of Surgery, University of Washington, Seattle, WA, USA
e-mail: kevin6@uw.edu

M. R. Flanagan
Breast Service, Department of Surgery, Memorial Sloan Kettering Cancer Center, New York, NY, USA
e-mail: mrf22@uw.edu

M. R. Kilgore
Department of Pathology, University of Washington, Seattle, WA, USA
e-mail: mrmk@uw.edu

B. O. Anderson (✉)
Department of Surgery, University of Washington, Seattle, WA, USA

Departments of Surgery and Global Health, University of Washington, Seattle, WA, USA

Surgery and Global Health Medicine, University of Washington, Seattle, WA, USA
e-mail: banderso@uw.edu

ILC   Invasive lobular carcinoma
LCIS   Lobular carcinoma in situ
LN   Lobular neoplasia
LOH   Loss of heterozygosity
NSABP   National Surgical Adjuvant Breast and Bowel Project
PLCIS   Pleomorphic lobular carcinoma in situ
PR   Progesterone receptor
RR   Risk ratio
SEER   Surveillance, Epidemiology, and End Results
SERM   Selective estrogen receptor modulator
SMMHC   Smooth muscle myosin heavy chain
SNP   Single nucleotide polymorphism
STAR   Study of Tamoxifen and Raloxifene
TDLU   Terminal duct lobular unit

Historical Background

The evolving management of lobular carcinoma in situ (LCIS) has been fueled by a long-standing debate regarding its natural history and biologic behavior. For 75 years, investigators have argued whether LCIS is a precursor lesion for invasive lobular carcinoma (ILC) or if it is merely a risk factor marking increased likelihood for breast cancer development but without a specific precursor role in the development of that disease. The first documented reference to an entity similar to LCIS was Ewing's 1919 description of an "atypical proliferation of acinar cells" [1]. The term "lobular carcinoma in situ" was first coined by Foote and Stewart in 1941 who further described the lesion as "noninfiltrative" but with "definitely cancerous cytology" [2]. In that era preceding mammographic screening and percutaneous biopsies when essentially all breast cancers were detected as palpable masses or thickenings, LCIS was only identified when it was seen in conjunction with clinically apparent invasive cancer. This association between LCIS and invasive cancer supported the argument that LCIS is itself a threatening malignant precursor. In 1952, Godwin reported a case of a woman with a prior excisional biopsy who presented 12 years later with a mass in the same location as her biopsy and was found to have ILC in her mastectomy specimen [3], leading many to conclude that LCIS should routinely be surgically resected to prevent malignant progression to life-threatening disease.

In the 1970s as more comprehensive data became available, studies challenged the LCIS precursor hypothesis by showing that malignant progression of LCIS is not inevitable and that subsequently diagnosed cancers are commonly at a different location in the breast from where LCIS had previously been diagnosed. Research showed that the increased breast cancer risk conveyed by LCIS could be anywhere in the breast or even in the contralateral breast rather than exclusively or primarily at the site where LCIS had previously been biopsied. In his classic 1971 textbook *Diseases of the Breast*, the acclaimed cancer surgeon and surgical pathologist

Cushman D. Haagensen firmly rejected the term LCIS as "a most unfortunate choice" because he believed it was leading surgeons to perform mastectomy unnecessarily. Haagensen felt it is "imperative that surgeons and pathologist distinguish this lesion from true breast carcinoma" and urged the adoption of the term "lobular neoplasia" in place of LCIS to help decrease the overdiagnosis and overtreatment of a disorder that he believed was not a true surgical disease [4].

Histopathology and Cytologic Features of Lobular Neoplasia

Today, the term lobular neoplasia (LN) is used to describe the spectrum of noninvasive epithelial proliferative changes within lobular acini of the breast terminal duct lobular unit (TDLU). As such, LN includes both atypical lobular hyperplasia (ALH) and LCIS. Thus, LN represents the full range of histologic findings of lobular acini filled with and distended by small round or polygonal, uniform, discohesive cells with features that cytologically resemble those seen in ILC but lack evidence of invasion or infiltration [2, 5, 6]. The distinction between ALH and LCIS is somewhat subjective, but in general LCIS is specifically defined as the filling and distension of more than half of the acinar units in the TDLU [7–9]. In situ lobular lesions with less than the 50% threshold or without distention are classified as ALH (Figs. 2.1 and 2.2).

Two epithelial cell types are usually noted to be present in LCIS. Type A cells are small, discohesive cells with scant cytoplasm; type B cells show more variation, abundant cytoplasm, and slightly larger nuclei. LCIS is usually low grade, strongly estrogen receptor (ER) and progesterone receptor (PR) positive, and HER2 negative [6]. Both ALH and LCIS are distinguished from in situ ductal proliferations (atypical ductal hyperplasia [ADH] and ductal carcinoma in situ [DCIS]) by the absence

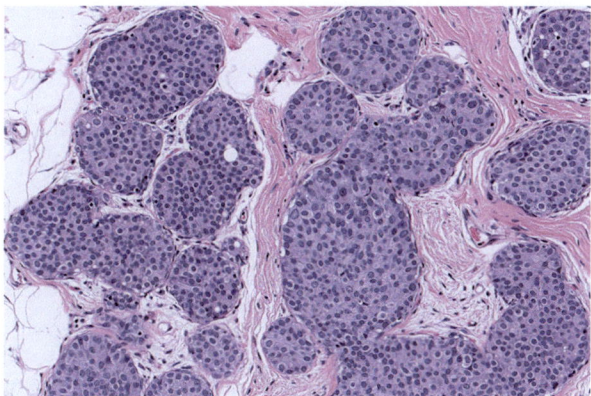

Fig. 2.1 Lobular carcinoma in situ (LCIS). Solid and monotonous proliferation of small cells with round-to-oval nuclei with homogeneous chromatin and inconspicuous to absent nucleoli. The proliferation involves and distends greater than 50% of the acini of this terminal duct lobular unit (TDLU). The morphology and extent of involvement fulfill the diagnostic criteria for classical lobular carcinoma in situ (LCIS)

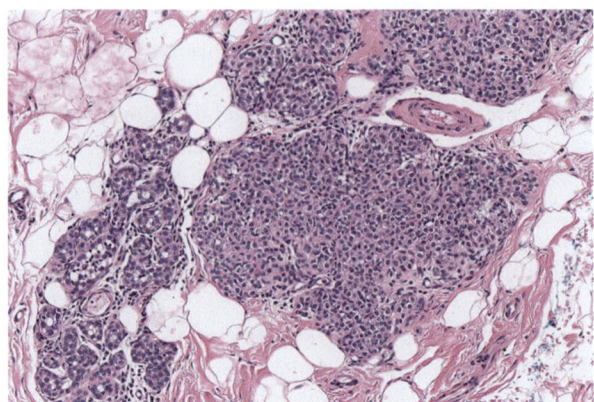

Fig. 2.2 Atypical lobular hyperplasia (ALH). Cells with similar cytologic features to those present in Fig. 2.1. The differentiating factor between LCIS (Fig. 2.1) and ALH (Fig. 2.2) is based solely on the extent of involvement of the TDLUs. An interpretation of ALH is made if either less than 50% of the acini are involved and distended or greater than 50% of the acini are involved but without distention. In Fig. 2.2, more than 50% of the acini are involved, but without distention, thus favoring an interpretation of ALH. The morphologic distinction between LCIS and ALH is somewhat arbitrary and open to interpretation

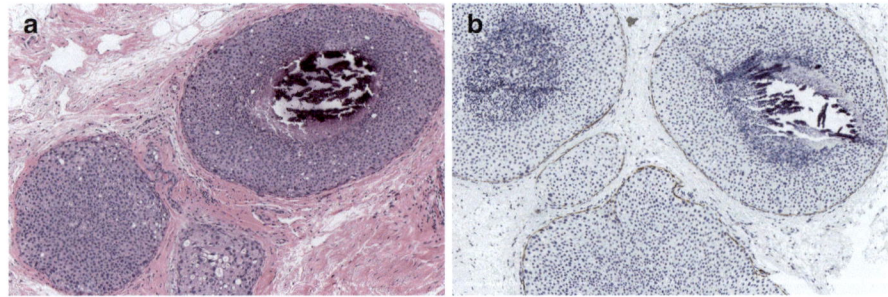

Fig. 2.3 (**a, b**) Pleomorphic LCIS (pLCIS). Solid proliferation of cells with high nuclear grade and pleomorphic cytomorphology. Central comedo-type necrosis is present in association with microcalcifications. The morphologic features on hematoxylin and eosin (H&E)-stained slides (**a**) are more reminiscent of high-grade ductal carcinoma in situ (DCIS); however, immunohistochemistry for E-cadherin reveals absence of membranous immunoreactivity (**b**). Taken together, the morphologic and immunohistochemical features are diagnostic of pleomorphic lobular carcinoma in situ (pLCIS)

of membranous E-cadherin staining, although aberrant E-cadherin staining has been reported in 0–9% of cases of LCIS [10]. A distinct subtype of LCIS that can resemble DCIS is pleomorphic LCIS (pLCIS), which shares many features of classical LCIS but is distinguished by the presence of high-grade, pleomorphic cytology that often has central comedo-type necrosis and associated microcalcifications (Figs. 2.3a, b). Absence of E-cadherin staining can help distinguish pLCIS from DCIS in challenging borderline cases.

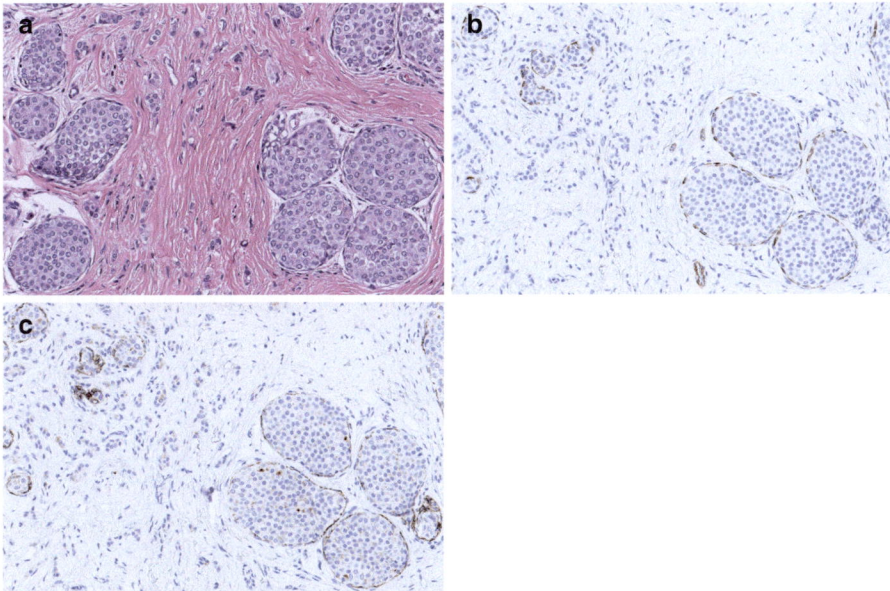

Fig. 2.4 (**a–c**) Invasive lobular carcinoma (ILC) arising in classical LCIS. Classical LCIS and associated single cells with low-grade cytomorphology infiltrating stroma in a linear and discohesive pattern (**a**). Immunohistochemistry (IHC) for smooth muscle myosin heavy chain (SMMHC) reveals immunoreactivity within the myoepithelial cells surrounding the foci of LCIS and absence in the infiltrative component (**b**), supporting an interpretation of in situ (LCIS) and invasive disease. IHC for E-cadherin (**c**) reveals absence of membranous immunoreactivity around both the in situ and invasive neoplastic cells, supporting an interpretation of lobular phenotype (invasive lobular carcinoma and LCIS). This intimate association of ILC and LCIS is morphologic evidence for a precursor lesion in this example

In situ lesions are distinguished from ILC by the lack of infiltration of neoplastic cells outside of the basement membrane and into the surrounding stroma. This interpretation can be supported by the absence of immunoreactive myoepithelial cells around neoplastic cells with immunohistochemical stains such as p63 and smooth muscle myosin heavy chain [11] (Fig. 2.4a–c).

Clinical Presentation and Epidemiology of Lobular Neoplasia

Clinically, LN most commonly presents as an asymptomatic lesion discovered incidentally in women aged 40–55 years during workup for another clinical or radiological indication. It has historically been reported to be found in 0.5–4% of excisional biopsies and 1.5% of core needle biopsies. LCIS rarely forms palpable masses and usually is mammographically occult. Thus, when microcalcifications are seen with LCIS, they generally are found in adjacent benign tissue separate from the lobular neoplastic architecture, making LCIS an incidental finding in the great majority of cases [12].

In an analysis of population-based registries of the National Cancer Institute's Surveillance, Epidemiology, and End Results (SEER) database from 1978 to 1998, Li and colleagues [13] found that LCIS incidence rates increased among women 40 years of age and older from 0.81 per 100,000 person-years in 1978–1980 to 3.19 per 100,000 person-years in 1996–1998. The highest incidence rate of LCIS in this dataset was 11.5 per 100,000 patient-years in women 50–59 years of age. In addition to the increasing rate of mammography, the authors hypothesized that combined hormone replacement therapy (HRT) may have contributed to the increase in LN given an increase in use of HRT during that time period. Subsequent studies have shown continued increases in LCIS diagnoses between 2000 and 2009 [14].

LCIS as an Invasive Cancer Risk Factor

Multicentricity and Bilaterality

Compared to the general population, women with LCIS have a 7–10-fold increased risk of future invasive breast carcinoma with a total lifetime risk of 1% per year [15], or about 7.7–26.3% in longer-term studies [16]. Studies from the 1970s demonstrated that the risk of future breast carcinoma was approximately equal in each breast after a diagnosis of LCIS. In one study in which routine contralateral breast biopsy was performed during initial surgery, 35% (9/26) of patients with LCIS were found to have bilateral carcinoma [17]. Table 2.1 summarizes the evidence for bilateral risk of future carcinoma after a diagnosis of LCIS. Across multiple studies, the rate of subsequent breast carcinomas was found to range from about 10% to 25% [18–24] over long-term follow-up, or 1–2% per year [17, 18]. Several early studies

Table 2.1 Studies demonstrating the incidence of subsequent invasive carcinoma in patients who underwent excision or partial mastectomy for LCIS

Study	Number	Mean follow-up (years)	Ipsilateral carcinoma N (%)	Contralateral carcinoma N (%)
Anderson, 1974 [61]	46 ipsilateral breasts, 52 contralateral breasts	16	9 (20%)	9 (17%)
Wheeler 1974 [7]	25 ipsilateral breasts, 34 contralateral breasts	15	1 (4%)	5 (15%)
Rosen, 1978 [62]	83 ipsilateral and contralateral breasts	24	18 (22%)	17 (20%)
Haagensen, 1978 [21]	257 ipsilateral breasts, 258 contralateral breasts	15	27 (11%)	27 (10%)
Page, 1991 [18]	39 ipsilateral and contralateral breasts	19	6 (15%)	4 (10%)
Bodian, 1996 [21]	236 patients	18	113 (48%)	92 (39%)
Fisher, 2004 [23]	180 patients	12	9 (5%)	10 (6%)
Chuba, 2005 [32]	350 patients	10	161 (46%)	189 (54%)

LCIS lobular carcinoma in situ

by Rosen and colleagues [16], Haagensen and colleagues [17], and Anderson and colleagues [20] examined patients in whom excisional biopsy was performed rather than mastectomy for LCIS. All of these studies noted an approximately equal percentage of subsequent carcinomas in the ipsilateral and contralateral breasts. More recent studies by Page and colleagues [15], as well as an analysis of the National Surgical Adjuvant Breast and Bowel Project (NSABP) B-17 study [22], supported the finding of comparable rates of future carcinoma in the ipsilateral and contralateral breast. One study even noted an increased incidence of contralateral over ipsilateral carcinoma [7]. In addition to the finding of bilateral risk of future carcinoma supporting the theory of LCIS as a risk factor lesion, Haagensen and colleagues [17] found that only 3 of 38 invasive carcinomas were believed to be derived from the lobular cells. Bodian and colleagues [22] examined 236 patients and showed that the risk of any invasive carcinoma was 12% at 10 years, 26% at 20 years, and 35% at 35 years, and of those who developed invasive carcinoma, the ipsilateral breast was involved only slightly more than the contralateral breast. Furthermore, 13% of those invasive carcinomas after LCIS were bilateral.

These data demonstrate that women with LCIS are at increased risk of breast carcinoma in the ipsilateral breast, but the incidence is lower than expected if LCIS were an obligate precursor of invasive carcinoma. In addition, the risk of breast carcinoma is evident in both the ipsilateral and contralateral breast. Taken together, the data found in Table 2.1 shows a similar risk of future carcinoma in the unaffected breast contralateral to the initial LCIS lesion and therefore supports the finding of LCIS as a risk factor for future carcinoma, rather than a direct precursor for carcinoma within the breast where the lesion was first identified.

Chemoprevention for LCIS

Noting that a large fraction of LCIS patients do not go on to form invasive breast cancer in the next one to two decades, Haagensen suggested that bilateral prophylactic mastectomy was an "excessively radical and unjustified form of treatment in terms of the relatively slight threat to life that lobular neoplasia presents" [21]. The management of LCIS then shifted away from mastectomy and has moved toward endocrine-based strategies for risk reduction. Several studies have shown that chemoprevention with selective estrogen receptor modulators (SERM) or aromatase inhibitors (AI) may reduce the risk of developing future invasive carcinoma.

In the 29-year prospective database study by King and colleagues [24], among women taking chemoprevention, the 10-year cumulative risk of breast carcinoma was reduced to 7% compared to 21% in women not taking chemoprevention. Chemoprevention was found to be the only clinical factor that reduced breast carcinoma risk. The International Breast Cancer Intervention Study (IBIS-I) was a randomized clinical trial that reported 7.0% rate of breast carcinoma in the tamoxifen group and 9.8% in the placebo group after a median follow-up of 16 years in women with increased risk of breast carcinoma, including family history, atypia, and LCIS. The NSABP-P1 study [25] randomized women at increased risk for breast carcinoma as defined by LCIS or Gail risk model criteria to either 5 years of tamoxifen or placebo. At the 7-year follow-up point, the rate of invasive carcinoma was reduced from 11.7 per 1000 women in the placebo group to 6.3 per 1000 women in the tamoxifen group. For this study, the risk ratio (RR) was 0.54 (95% CI 0.27–1.02). The Study of Tamoxifen and Raloxifene (STAR) trial [26] demonstrated that among postmenopausal women, both tamoxifen and another SERM, raloxifene, were equivalent in reducing the risk of invasive breast carcinoma. With respect to atypical lesions, 9% of patients in the study had LCIS and 23% had either ADH or ALH. Invasive events did not differ depending on tamoxifen or raloxifene treatment. AI therapy as exemestane in the MAP.3 trial or anastrozole in the IBIS-II trial in postmenopausal women was also found to reduce the incidence of breast cancers, with reduction specifically in patients with prior LN [27, 28]. In a large retrospective study, Coopey and colleagues [29] evaluated the effect of chemoprevention on women with atypical breast lesions (ADH, ALH, LCIS) and, at 10 years, found a decrease in invasive breast cancers from 32% to 10% with the use of chemoprevention. Therefore, given the increased risk of breast carcinoma in both breasts for women diagnosed with LCIS, consideration of chemoprevention with a SERM or AI is recommended [30] (Table 2.2).

Table 2.2 Summary of evidence for chemoprevention trials for LCIS

Study	Patients	Follow-up (years)	Agents	Results
Randomized controlled trials				
IBIS-I [63]	7154 women	16	Tamoxifen vs. placebo	HR = 0.71 (95% CI 0.60–0.83) in tamoxifen group vs placebo
NSABP-P1 [25]	14,453 women, 411 with LCIS	4.5	Tamoxifen vs. placebo	RR = 0.44 (95% CI 0.16–1.06) in tamoxifen vs placebo group
STAR P-2 [26]	20,616 women	6	Tamoxifen vs. raloxifene	Both agents equivalent in reducing breast cancer risk, breast cancer event rates similar in women with LCIS and did not differ by treatment
MAP.3 [27]	4560 women total, 373 with LN	2.9	Exemestane vs. placebo	HR = 0.61 (95% CI 0.20–1.82) for women with history of LN
IBIS-II [28]	3864 women total, 344 with LN	7	Anastrozole vs. placebo	HR = 0.31 (95% CI 0.12–0.84) for women with history of LN
Retrospective cohort studies				
Coopey [29]	2938 women with atypical lesions	5.7	Tamoxifen, raloxifene, exemestane	After 10 years, breast cancer rate reduced from 32% in no chemoprevention group to 10% in chemoprevention group
King [24]	1004 women	6.8	Chemoprevention not specified	HR 0.27 (95% CI 0.15–0.50) in women taking chemoprevention vs no chemoprevention

HR hazard ratio, *RR* risk ratio, *CI* confidence interval, *LCIS* lobular carcinoma in situ, *ILC* invasive lobular carcinoma, *NSABP* National Surgical Adjuvant Breast and Bowel Project, *IBIS* International Breast Cancer Intervention Study, *STAR*, Study of Tamoxifen and Raloxifene

LCIS as an Invasive Cancer Precursor

Ipsilateral Breast Carcinoma Risk

Although a portion of future invasive breast carcinomas following a diagnosis of LCIS are discovered at a site other than the original LCIS, there is evidence that risk may still be present at the breast of the initial lesion. Hutter and Foote [19] also provided early evidence supporting the theory of LCIS as a precursor lesion when they demonstrated subsequent invasive carcinoma in 25% (10/40) of patients with prior ipsilateral LCIS at follow-up ranging from 4 to 24 years. A retrospective study of 252 women demonstrated that following a diagnosis of ALH, the ipsilateral breast is 3 times more likely to develop invasive breast carcinoma than the contralateral breast [31]. Table 2.3 summarizes studies that demonstrate a greater rate of ipsilateral carcinoma following the finding of LCIS. In brief, large studies including a Danish nationwide prospective study [26], the SEER database [27], and the 29-year experience at Memorial Sloan Kettering Cancer Center [18] found that the rate of ipsilateral carcinoma was higher than the rate of contralateral carcinoma following a prior finding of LCIS. In particular, the SEER study by Li and colleagues [27] found not only that the rate of carcinoma was higher for the ipsilateral versus contralateral breast but also that the rate of ipsilateral carcinoma after LCIS was higher than the rate of ipsilateral carcinoma after DCIS. This data suggests that LCIS may be more than a risk factor for future invasive carcinoma.

Invasive Lobular Carcinoma at the Site of LCIS

If LCIS were a precursor to invasive carcinoma, it would be expected that the carcinoma would be more likely to be lobular than ductal as the noninvasive in situ lesion progresses and gains invasive capability. This finding has been confirmed in multiple studies that investigated the histology and laterality of subsequent breast carcinomas following biopsies showing LCIS. Although the 12-year follow-up analysis of the NSABP B-17 trial by Fisher and colleagues [23] found comparable rates of

Table 2.3 Studies showing high association of invasive carcinoma at the site of LCIS

Study	Findings
Otteson, 2000 [64]	Out of 100 women with LCIS, 18 developed invasive carcinoma. 16/18 (89%) were ipsilateral to LCIS, and 2/18 (11%) were contralateral
Li, 2006 [33]	Analysis of the SEER database revealed a rate of ipsilateral carcinoma was 7.3/1000 person-years and 5.2/1000 person-years for contralateral in women with LCIS. The rate of ipsilateral carcinoma was 35% higher than the rate of ipsilateral carcinoma for DCIS
King, 2015 [24]	150 women developed breast carcinoma out of 1004 with LCIS over 29-year experience. 94/150 (63%) of subsequent breast carcinomas were ipsilateral to the LCIS, 38/150 (25%) were contralateral, and the remainder were bilateral

LCIS lobular carcinoma in situ, *DCIS* ductal carcinoma in situ *ILC* invasive lobular carcinoma

Table 2.4 Comparison of invasive carcinoma histology following LCIS

Study	Findings
Fisher, 2004 [23]	8/9 (89%) ipsilateral invasive carcinomas were ILC in histology
Chuba, 2005 [32]	ILC more likely the histology of invasive carcinoma following LCIS (23%) than for invasive carcinoma without history of LCIS (6%)
Li, 2006 [33]	ILC was 5.3 times more likely to be found in LCIS patients than DCIS patients
Wallace, 2014 [34]	46% of ILC had associated LCIS
King, 2015 [24]	ILC and IDC after LCIS were equivalent

LCIS lobular carcinoma in situ, *ILC* invasive lobular carcinoma, *DCIS* ductal carcinoma in situ

invasive carcinoma in the ipsilateral and contralateral breasts, almost all of the invasive ipsilateral breast tumor recurrences were lobular histology. In the previously mentioned study by Chuba and colleagues [32], the histology of invasive carcinoma after LCIS was almost four times more likely to be ILC compared to primary breast carcinoma. Concurrent with the increased incidence of ILC, there was an associated decrease in IDC from 71% of primary invasive breast carcinomas to 50% of invasive breast carcinomas among patients with a history of LCIS. Li and colleagues [33] demonstrated that patients with LCIS were 5.3-fold more likely to be diagnosed with ILC compared to patients with DCIS. In a retrospective review of 148 cases with ILC or LCIS, Wallace and colleagues [34], for example, found that LCIS was frequently found in the vicinity associated with lobular carcinoma. In addition to the aforementioned studies, several others summarized in Table 2.4 show high rate of lobular histology of carcinoma following LCIS. Hence, the higher incidence of lobular histology of future carcinoma compared to the incidence of ILC in a population without LCIS suggests a relationship that ILC in some cases may have resulted from LCIS.

Genomic Similarities of LCIS and ILC

LCIS and ILC share many similarities both at the genotypic and phenotypic level. The classical types of both LCIS and ILC are usually ER/PR positive and HER2 negative. In addition to overlapping prognostic/predictive marker expression, a hallmark feature of both LCIS and ILC is the lack of E-cadherin expression on the cell surface, with aberrant expression noted in 0–9% of LCIS cases [10, 35]. While not strictly diagnostic of LCIS compared to DCIS because of aberrant expression patterns, the absence of membranous E-cadherin staining by IHC is a notable difference between the two entities [36]. At a genomic level, the gene for E-cadherin, CDH1, is located on chromosome 16q. CDH1 is frequently found to contain mutations and loss of heterozygosity (LOH) in both LCIS and ILC, but not IDC [37–40]. In addition to similar genomic and molecular profiles in LCIS and ILC with respect to E-cadherin expression, several other genomic alterations are noted to be similar in both entities. LOH is the loss of a normal allele on a cell which increases the risk of malignant transformation from potential loss of a tumor suppression gene. LOH on chromosome 16q has also been noted to be present by comparative genomic hybridization (CGH) in both ALH and LCIS lesions, suggesting a potential evolutionary link along the spectrum of LN [41]. LOH analysis at several additional chromosomal areas in addition to chromosome 16q, such as 17p, 17q, and 13q, demonstrates a monoclonal or neoplastic proliferation rather than a hyperplastic proliferation [42]. LOH has also been found at chromosome 11q13 in about 50% of cases of LCIS associated with ILC but with much lower frequency of LOH in cases of pure LCIS without ILC. Thus, LOH at this site may have also contributed to progression to invasion in those cases [43].

Several CGH and array CGH studies have been performed analyzing the clonality of LCIS and synchronous ILC. A series of 24 patients found frequent gain of 1q, loss of 16q, and loss of 11q suggesting clonality between LCIS and synchronous ILC in their samples [44]. Buerger and colleagues [45] found similarities of LCIS with DCIS on CGH analysis, including gains at 1q and losses at 16q. Another study of LCIS and adjacent ILC performed by Morandi and colleagues also demonstrated clonality in 7 out of 12 cases by CGH and 8 out of 12 cases by mitochondrial DNA and again demonstrated LOH at chromosome 16q [46]. Examining matched LCIS and synchronous invasive lesions, Andrade and colleagues [47] performed single nucleotide polymorphism (SNP) DNA microarrays and found that the majority (41%) were clonally related, with an additional 29% that were suggestive of clonality but equivocal. Begg and colleagues [48] performed whole-exome sequencing on fresh-frozen samples and by this technique also demonstrated clonal relatedness of LCIS and invasive breast carcinomas including both ILC and DCIS. The most frequent mutations were found in the genes CDH1 and PIK3CA. Parallel sequencing analysis found that shared mutations at one or both of these two sites were present in both LCIS and synchronous ILC [49]. Together (Table 2.5), these studies investigating genetic changes by multiple genomic techniques, including LOH analysis, CGH analysis, and whole genome and parallel sequencing analysis, suggest that LCIS is clonal and neoplastic, potentially indicating a non-obligate precursor for invasive disease.

Table 2.5 Summary of genetic data for LCIS and ILC

Study	Findings
Vos [37], Droufakou [38], Huiping [39], de Leeuw [40]	Decreased expression, LOH, and mutations of E-cadherin gene (*CDH1*) similar between LCIS and ILC
Lakhani [42]	LOH at chromosome 16q (also the location of E-cadherin gene), 17p, 17q, and 13q
Nayar [43]	11q13 in about 50% of cases of LCIS associated with ILC
Hwang [44], Morandi [46], Andrade [47]	CGH (showing gain at chromosome 1q, loss at 16q), SNP, and mitochondrial DNA analysis indicating high degree of clonality between LCIS and invasive carcinoma
Begg [48], Sakr [49]	Whole genome sequencing and parallel sequencing analysis demonstrate clonality and shared mutations of *CDH1* and *PIK3CA* genes

LCIS lobular carcinoma in situ, *ILC* invasive lobular carcinoma, *LOH* loss of heterozygosity, *CGH* comparative genomic hybridization, *SNP* single nucleotide polymorphism

Pleomorphic LCIS

Pleomorphic LCIS (pLCIS) is a distinct histopathologic subtype of LCIS that is typically considered to have a more aggressive biology than classical type LCIS. It also has a high rate of concurrent invasive carcinoma, with multiple studies demonstrating 17–66% of cases of pLCIS present in association with adjacent invasive carcinoma, predominantly ILC. Furthermore, up to 40% of cases of PLCIS have concurrent DCIS [50–59]. In total, these retrospective studies represent a total of 121 cases of pLCIS with an average of 15% concurrent DCIS and 40% concurrent invasive carcinoma, mostly ILC but also including IDC [60]. The recurrence rate of subsequent invasive carcinoma is reported to range from 0% to 12% [60]. Given the especially high rate of concurrent DCIS and invasive carcinoma, pLCIS is generally managed differently from classical LCIS with surgical excision [30].

Summary

LCIS lies on a spectrum of proliferative changes within the TDLU with intermediate risk between ALH and ILC. ALH and LCIS are often described collectively as LN, largely because the diagnostic criteria that distinguish these entities are somewhat subjective and open to interpretation. When first discovered, LN was considered to be a direct precursor to invasive carcinoma thought to be best treated by mastectomy. With additional data supporting the increased bilateral risk of subsequent invasive carcinoma, the view of LN changed toward that of a risk factor or a lesion that confers risk of future invasive carcinoma to both breasts. Genomic evidence now supports LN as having findings similar to invasive carcinoma, signifying LCIS as a precursor of invasive carcinoma. The current model now describes LCIS as both a risk factor and non-obligate precursor (Table 2.6).

Table 2.6 Summary of factors supporting LCIS as either risk factor lesion versus precursor lesion

LCIS as a risk factor	LCIS as a precursor
Carcinoma risk is bilateral	Similar morphology of LCIS to ILC
Only 15% of patients develop invasive carcinoma	LN present in 90% of ILC
50% of carcinomas are ductal	*CDH1* gene mutation common to LCIS and ILC
ADH and DCIS are also frequently present	CGH and LOH data with similar loss at 16q and gain at 1q between LCIS and ILC

LCIS lobular carcinoma in situ, *ILC* invasive lobular carcinoma, *ADH* atypical ductal hyperplasia, *DCIS* ductal carcinoma in situ, *CGH* comparative genomic hybridization, *LOH* loss of heterozygosity

References

1. Ewing J. Neoplastic diseases. 1st ed. Philadelphia: W.B. Saunders; 1919.
2. Foote FJ, Stewart FW. Lobular carcinoma in situ: a rare form of mammary carcinoma. Am J Pathol. 1941;17(4):491–6.
3. Godwin J. Chronology of lobular carcinoma of the breast: report of a case. Cancer. 1952;5(2):259–66.
4. Haagensen CD. Lobular neoplasia. In: Haagensen CD, editor. Diseases of the breast. 2nd ed. Philadelphia: W.B Saunders; 1971. p. 503.
5. Arpino G, Allred DC, Mohsin SK, Weiss HL, Conrow D, Elledge RM. Lobular neoplasia on core-needle biopsy – clinical significance. Cancer. 2004;101(2):242–50.
6. Frykberg ER. Lobular carcinoma in situ of the breast. Breast J. 1999;5(5):296–303.
7. Wheeler JE, Enterline HT, Roseman JM, Tomasulo JP, McIlvaine CH, Fitts WT, et al. Lobular carcinoma in situ of the breast. Long-term followup. Cancer. 1974;34(3):554–63.
8. Shin SJ, Rosen PP. Excisional biopsy should be performed if lobular carcinoma in situ is seen on needle core biopsy. Arch Pathol Lab Med. 2002;126(6):697–701.
9. Page DL, Dupont WD, Rogers LW, Rados MS. Atypical hyperplastic lesions of the female breast. A long-term follow-up study. Cancer. 1985;55(11):2698–708.
10. Canas-Marques RSS. E-cadherin immunohistochemistry in breast pathology: uses and pitfalls. Histopathology. 2016;68(1):57–69.
11. Zaha D. Significance of immunohistochemistry in breast cancer. World J Clin Oncol. 2014;5(3):382–92.
12. Beute BJ, Kalisher L, Hutter RV. Lobular carcinoma in situ of the breast: clinical, pathologic, and mammographic features. AJR Am J Roentgenol. 1991;157(2):257–65.
13. Li C, Anderson B, Daling J, Moe R. Changing incidence of lobular carcinoma in situ of the breast. Breast Cancer Res Treat. 2002;75(3):259–68.
14. Portschy PR, Marmor S, Nzara R, Virnig BA, Tuttle TM. Trends in incidence and management of lobular carcinoma in situ: a population-based analysis. Ann Surg Oncol. 2013;20(10):3240–6.
15. King TA, Reis-Filho JS. Lobular Neoplasia. Surg Oncol Clin N Am. 2014;23(3):487–503.
16. Afonso N, Bouwman D. Lobular carcinoma in situ. Eur J Cancer Prev Off J Eur Cancer Prev Organ. 2008;17(4):312–6.
17. Urban JA. Bilaterality of cancer of the breast. Biopsy of the opposite breast. Cancer. 1967;20(11):1867–70.
18. Page DL, Kidd TE, Dupont WD, Simpson JF, Rogers LW. Lobular neoplasia of the breast: higher risk for subsequent invasive cancer predicted by more extensive disease. Hum Pathol. 1991;22(12):1232–9.
19. Hutter R, Foote F. Lobular carcinoma in situ: long term follow up. Cancer. 1969;24(5):1081–5.
20. Anderson JA. Lobular carcinoma in situ. A histological study of 52 cases. Acta Pathol Microbiol Scand A. 1974;82(6):735–41.
21. Haagensen CD, Lane N, Lattes R, Bodian C. Lobular neoplasia (so-called lobular carcinoma in situ) of the breast. Cancer. 1978;42(2):737–69.
22. Bodian CA, Perzin KH, Lattes R. Lobular neoplasia. Long term risk of breast cancer and relation to other factors. Cancer. 1996;78(5):1024–34.
23. Fisher ER, Land SR, Fisher B, Mamounas E, Gilarski L, Wolmark N. Pathologic findings from the National Surgical Adjuvant Breast and Bowel Project: twelve-year observations concerning lobular carcinoma in situ. Cancer. 2004;100(2):238–44.
24. King TA, Pilewskie M, Muhsen S, Patil S, Mautner SK, Park A, et al. Lobular carcinoma in situ: a 29-year longitudinal experience evaluating clinicopathologic features and breast cancer risk. J Clin Oncol. 2015;33(33):3945–52.

25. Fisher B, Costantino JP, Wickerham DL, Cecchini RS, Cronin WM, Robidoux A, et al. Tamoxifen for the prevention of breast cancer: current status of the National Surgical Adjuvant Breast and Bowel Project P-1 study. JNCI: J Natl Cancer Inst. 2005;97(22):1652–62.
26. Vogel VG, Costantino JP, Wickerham DL, Cronin WM, Cecchini RS, Atkins JN, et al. Update of the National Surgical Adjuvant Breast and Bowel Project Study of Tamoxifen and Raloxifene (STAR) P-2 trial: preventing breast cancer. Cancer Prev Res (Phila). 2010;3(6):696–706.
27. Goss PE, Ingle JN, Alés-Martínez JE, Cheung AM, Chlebowski RT, Wactawski-Wende J, et al. Exemestane for breast-cancer prevention in postmenopausal women. N Engl J Med. 2011;364(25):2381–91.
28. Cuzick J, Sestak I, Forbes JF, Dowsett M, Knox J, Cawthorn S, et al. Anastrozole for prevention of breast cancer in high-risk postmenopausal women (IBIS-II): an international, double-blind, randomised placebo-controlled trial. Lancet. 2014;383(9922):1041–8.
29. Coopey SB, Mazzola E, Buckley JM, Sharko J, Belli AK, Kim EMH, et al. The role of chemoprevention in modifying the risk of breast cancer in women with atypical breast lesions. Breast Cancer Res Treat. 2012;136(3):627–33.
30. NCCN. Breast cancer (Version 2.2017) [Available from: https://www.nccn.org/professionals/physician_gls/pdf/breast.pdf
31. Page DL, Schuyler PA, Dupont WD, Jensen RA, Plummer WD, Simpson JF. Atypical lobular hyperplasia as a unilateral predictor of breast cancer risk: a retrospective cohort study. Lancet. 2003;361(9352):125–9.
32. Chuba PJ, Hamre MR, Yap J, Severson RK, Lucas D, Shamsa F, et al. Bilateral risk for subsequent breast cancer after lobular carcinoma-in-situ: analysis of surveillance, epidemiology, and end results data. J Clin Oncol. 2005;23(24):5534–41.
33. Li CI, Malone KE, Saltzman BS, Daling JR. Risk of invasive breast carcinoma among women diagnosed with ductal carcinoma in situ and lobular carcinoma in situ, 1988-2001. Cancer. 2006;106(10):2104–12.
34. Wallace AS, Xiang D, Hockman L, Arya M, Jeffress J, Wang Z, et al. Synchronous lobular carcinoma in situ and invasive lobular cancer: marker or precursor for invasive lobular carcinoma. Eur J Surg Oncol. 2014;40(10):1245–9.
35. Acs G, Lawton TJ, Rebbeck TR, LiVolsi VA, Zhang PJ. Differential expression of E-cadherin in lobular and ductal neoplasms of the breast and its biologic and diagnostic implications. Am J Clin Pathol. 2001;115(1):85–98.
36. Dabbs DJ, Schnitt SJ, Geyer FC, Weigelt B, Baehner FL, Decker T, et al. Lobular neoplasia of the breast revisited with emphasis on the role of E-cadherin immunohistochemistry. Am J Surg Pathol. 2013;37(7):e1–11.
37. Vos CB, Cleton-Jansen AM, Berx G, de Leeuw WJ, ter Haar NT, van Roy F, et al. E-cadherin inactivation in lobular carcinoma in situ of the breast: an early event in tumorigenesis. Br J Cancer. 1997;76(9):1131–3.
38. Droufakou S, Deshmane V, Roylance R, Hanby A, Tomlinson I, Hart IR. Multiple ways of silencing E-cadherin gene expression in lobular carcinoma of the breast. Int J Cancer. 2001;92(3):404–8.
39. Huiping C, Sigurgeirsdottir JR, Jonasson JG, Eiriksdottir G, Johannsdottir JT, Egilsson V, et al. Chromosome alterations and E-cadherin gene mutations in human lobular breast cancer. Br J Cancer. 1999;81(7):1103–10.
40. de Leeuw WJ, Berx G, Vos CB, Peterse JL, van de Vijver MJ, Litvinov S, et al. Simultaneous loss of E-cadherin and catenins in invasive lobular breast cancer and lobular carcinoma in situ. J Pathol. 1997;183(4):404–11.
41. Mastracci TL, Boulos FI, Andrulis IL, Lam WL. Genomics and premalignant breast lesions: clues to the development and progression of lobular breast cancer. Breast Cancer Res. 2007;9(6):215.
42. Lakhani SR, Collins N, Sloane JP, Stratton MR. Loss of heterozygosity in lobular carcinoma in situ of the breast. Clin Mol Pathol. 1995;48(2):M74–8.

43. Nayar RZ, Zhengping, Merino M, Silverberg S. Loss of heterozygosity on chromosome 11q13 in lobular lesions of the breast using tissue microdissection and polymerase chain reaction. Hum Pathol. 1997;28(3):277–82.
44. Hwang ES, Nyante SJ, Yi Chen Y, Moore D, DeVries S, Korkola JE, et al. Clonality of lobular carcinoma in situ and synchronous invasive lobular carcinoma. Cancer. 2004;100(12):2562–72.
45. Buerger H, Simon R, Schäfer KL, Diallo R, Littmann R, Poremba C, et al. Genetic relation of lobular carcinoma in situ, ductal carcinoma in situ, and associated invasive carcinoma of the breast. Mol Pathol. 2000;53(3):118–21.
46. Morandi L, Marucci G, Foschini MP, Cattani MG, Pession A, Riva C, et al. Genetic similarities and differences between lobular in situ neoplasia (LN) and invasive lobular carcinoma of the breast. Virchows Arch. 2006;449(1):14–23.
47. Andrade VP, Ostrovnaya I, Seshan VE, Morrogh M, Giri D, Olvera N, et al. Clonal relatedness between lobular carcinoma in situ and synchronous malignant lesions. Breast Cancer Res. 2012;14(4):R103.
48. Begg CB, Ostrovnaya I, Carniello JVS, Sakr RA, Giri D, Towers R, et al. Clonal relationships between lobular carcinoma in situ and other breast malignancies. Breast Cancer Res. 2016;18(1):66.
49. Sakr RA, Schizas M, Carniello JVS, Ng CKY, Piscuoglio S, Giri D, et al. Targeted capture massively parallel sequencing analysis of LCIS and invasive lobular cancer: repertoire of somatic genetic alterations and clonal relationships. Mol Oncol. 2015;10(2):360–70.
50. Carder PJ, Shabaan A, Alizadeh Y, Kumarasuwamy V, Liston JC, Sharma N. Screen-detected pleomorphic lobular carcinoma in situ (PLCIS): risk of concurrent invasive malignancy following a core biopsy diagnosis. Histopathology. 2010;57(3):472–8.
51. Chivukula M, Haynik DM, Brufsky A, Carter G, Dabbs DJ. Pleomorphic lobular carcinoma in situ (PLCIS) on breast core needle biopsies: clinical significance and immunoprofile. Am J Surg Pathol. 2008;32(11):1721–6.
52. Fasola C, Jensen K, Horst K. Local regional recurrence among patients with pleomorphic lobular carcinoma in situ: is there a role for radiation therapy? Int J Radiat Oncol Biol Phys. 2012;84(3):S238.
53. Morris K, Howe M, Kirwan C, Harvey J. Clinical and phenotypic characteristics of core biopsy diagnosed pleomorphic lobular carcinoma-in-situ in a UK population (PLCIS). Eur J Surg Oncol. 2013;39(5):484.
54. Niell B, Specht M, Gerade B, Rafferty E. Is excisional biopsy required after a breast core biopsy yields lobular neoplasia? AJR Am J Roentgenol. 2012;199(4):929–35.
55. Lavoué V, Graesslin O, Classe JM, Fondrinier E, Angibeau H, Levêque J. Management of lobular neoplasia diagnosed by core needle biopsy: study of 52 biopsies with follow-up surgical excision. Breast. 2007;16(5):533–9.
56. Georgian-Smith D, Lawton TJ. Calcifications of lobular carcinoma in situ of the breast: radiologic-pathologic correlation. AJR Am J Roentgenol. 2001;176:1255–9.
57. Mahoney MC, Robinson-Smith TM, Shaughnessy EA. Lobular neoplasia at 11-gauge vacuum-assisted stereotactic biopsy: correlation with surgical excisional biopsy and mammographic follow-up. AJR Am J Roentgenol. 2006;187(4):949–54.
58. Purdie CA, McLean D, Stormonth E, Macaskill EJ, McCullough JB, Edwards SL, Brown DC, Jordan LB. Management of in situ lobular neoplasia detected on needle core biopsy of breast. J Clin Pathol. 2010;63(11):987–93.
59. Flanagan MR, Rendi MH, Calhoun KE, Anderson BO, Javid SH. Pleomorphic lobular carcinoma in situ: radiologic-pathologic features and clinical management. Ann Surg Oncol. 2015;22(13):4263–9.
60. Wazir U, Wazir A, Wells C, Mokbel K. Pleomorphic lobular carcinoma in situ: current evidence and a systemic review. Oncol Lett. 2016;12(6):4863–8.
61. Anderson JA. Multicentric and bilateral appearance of lobular carcinoma in situ of the breast. Acta Pathol Microbiol Scand A. 1974;82(6):730–4.

62. Rosen PP, Lieberman PH, Braun DWJ, Kosloff C, Adair F. Lobular carcinoma in situ of the breast. Detailed analysis of 99 patients with average follow-up of 24 years. Am J Surg Pathol. 1978;2(3):225–51.
63. Cuzick J, Sestak I, Cawthorn S, Hamed H, Holli K, Howell A, et al. Tamoxifen for prevention of breast cancer: extended long-term follow-up of the IBIS-I breast cancer prevention trial. Lancet Oncol. 2015;16(1):67–75.
64. Ottesen GL, Graverson HP, Blichert-Toft M, Christensen IJ, Andersen JA. Carcinoma in situ of the female breast. 10 year follow-up results of a prospective nationwide study. Breast Cancer Res Treat. 2000;62(3):197–210.

Ductal Carcinoma In Situ: Risk Factor or Cancer

Nicci Owusu-Brackett and Funda Meric-Bernstam

Introduction

Ductal carcinoma in situ (DCIS or stage 0 breast cancer) is defined as a group of malignant-appearing cells within the breast ducts. The diagnosis has increased with the widespread adoption of screening mammography. Currently, DCIS accounts for 25% of breast cancers diagnosed in the United States and 20% of breast cancers detected with screening mammography [1, 2].

The risk of DCIS increases with age, and it is rare in women younger than 40, the age to begin mammographic screening in women of average risk of breast cancer. Other risk factors for DCIS include family history of breast cancer, late age at first birth, obesity, increased bone density, and nulliparity [3–7]. In addition, deleterious mutations in BRCA1 and BRCA2 genes result in inherited breast-ovarian cancer syndrome, where DCIS frequently occurs at a younger age in women with inherited BRCA mutations.

N. Owusu-Brackett
Department of Surgical Oncology, The University of Texas MD Anderson Cancer Center, Houston, TX, USA
e-mail: owusubracket@uthscsa.edu

F. Meric-Bernstam (✉)
Department of Surgical Oncology, The University of Texas MD Anderson Cancer Center, Houston, TX, USA

Department of Breast Surgical Oncology, The University of Texas MD Anderson Cancer Center, Houston, TX, USA

Department of Investigational Cancer Therapeutics (Phase I Clinical Trials Program), The University of Texas MD Anderson Cancer Center, Houston, TX, USA

Institute of Personalized Cancer Therapy, The University of Texas MD Anderson Cancer Center, Houston, TX, USA
e-mail: fmeric@mdanderson.org

There are no specific clinical manifestations of DCIS as more than 90% of DCIS cases are detected on imaging [8]. In the modern era, clustered calcifications in one area of the breast are often seen on mammography. Prior to routine screening mammography, patients typically presented with a palpable mass, Paget's disease, or nipple discharge [9, 10]. Of note, MRI may be more sensitive than mammogram for detection of DCIS; however, it can lack specificity. Mammographic patterns of microcalcifications such as linear branching and fine, granular calcifications are associated with different types of DCIS. While there are a variety of appearances of DCIS, all are confined to the breast duct, with the presence of malignant-appearing cells confined to the ductal lumen the hallmark of DCIS.

Sampling of the abnormal lesion or calcifications through core needle biopsy (preferably) or excisional biopsy is required to diagnose DCIS. The spectrum of DCIS histologic architectural subtypes includes micropapillary, cribriform, solid, comedo, and papillary with uniform cells growing from the duct wall (papillary), bridging the duct (cribriform), or filling the entire duct (solid). DCIS is also classified by nuclear grade ranging from low-grade, uniform-appearing nuclei to high-grade, large, and pleomorphic nuclei with or without necrosis within the duct. Histology and nuclear grade are prognostic and predictive factors that provide insight into the likelihood of progression, recurrence, and/or response to treatment in addition to size and estrogen receptor status of DCIS. These prognostic and predictive factors are important because DCIS can be associated with an increased risk of invasive breast cancer.

DCIS is considered a noninvasive or preinvasive breast cancer because the cells have yet to breach the ductal basement membrane to invade into the surrounding breast tissue, which differentiates it from invasive cancer. While not invasive in and of itself, DCIS is associated with an increased risk of invasive breast cancer. The fact that not all patients with DCIS progress to invasive cancer, along with an inability to reliably predict who will progress to invasion, has led to debate as to whether DCIS is simply a risk factor, or represents early cancer, and whether we should alter our locoregional management approach to this disease.

To acquire the traits to enable them to become tumorigenic and malignant, normal cells must undergo a process of tumor pathogenesis. Hanahan described eight biological capabilities acquired during the development of human tumors that enable tumor growth and metastatic dissemination: sustaining proliferative signaling, evading growth suppressors, resisting cell death, enabling replicative immortality, inducing angiogenesis, activating invasion and metastasis, reprogramming of energy metabolism, and evading immune destruction [11]. Normal cells maintain tissue architecture, function, and cell number via tight control of growth-promoting signals that regulate progression through the cell growth-and-division cycle. Somatic mutations that activate downstream pathways and defects in negative feedback mechanisms that attenuate proliferative signaling deregulate the controlled production and release of these growth-promoting signals allowing tumor cells to sustain chronic proliferation. In addition to sustaining growth signals, tumor cells must evade growth suppressors, avoid immune destruction, and resist cell death. To develop into large tumors, cancer cells require unlimited replicative potential for which nutrients, oxygen, and the removal of metabolic waste and carbon dioxide are necessary. Cancer cells induce angiogenesis to provide these metabolic needs in addition to adjusting their energy metabolism to fuel cell growth. Furthermore, genomic instability and mutations with tumor-promoting inflammation help promote tumorigenesis. As tumors develop, the cancer cells invade local tissue and then nearby the blood and lymphatic vessels. The cells later escape the vessels into distant tissues where they continue unlimited growth into macroscopic tumors. Talmadge and Fidler described these last steps as the invasion-metastasis cascade [12]. These eight hallmarks are integral to the pathogenesis of cancer and cancer metastasis, and all of these hallmarks exist in DCIS with the exception of angiogenesis and invasion/metastasis, which occur upon progression of DCIS to invasive cancer.

Progression of DCIS to Invasive Cancer

While DCIS has historically been surgically removed with breast-conserving surgery or mastectomy, information regarding the natural history of untreated disease is difficult to determine, although laboratory data and retrospective clinical studies can provide insight.

Holland demonstrated that estrogen receptor (ER)-negative comedo DCIS in xenograft mice had a faster proliferative rate than ER-positive noncomedo DCIS [13]. Estrogen treatment of xenograft-bearing mice did not affect the high level of cell proliferation in ER-negative comedo DCIS specimen but did increase levels of proliferation in ER-positive specimens; however, cell proliferation in ER-positive specimens with estrogen treatment did not reach the levels of proliferation in ER-negative DCIS specimens. Furthermore, in response to the NSABP B-24 trial, Gandhi evaluated the effect of antiestrogen treatment with fulvestrant on apoptosis or proliferation in ER-negative and ER-positive DCIS xenografts [14]. No effects of antiestrogen therapy were seen in ER-negative DCIS lesions, while no effect on proliferation but increased apoptosis was seen in ER-positive DCIS xenografts due to antiestrogen therapy, thus illustrating similarities in the biology of invasive disease and DCIS. In addition, Duru demonstrated in vitro and in vivo that DCIS can transition to invasive ductal carcinoma through increased activation of the OCT4/SOX2/lincRNA-RoR signaling axis as well as increased expression of K14, ARF6, and miR-10b [15]. Further evidence can be seen from retrospective clinical studies.

Mommers detected progressive changes in nuclear morphological and subvisual chromatin distribution features in the spectrum from intraductal proliferation to invasive cancer through evaluation of hyperplastic lesions, DCIS, and invasive cancer with image cytometry [16]. Larger and more pleomorphic nuclei with altered nuclear chromatin evidenced by reduced area of high-density chromatin, decreased contrast, increased fractal area, and increased optical intensity were found in more advanced lesions. In the DCIS and invasive carcinoma groups, significant differences in the feature values were noted between the poorly and well-differentiated

Table 3.1 Results of untreated ductal carcinoma in situ

Author	Number of patients that developed invasive breast carcinoma	Total number of patients
Dean [18]	6 (75%)	8
Haagensen [19]	8 (73%)	11
Rosen [20]	8 (53%)	15
Kraus [21]	2 (50%)	4
Page [22, 23]	9 (32%)	28
Millis [24]	2 (25)	8
Farrow [25]	5 (20%)	25
Eusebi [26]	11 (14%)	80

lesions, while the well-differentiated DCIS nuclei and well-differentiated invasive cancer were comparable. Similarly, the feature values for poorly differentiated invasive cancer were comparable to those of poorly differentiated DCIS.

Additionally, Leonard and Swain reviewed eight studies of patients misdiagnosed with benign breast disease. The patients received no treatment and were found subsequently to have DCIS on biopsy [17]. The rates of progression from DCIS to invasive cancer (as summarized in Table 3.1) ranged from 14% to 73% with an average rate of 43% from all the studies. In addition, Hernandez compared 13 cases of DCIS and synchronously diagnosed adjacent invasive carcinomas [18]. Pairwise analysis of each matched pair occasionally revealed important differences; however, overall pairs did not show significant differences in terms of copy number aberrations and mutations in known cancer genes when analyzed as a group. Matched DCIS and adjacent invasive breast carcinomas had a remarkably similar genomic profile, which supports the hypothesis that DCIS progressed to invasive cancer and suggests that the observed differences may be drivers of this progression. Buerger had similar results after performing comparative genomic hybridization (CGH) analysis on 38 DCIS specimens [19]. Analysis of five of six adjacent invasive breast cancer demonstrated genetic alterations almost identical to their corresponding DCIS counterpart, while one specimen revealed additional aberrations. Common alterations included 1q gains, amplifications of 17q12 and 11q13, and a whole-arm gain of 17q. Loss of 11q was suggested as a step in the progression from DCIS to invasive cancer. This data characterizes DCIS as a precursor of invasive breast carcinoma. Similarly, Burkhardt et al. [20] found no statistical significant differences between the amplification rates of HER2, ESR1, CCND1, and MYC when fluorescence in situ hybridization (FISH) was performed on DCIS and invasive breast carcinoma specimens [20]. This further supports the theory of progression of DCIS to invasive cancer.

Of note, non-genetic drivers of progression such as tumor microenvironment or stroma have been suggested. Elevated stromal cell expression of lysyl oxidases, an extracellular matrix-modifying enzyme, has been linked to invasion and metastasis [21, 22]. In addition, increased expression of COX-2 in tumor epithelial cells resulted in increased invasion in a DCIS xenograft model by stromal fibroblasts

[23]. Loss of the suppressive environment of the normal myoepithelium in addition to the loss of the secretion of protease inhibitors such as Maspin by the myoepithelial cells has been reported to contribute to progression of DCIS [24–26]. Furthermore, epigenetic alterations such as changes in histone modifications have been implicated in the epithelial-to-mesenchymal transition and reported to be associated with progression to invasive disease [27, 28].

Furthermore, similar molecular profiles between DCIS and invasive cancer also suggest progression. ER is frequently expressed in DCIS and invasive cancer. Zafrani noted higher levels of ER expression in less aggressive DCIS (increased differentiation and absence of necrosis) [29], while similar findings were noted for progesterone receptor expression. These findings support a common origin and that there can be progression of DCIS to invasive cancer.

Finally, Duffy obtained aggregate data for screen-detected cancers from 84 local screening units within 11 regional Quality Assurance Reference Centres in the National Health Service Breast Screening Programme [30]. This study found that for every three screen-detected cases of DCIS, there was one fewer invasive interval cancer in the next 3 years. This suggests not only that DCIS develops into invasive cancer but also that detection and treatment of DCIS is worthwhile in the prevention of future invasive disease.

Coexistence of DCIS and Invasive Cancer

While the development of invasive cancer from DCIS is a significant concern, some patients already have invasive disease at the time of diagnosis of their DCIS, a fact that is important to acknowledge as surgical nonintervention trials are being developed.

Field cancerization describes the association of invasive cancer with a surrounding area of in situ carcinoma [31], and clinical studies support the application of this concept to the breast. Dominguez performed a review of 177 patients with preoperative diagnoses of DCIS without invasion or microinvasion who underwent sentinel lymph node biopsies and mastectomies [32]. Invasive carcinoma was identified in 20 of 179 mastectomy specimens (11%). In 2016, Pilewskie evaluated 233 patients who underwent completion mastectomy for DCIS [33] and found that 9% of patients were upgraded on final pathology to invasive carcinoma. In a separate study, Pilewskie studied the incidence of synchronous invasive carcinoma in 296 patients and found that 20% of the patients had invasive carcinoma with heterogeneous grade, size, and receptor status at excision [34]. Evans reviewed 61 screen-detected grade 3 invasive breast tumors and found the presence of DCIS in 48 specimens (78.7%) [35]. In a larger study, Abdel-Fattah reported the presence of concurrent DCIS in 89% of 147 invasive breast cancer specimens reviewed [36]. Finally, Doebar found that 22% ($n = 34$) of 155 patients they identified with a preoperative diagnosis of DCIS upstaged to invasive breast cancer [37]. This study identified mass lesion on mammography, moderate to severe periductal inflammation, periductal loss of decorin expression, young age (≤40 years), and palpability as risk factors significantly associated with upstaging. The data supports that some patients with DCIS alone on biopsy already have invasive cancer, and most surgeons routinely perform sentinel lymph node biopsy in cases of mastectomies for DCIS to address this possibility of upstaging on final pathology.

Recurrence of DCIS

Current standard therapeutic options for DCIS include excision, excision with adjuvant endocrine or radiation therapy or both, and mastectomy. As previously mentioned, the diagnosis of DCIS has increased with adoption of screening mammography. The outcome of patients with DCIS is in general favorable, so there is much controversy about the need for therapy for DCIS and concern that DCIS is being overdiagnosed and overtreated. With this in mind, efforts are underway to determine which patient populations can be managed with observation alone and will be discussed in later chapters.

Muhsen hypothesized that patients with minimal-volume DCIS, which is defined as disease completely excised by core biopsy, would have a low risk for local recurrence after breast-conserving surgery and no adjuvant therapy if in fact their minimal-volume disease was a breast cancer risk factor and not a precursor lesion [38]. In addition, they hypothesized that risk of events in ipsilateral (IBE) and contralateral breast (CBE) would be similar. Among the 290 women evaluated with minimal-volume DCIS, 178 did not receive adjuvant therapy following breast-conserving surgery. The 10-year rate of ipsilateral breast events was higher than that of contralateral breast events at 14.5% compared to 2.7%. The rate of recurrence suggests that even minimal-volume DCIS is clinically relevant disease, while the greater risk of IBE than CBE supports DCIS as a precursor to invasive cancer rather than a risk marker.

Similarly, Wong hypothesized that wide local excision of DCIS with margins ≥1 cm would be sufficient therapy for small, grade 1 or 2 DCIS with a mammographic extent of ≤2.5 cm [39]. 158 patients were accrued in the study, and the observed 5-year rate of ipsilateral local recurrence was 12%. Of note, nine patients had recurrence of DCIS, while four had recurrence with invasive disease. The Eastern Cooperative Oncology Group (ECOG) 5194 DCIS single-arm prospective trial reported similar local failure rates of 10.5% in a low-risk DCIS cohort at the 7-year follow-up after breast-conserving surgery [40], while Pilewskie reported a comparable 10-year IBE rate of 12.1% [41].

While the treatment of DCIS may prevent development of invasive breast cancer, some patients will recur after surgery alone or with surgery and radiation. Much effort has gone into identifying which patients will recur. Rudloff built ten clinical, pathologic, and treatment variables into a nomogram to estimate the risk of ipsilateral breast tumor recurrence following treatment of DCIS with breast-conserving surgery [42]. Absence of adjuvant radiation or endocrine therapy, positive or close margin status, greater than three excisions and age at surgery were associated with

Table 3.2 Predictors of recurrence

Young age [35]
Tumor size [35]
Tumor grade [35]
Tumor subtype (estrogen receptor, progesterone receptor, human epidermal growth factor receptor 2) [35]
Molecular features (e.g., recurrence score, ductal carcinoma in situ score, decision score) [43–45]
Treatment (surgery type) [35]
Treatment (radiotherapy) [35]
Margin width [35]

significantly increased risk of ipsilateral breast tumor recurrence. A total of 11% ($n = 202$) of the 1868 patients within this study had recurrence, with 7% (122) recurring with DCIS and 4% ($n = 80$) with invasive disease.

It is also believed that molecular variables can be used to predict recurrence risk.

Benson and Wishart described the integration of molecular risk factors such as tumor subtype (ER, PR, HER2 statuses), indicators of proliferative activity (Ki67), and DCIS recurrence score with conventional histopathological and host risk factors such as treatment (surgery and radiotherapy), margin width, tumor size, tumor grade, and young age for more accurate prediction of invasive recurrence risk (as summarized in Table 3.2) [43]. Solin performed an Oncotype DX breast cancer assay for patients with DCIS treated with surgical excision without radiation [44]. The association of the DCIS score with the risk of developing an ipsilateral breast carcinoma was analyzed. The 10-year risks of developing any ipsilateral breast event for low-, intermediate-, and high-risk DCIS groups were 10.6%, 26.7%, and 25.9%, while the 10-year risks of developing an invasive ipsilateral breast event were 3.7%, 12.3%, and 19.2%, respectively. It does appear that the multigene DCIS score can be used a variable to predict risk of local recurrence independent of traditional clinical and pathologic factors.

Wärnberg validated a DCIS biologic signature for predictive utility in the SweDCIS trial [45]. 1046 women treated with breast cancer surgery (BCS) were randomized to adjuvant radiotherapy (RT) or no RT, and the 10-year benefit of RT on ipsilateral breast event and invasive breast cancer risks were assessed. The biologic signature along with clinical factors (age, margin, palpability, and size) was used to calculate continuous decision scores in 584 women. Patients with a score greater than three were defined as an elevated risk group. Analysis of decision score and radiotherapy interaction was significant for 10-year invasive breast cancer risk and ipsilateral breast events. In addition, stratification of patients into clinically relevant cohorts based on their decision scores (low and elevated risk) allowed the prediction of the RT benefit for ipsilateral breast events with significance. The patients with elevated risk were noted to have a 10-year benefit of RT with an absolute risk reduction of 9% for IBC, while no significant RT benefit was observed in the low-risk groups. Thus, this signature was able to identify a high-risk population that benefits from radiation therapy and a low-risk population that does not.

DCIS-Associated Mortality

Even at advanced centers, some patients who present with DCIS ultimately die from their disease, with mortality associated with DCIS due generally to recurrence as invasive disease. Roses identified 25 patients with distant breast cancer metastases after a diagnosis of pure DCIS from 2449 patients with a diagnosis of pure DCIS within the MD Anderson Breast Cancer Management System database [46]. While most patients (64%) with distant breast cancer metastases had preceding locoregional recurrence, 36% ($n = 9$) of patients with distant metastases did not. This suggests that in rare cases, recurrence as invasive disease is not required for DCIS-associated mortality. In addition, Narod reviewed a database of 108,196 women diagnosed with DCIS and found an overall breast cancer-specific mortality rate of 3.3% at 20 years [47]. The risk of dying from breast cancer increased after ipsilateral recurrence of invasive breast cancer; however, 517 patients died without having an invasive episode in either breast prior to death. These reports suggest that some patients with DCIS had invasive disease that was not diagnosed at the onset, likely due to limitation of tissue sampling.

Survival Benefit

Further need to treat DCIS as cancer is evidenced by the survival benefit observed with traditional management of DCIS with surgery and radiotherapy. Sagara performed a retrospective longitudinal cohort study using the Surveillance, Epidemiology, and End Results (SEER) database and identified 57,222 patients diagnosed with DCIS [48]. 1169 (2%) cases were managed without surgery, while 56,053 (98%) were managed with surgery. There were 576 (1%) breast cancer-specific deaths at the median follow-up of 72 months. The 10-year breast cancer-specific survival was 93.4% for the non-surgery cohort compared to 98.5% for the surgery cohort; however, the degree of survival benefit for the surgically managed patients differed depending on nuclear grade. For the low-grade DCIS patients, the survival benefit between the surgery and non-surgery groups was not significant. There was a significant difference in the survival benefits between the two cohorts of the intermediate- and high-grade DCIS patients. Of note, all patients within in the study had removal of some or all of the DCIS due to core or excisional biopsies [49]. Therefore, one could conclude that minimal or incomplete excision of low-grade DCIS may be sufficient to prevent death, while a more extensive excision is required for intermediate- and high-grade DCIS.

Subsequently, Sagara studied the survival benefit of the addition of radiotherapy (XRT) after breast-conserving surgery for DCIS [50]. 32,144 patients were identified from the SEER database. 20,329 patients received radiotherapy treatments, while 11,815 patients did not. 304 breast cancer-specific deaths occurred at the median follow-up of 96 months. The 10-year breast cancer-specific mortality at 10 years was 1.8% in the radiotherapy group and 2.1% in the non-radiotherapy group, although the difference observed between the two groups was not statistically significant. Age, tumor size, and nuclear grade were effect modifiers of radiotherapy for breast cancer mortality. Significant survival benefit in the XRT group was observed in patients with younger age, larger tumor size, and higher nuclear grade. In addition, the magnitude of the improved survival of XRT-managed patients was significantly correlated with the patient prognostic score for DCIS, which is determined by patient age, tumor size, and tumor histology [51]. Older patients with smaller and lower-grade tumors received lower prognostic scores. Patients with low scores (0 or 1) received no survival benefit, while those with higher scores (4 or 5) had an almost 70% reduction in breast cancer-specific mortality. Therefore, surgical treatment of DCIS with adjuvant therapies depending on risk factors provides a survival benefit.

Four prospective trials were designed to determine the effectiveness of breast-conserving surgery and adjuvant radiation therapy compared to only breast-conserving surgery in patients with DCIS [52–55] and are described in greater detail in later chapters. In addition, the Radiation Therapy Oncology Group 9804 study (RTOG9804) designed a prospective randomized trial in women with "good-risk" DCIS, defined as mammographically detected low- or intermediate-grade DCIS, measuring less than 2.5 cm with margins ≥3 mm [56]. RTOG 9804 evaluated the benefit of adjuvant radiotherapy following breast-conserving surgery in "good-risk" DCIS patients and also investigated whether clinical pathologic criteria could be used to define which cohort of DCIS patients would be expected to have a low risk for recurrence without radiation therapy in the first 7 years following breast-conserving surgery. The trial included 638 patients and reported a 7-year local failure rate of 0.9% in the radiotherapy arm compared to 6.7% in the observation cohort.

Finally, Muhsen evaluated the effect of adjuvant radiation in their retrospective review of 290 patients with minimal-volume DCIS [38]. They noted that women with intermediate- or high-risk DCIS were more likely to receive radiation. Adjuvant radiation was at the discretion of the treating physicians; therefore, the increase use of radiation in intermediate- and high-risk DCIS patients reflected the perception of recurrence risk. Despite the fact that the subset of patients receiving radiation had a higher recurrence risk, the radiotherapy subset had a nearly significant lower rate of IBE compared to the IBE rate of those who did not receive radiation. This demonstrates that even those with minimal-volume DCIS benefit from adjuvant radiation. The lower IBE risk compared to the CBE in the radiation subset while the IBE risk was greater in the non-radiation subset further supports the benefit of radiation. Recent interest has increased in less invasive therapies for DCIS by eliminating adjuvant radiation or endocrine therapy or surgery. Primary focus has been on patients perceived to have a minimal risk or recurrence. The Muhsen study confirms that even patients with perceived low risk (low grade and minimal volume) of recurrence benefit from managing DCIS as a precursor to invasive disease rather than a risk marker. Treatment needs to be personalized, and better predictors of outcome need to be developed and tested in clinical trials to better implement therapeutic decision-making.

Conclusion

The ability of DCIS to progress to invasive cancer, harbor concurrent invasive disease, recur after treatment, and cause distant metastases and death defines DCIS as a cancer; however, not all DCIS will behave this way. Studies to identify potential markers of progression to invasive disease and local recurrence are ongoing. Unfortunately, we have yet to establish biomarkers to predict outcome of DCIS. Due to the unknowns regarding who will progress, who will have synchronous invasive cancer, and who will recur, as well as the various clinical outcomes of DCIS, management of DCIS needs to be personalized for each individual based on patient factors such as age and race; histopathologic factors such as grade, size, necrosis, and receptor status; and genetics with oncotype DCIS. Because DCIS is a spectrum with varying malignant potentials, further clinical trials are needed to determine better predictors of outcome.

References

1. Siegel R, Naishadham D, Jemal A. Cancer statistics, 2013. CA Cancer J Clin. 2013;63(1):11–30.
2. Ernster VL, Ballard-Barbash R, Barlow WE, Zheng Y, Weaver DL, Cutter G, et al. Detection of ductal carcinoma in situ in women undergoing screening mammography. J Natl Cancer Inst. 2002;94(20):1546–54.
3. Schwartz GF, Solin LJ, Olivotto IA, Ernster VL, Pressman PI. Consensus conference on the treatment of in situ ductal carcinoma of the breast, April 22–25, 1999. Cancer. 2000;88(4):946–54.
4. Barclay J, Ernster V, Kerlikowske K, Grady D, Sickles EA. Comparison of risk factors for ductal carcinoma in situ and invasive breast cancer. J Natl Cancer Inst. 1997;89(1):76–82.
5. Claus EB, Stowe M, Carter D. Family history of breast and ovarian cancer and the risk of breast carcinoma in situ. Breast Cancer Res Treat. 2003;78(1):7–15.
6. Claus EB, Stowe M, Carter D. Breast carcinoma in situ: risk factors and screening patterns. J Natl Cancer Inst. 2001;93(23):1811–7.
7. Claus EB, Petruzella S, Matloff E, Carter D. Prevalence of BRCA1 and BRCA2 mutations in women diagnosed with ductal carcinoma in situ. JAMA. 2005;293(8):964–9.
8. Siegel R, Ward E, Brawley O, Jemal A. Cancer statistics, 2011: the impact of eliminating socioeconomic and racial disparities on premature cancer deaths. CA Cancer J Clin. 2011;61(4):212–36.
9. Richards T, Hunt A, Courtney S, Umeh H. Nipple discharge: a sign of breast cancer? Ann R Coll Surg Engl. 2007;89(2):124–6.
10. Günhan-Bilgen I, Oktay A. Paget's disease of the breast: clinical, mammographic, sonographic and pathologic findings in 52 cases. Eur J Radiol. 2006;60(2):256–63.
11. Hanahan D, Weinberg RA. Hallmarks of cancer: the next generation. Cell. 2011;144(5):646–74.
12. Talmadge JE, Fidler IJ. AACR centennial series: the biology of cancer metastasis: historical perspective. Cancer Res. 2010;70(14):5649–69.
13. Holland PA, Knox WF, Potten CS, Howell A, Anderson E, Baildam AD, et al. Assessment of hormone dependence of comedo ductal carcinoma in situ of the breast. J Natl Cancer Inst. 1997;89(14):1059–65.
14. Gandhi A, Holland PA, Knox WF, Potten CS, Bundred NJ. Effects of a pure antiestrogen on apoptosis and proliferation within human breast ductal carcinoma in situ. Cancer Res. 2000;60(15):4284–8.
15. Duru N, Gernapudi R, Lo PK, Yao Y, Wolfson B, Zhang Y, et al. Characterization of CD49f+/CD44+/CD24- single cell derived stem cell population in basal-like DCIS cells. Oncotarget. 2016;7(30):47511–25.

16. Mommers EC, Poulin N, Sangulin J, Meijer CJ, Baak JP, van Diest PJ. Nuclear cytometric changes in breast carcinogenesis. J Pathol. 2001;193(1):33–9.
17. Leonard G, Swain SM. Ductal carcinoma in situ, complexities and challenges. J Natl Cancer Inst. 2004;96(12):906–20.
18. Dean L, Geschickter CF. Comedo carcinoma of the breast. Archaeology. 1938;36:225–34.
19. Haagensen CD, Lane N, Lattes R. Neoplastic proliferation of the epithelium of the mammary lobules: adenosis, lobular hyperplasia, and small cell carcinoma. Surg Clin North Am. 1972;52:497–524.
20. Rosen PP, Braun DW Jr, Kinne DE. The clinical significance of preinvasive breast carcinoma. Cancer. 1980;46(4 Suppl):919–25.
21. Kraus FT, Neubecker RD. The differential diagnosis of papillary tumors of the breast. Cancer. 1962;15(3):444–55.
22. Page DL, Dupont WD, Rogers LW, Landenberger M. Intraductal carcinoma of the breast: follow up after biopsy only. Cancer. 1982;49(4):751–8.
23. Page DL, Dupont WD, Rogers LW, Jensen RA, Schuyler PA. Continued local recurrence of carcinoma 15–25 years after a diagnosis of low grade ductal carcinoma in situ of the breast treated only by biopsy. Cancer. 1995;76(7):1197–200.
24. Millis RR, Thynne GS. In situ intraduct carcinoma of the breast: a long term follow-up study. Br J Surg. 1975;62:957–62.
25. Farrow JH. Current concepts in the detection and treatment of the earliest of the early breast cancers. Cancer. 1970;25(2):468–77.
26. Eusebi V, Feudale E, Foschini MP, Micheli A, Conti A, Riva C, et al. Long-term follow-up of in situ carcinoma of the breast. Semin Diagn Pathol. 1994;11(3):223–35.
27. Hernandez L, Wilkerson PM, Lambros MB, Campion-Flora A, Rodrigues DN, Gauthier A, et al. Genomic and mutational profiling of ductal carcinomas in situ and matched adjacent invasive breast cancers reveals intra-tumour genetic heterogeneity and clonal selection. J Pathol. 2012;227(1):42–52.
28. Buerger H, Otterbach F, Simon R, Poremba C, Diallo R, Decker T, et al. Comparative genomic hybridization of ductal carcinoma in situ of the breast-evidence of multiple genetic pathways. J Pathol. 1999;187(4):396–402.
29. Burkhardt L, Grob TJ, Hermann I, Burandt E, Choschzick M, Janicke F, et al. Gene amplification in ductal carcinoma in situ of the breast. Breast Cancer Res Treat. 2010;123(3):757–65.
30. Barker HE, Chang J, Cox TR, Lang G, Bird D, Nicolau M, et al. LOXL2-mediated matrix remodeling in metastasis and mammary gland involution. Cancer Res. 2011;71(5):1561–72.
31. Levental KR, Yu H, Kass L, Lakins JN, Egeblad M, Erler JT, et al. Matrix crosslinking forces tumor progression by enhancing integrin signaling. Cell. 2009;139(5):891–906.
32. Hu M, Peluffo G, Chen H, Gelman R, Schnitt S, Polyak K. Role of COX-2 in epithelial-stromal cell interactions and progression of ductal carcinoma in situ of the breast. Proc Natl Acad Sci U S A. 2009;106(9):3372–7.
33. Place AE, Jin Huh S, Polyak K. The microenvironment in breast cancer progression: biology and implications for treatment. Breast Cancer Res. 2011;13(6):227.
34. Barsky SH, Karlin NJ. Myoepithelial cells: autocrine and paracrine suppressors of breast cancer progression. J Mammary Gland Biol Neoplasia. 2005;10(3):249–60.
35. Barsky SH, Karlin NJ. Mechanisms of disease: breast tumor pathogenesis and the role of the myoepithelial cell. Nat Clin Pract Oncol. 2006;3(3):138–51.
36. McDonald OG, Wu H, Timp W, Doi A, Feinberg AP. Genome-scale epigenetic reprogramming during epithelial-to-mesenchymal transition. Nat Struct Mol Biol. 2011;18(8):867–74.
37. Knudsen ES, Ertel A, Davicioni E, Kline J, Schwartz GF, Witkiewicz AK. Progression of ductal carcinoma in situ to invasive breast cancer is associated with gene expression programs of EMT and myoepithelial. Breast Cancer Res Treat. 2012;133(3):1009–24.
38. Zafrani B, Leroyer A, Fourqurt A, Laurent M, Trophilme D, Validire P, et al. Mammographically-detected ductal in situ carcinoma of the breast analysed with a new classification. A study of 127 cases: correlation with estrogen and progesterone receptors, p53 and c-erbB-2 proteins, and proliferative activity. Semin Diagn Pathol. 1994;11(3):208–14.

39. Duffy SW, Dibden A, Michalopoulos D, Offman J, Parmar D, Jenkins J, et al. Screen detection of ductal carcinoma in situ and subsequent incidence of invasive interval breast cancers: a retrospective population-based study. Lancet Oncol. 2016;17(1):109–14.
40. Slaughter DP, Southwick HW, Smejkal W. Field cancerization in oral stratified squamous epithelium; clinical implications of multicentric origin. Cancer. 1953;6(5):963–8.
41. Dominguez FJ, Golshan M, Black DM, Hughes KS, Gadd MA, Christian R, et al. Sentinel node biopsy is important in mastectomy for ductal carcinoma in situ. Ann Surg Oncol. 2008;15(1):268–73.
42. Pilewskie M, Karsten M, Radosa J, Eaton A, Kig TA. Is sentinel lymph node biopsy indicated at completion mastectomy for ductal carcinoma in situ? Ann Surg Oncol. 2016;23(7):2229–34.
43. Pilewskie M, Stempel M, Rosenfeld H, Eaton A, Van Zee KJ. Do LORIS trial eligibility criteria identify a ductal carcinoma in situ patient population at low risk of upgrade to invasive carcinoma? Ann Surg Oncol. 2016;23(11):3487–93.
44. Evans AJ, Pinder SE, Snead DR, Wilson AR, Ellis IO, Elston CW. The detection of ductal carcinoma in situ at mammographic screening enables the diagnosis of small, grade 3 invasive tumours. Br J Cancer. 1997;75(4):542–4.
45. Abdel-Fatah TM, Powe DG, Hodi Z, Lee AH, Reis-Filho JS, Ellis IO. High frequency of coexistence of columnar cell lesions, lobular neoplasia, and low grade ductal carcinoma in situ with invasive tubular carcinoma and invasive lobular carcinoma. Am J Surg Pathol. 2007;31(3):417–26.
46. Doebar SC, de Monyé C, Stoop H, Rothbarth J, Willemsen SP, van Deurzen CH. Ductal carcinoma in situ diagnosed by breast needle biopsy: predictors of invasion in the excision specimen. Breast. 2016;27:15–21.
47. Muhsen S, Barrio AV, Miller M, Olcese C, Patil S, Morrow M, Van Zee KJ. Outcomes for women with minimal-volume ductal carcinoma in situ completely excised at core biopsy. Ann Surg Oncol. 2017;24(13):3888–95.
48. Wong JS, Chen YH, Gadd MA, Gelman R, Lester SC, Schnitt SJ, et al. Eight-year update of a prospective study of wide excision alone for small low- or intermediate-grade ductal carcinoma in situ (DCIS). Breast Cancer Res Treat. 2014;143(2):343–50.
49. Hughes LL, Wang M, Page DL, Gray R, Solin LJ, Davidson NE, et al. Local excision alone without irradiation for ductal carcinoma in situ of the breast: a trial of the Eastern Cooperative Oncology Group. J Clin Oncol. 2009;27(32):5319–24.
50. Pilewskie M, Olcese C, Patil S, Van Zee KJ. Women with low-risk DCIS eligible for the LORIS trial after complete surgical excision: how low is their risk after standard therapy? Ann Surg Oncol. 2016;23(13):4253–61.
51. Rudloff U, Jacks LM, Goldberg JI, Wynveen CA, Brogi E, Patil S, et al. Nomogram for predicting the risk of local recurrence after breast-conserving surgery for ductal carcinoma in situ. J Clin Oncol. 2010;28(23):3762–9.
52. Benson JR, Wishart GC. Predictors of recurrence for ductal carcinoma in situ after breast-conserving surgery. Lancet Oncol. 2013;14(9):e348–57.
53. Solin LJ, Gray R, Baehner FL, Butler SM, Hughes LL, Yoshizawa C, et al. A multigene expression assay to predict local recurrence risk for ductal carcinoma in situ of the breast. J Natl Cancer Inst. 2013;105(10):701–10.
54. Wärnberg F, et al. Abstract GS5-08: A validation of DCIS biological risk profile in a randomised study for radiation therapy with 20 year follow-up (SweDCIS). Cancer Research, 2018;78(4 Supplement):p. GS5-08-GS5-08.
55. Roses RE, Arun BK, Lari SA, Mittendorf EA, Lucci A, Hunt KK, et al. Ductal carcinoma-in-situ of the breast with subsequent distant metastasis and death. Ann Surg Oncol. 2011;18(10):2873–8.
56. Narod SA, Igbal J, Giannakeas V, Sopik V, Sun P. Breast cancer mortality after a diagnosis of ductal carcinoma in situ. JAMA Oncol. 2015;1(7):888–96.
57. Sagara Y, Mallory MA, Wong S, Aydogan F, DeSantis S, Barry WT, et al. Survival benefit of breast surgery for low-grade ductal carcinoma in situ: a population-based cohort study. JAMA Surg. 2015;150(8):739–45.

58. Hughes K. DCIS does not need treatment... really? Breast Cancer Res Treat. 2015;154(1):1–4.
59. Sagara Y, Freedman RA, Vaz-Luis I, Malloy MA, Wong SM, Aydogan, et al. Patient prognostic score and associations with survival improvement offered by radiotherapy after breast-conserving surgery for ductal carcinoma in situ: a population-based longitudinal cohort study. J Clin Oncol. 2016;34(11):1190–6.
60. Smith GL, Smith BD, Hafty BG. Rationalization and regionalization of treatment for ductal carcinoma in situ of the breast. Int J Radiat Oncol Biol Phys. 2006;65(5):1397–403.
61. Fisher B, Dignam J, Wolmark N, Mamounas E, Costantino J, Poller W, et al. Lumpectomy and radiation therapy for the treatment of intraductal breast cancer: findings from the National Surgical Adjuvant Breast and Bowel Project B-17. J Clin Oncol. 1998;16(2):441–52.
62. Julien JP, Bijker N, Fentimen IS, Peterse JL, Delledonne V, Rouanet P, et al. Radiotherapy in breast conserving treatment for ductal carcinoma in situ: first results of the EORTC randomized phase III trial 10853—EORTC Breast Cancer Cooperative Group and EORTC Radiotherapy Group. Lancet. 2000;355:528–33.
63. Emdin SO, Granstrand B, Ringberg A, Sandelin K, Arnesson LG, Nordgren H, et al. SweDCIS: radiotherapy after sector resection for ductal carcinoma in situ of the breast—results of a randomized trial in a population offered mammography screening. Acta Oncol. 2006;45:536–43.
64. Houghton J, George WD, Cuzick J, Duggan C, Fentiman IS, Spittle M, et al. Radiotherapy and tamoxifen in women with completely excised ductal carcinoma in situ of the breast in the UK, Australia and New Zealand: randomized controlled trial. Lancet. 2003;362(9378):95–102.
65. McCormick B, Winter K, Hudis C, Kuerer HM, Rakovitch E, Smith BL, et al. RTOG 9804: a prospective randomized trial for good-risk ductal carcinoma in situ comparing radiotherapy with observation. J Clin Oncol. 2015;33(7):709–15.

Diagnostic Management of Papillomas, Radial Scars, and Flat Epithelial Atypia: Core Biopsy Alone Versus Core Biopsy Plus Excision

4

George Z. Li, Beth T. Harrison, and Faina Nakhlis

Introduction

Intraductal papillomas, radial scars, and flat epithelial atypia (FEA) are common benign breast lesions. This chapter will examine each of these three lesions and discuss the literature supporting core biopsy alone versus core biopsy plus excision. An important factor to consider in the management of any benign breast lesion diagnosed on core biopsy is the "upgrade rate" from a benign diagnosis on core biopsy to an in situ or invasive breast carcinoma diagnosis on subsequent surgical excision. The upgrade rates reported on excision of intraductal papillomas, radial scars, and FEA range widely, as the evidence is based on retrospective studies with varying sample sizes. This makes patient counseling challenging, and, as such, the decision to proceed with an excisional biopsy as a more definitive diagnostic procedure should be made in a multidisciplinary fashion with a radiologist and a pathologist.

An additional factor that plays a significant role in management decisions is the concept of radiographic-pathologic concordance, which is based on the Breast Imaging-Reporting and Data System (BI-RADS) classification [1]. A BI-RADS 1-3 designation implies that a benign core biopsy diagnosis is satisfactory and no further diagnostic intervention is needed. In contrast, a benign core biopsy diagnosis of a lesion with a BI-RADS classification of 4 or greater could raise concern for an insufficiently sampled malignancy. In 1996, the National Cancer Institute introduced the "triple test" for establishing concordance, which states that an excisional biopsy should be performed if there are any inconsistencies between clinical,

G. Z. Li · F. Nakhlis (✉)
Department of Surgery, Brigham and Women's Hospital, Boston, MA, USA
e-mail: gzli@partners.org; fnakhlis1@bwh.harvard.edu

B. T. Harrison
Department of Pathology, Brigham and Women's Hospital, Boston, MA, USA
e-mail: bharrison3@bwh.harvard.edu

© Springer International Publishing AG, part of Springer Nature 2018
F. Amersi, K. Calhoun (eds.), *Atypical Breast Proliferative Lesions and Benign Breast Disease*, https://doi.org/10.1007/978-3-319-92657-5_4

imaging, and pathological findings [2]. Evaluation of concordance can be somewhat subjective and requires a careful discussion with both the radiologist and the pathologist, but several confirmatory steps can help. For image-guided core biopsies, real-time images documenting the biopsy needle traversing the lesion of interest and adequately sampling it should be obtained during the procedure. In addition, for core biopsies of calcifications, radiographs of the specimen should be obtained to confirm that the targeted calcifications are present within the specimen. Additionally, the pathologist should histologically confirm the presence of calcifications to ensure that the lesion of interest has been sufficiently sampled [3].

Intraductal Papillomas

Intraductal papillomas are common lesions that account for at least 10% of benign breast disease. They are classified as solitary or multiple papillomas, and solitary papillomas are further subclassified as benign solitary intraductal papillomas and atypical papillomas [4]. Benign solitary intraductal papillomas are not associated with any malignancy, atypia, or other high-risk lesions, while atypical papillomas are associated with atypia, most commonly atypical ductal hyperplasia (ADH) [5, 6].

Clinically, papillomas can present with pathologic (bloody or serous) nipple discharge and/or a palpable mass but can also be asymptomatic and only discovered by screening mammography or as an incidental histological finding on a breast biopsy for another indication. Solitary papillomas tend to be subareolar, while multiple papillomas may present in more peripheral regions of the breast [4]. Mammography may demonstrate a circumscribed mass with or without calcifications (Fig. 4.1a), and ultrasound may show an intraductal mass (Fig. 4.1b).

Histologically, an intraductal papilloma appears as an intraductal proliferation composed of luminal epithelial cells and myoepithelial cells surrounding fibrovascular stalks (Fig. 4.1c). A variant of note is the sclerosing papilloma, which is characterized by stromal sclerosis that imparts the lesion with an irregular border. Papillomas may be involved by proliferative epithelial changes, including usual ductal hyperplasia (UDH), ADH, or ductal carcinoma in situ (DCIS). The term "atypical papilloma" refers to a papilloma with some degree of cytologic and/or architectural atypia, frequently sufficient for a diagnosis of ADH (Fig. 4.1d). An estimated 15% of ADH arises in association with a papilloma [4]. It is important to distinguish intraductal papillomas from papillary carcinoma, including intraductal ("papillary DCIS"), encapsulated, and solid forms. The diagnosis is facilitated by the use of immunohistochemical stains for myoepithelial markers (e.g., p63, smooth muscle myosin heavy chain, calponin), which highlight an intact myoepithelial cell layer in the fronds of a papilloma, in contrast to its absence in the those of papillary carcinoma.

The existing literature addressing the management of intraductal papillomas on core biopsy has shown conflicting results. A meta-analysis of 34 studies reported an upgrade rate of approximately 16% for 2236 papillary lesions diagnosed on core biopsy [7]. These studies are retrospective in nature, and the details regarding the

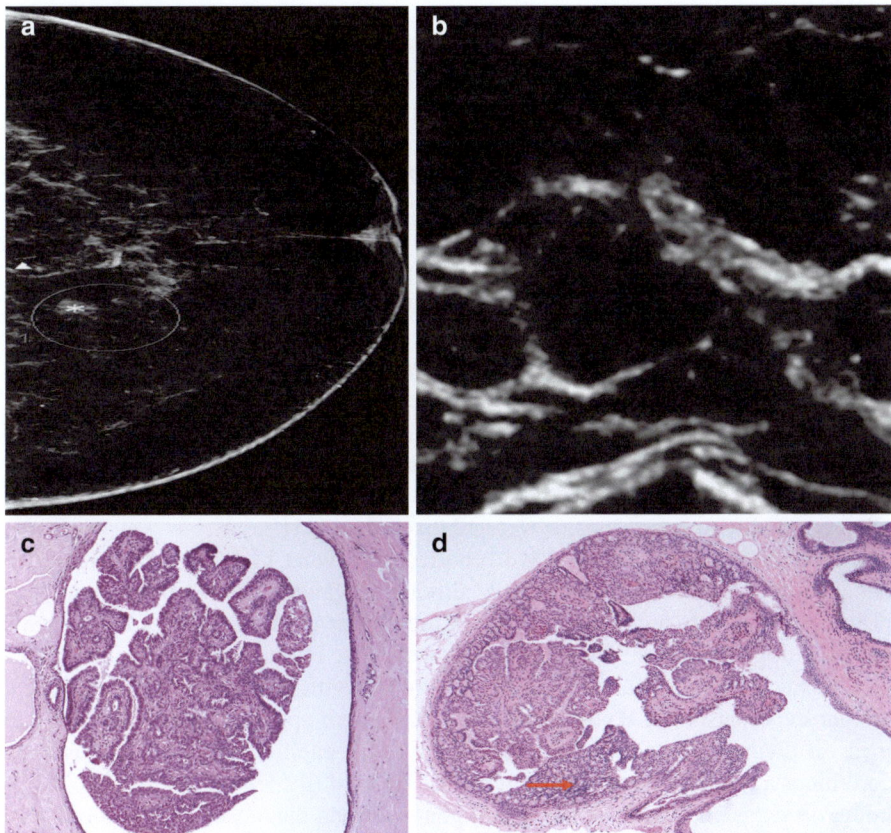

Fig. 4.1 (a) An intraductal papilloma presenting as a mammographic mass. (b) A hypoechoic mass corresponding to the mammographic finding in panel a. (c) An intraductal papilloma without atypia. (d) An intraductal papilloma with atypical ductal hyperplasia pointed by red arrow. (Courtesy of Dr. B. T. Harrison)

imaging characteristics and the clinical circumstances surrounding the decision to excise are incomplete. Nevertheless, based on this relatively high upgrade rate, some groups advocate for surgical excision of all intraductal papillomas found on core biopsy.

However, there is growing evidence that a "one size fits all" approach may not be appropriate for the management of papillary lesions diagnosed on core biopsy. In particular, benign solitary intraductal papillomas seem to have a much lower upgrade rate than other papillomas. Pareja et al. retrospectively examined 171 patients, all of whom had radiologic-pathologic concordance and no atypia or malignancy on core biopsy, and found a low upgrade rate of 2.3% (4/171) in this selected population [8]. Of the four malignancies, one was a DCIS involving the papilloma, while the other three (two invasive lobular carcinomas and one DCIS) were more than 8 mm away from the index papillary lesion, suggesting that the papilloma may have been incidental and unrelated to the adjacent carcinomas in these cases. Another retrospective study included 224 patients with a core biopsy diagnosis of benign solitary intraductal papilloma; 77 patients underwent surgical excision with a 0% upgrade rate, and 100 patients were observed with no imaging changes detected at a mean follow-up of 36 months [9].

In contrast, atypical papillomas and palpable papillomas have much higher upgrade rates. Sydnor et al. reported an upgrade rate of 67% (10/15) for atypical papillomas, in contrast to a 3% upgrade rate for papillomas without atypia (1/38), although the diagnosis on excision for the one upgraded lesion in the latter group was actually a lobular carcinoma in situ (LCIS), the latter not considered a true upgrade as this is a high-risk lesion but not a malignancy [10]. Another retrospective series of 97 patients with intraductal papillomas on core biopsy found a 6% upgrade rate to DCIS (two patients) or invasive cancer (one patient) for papillomas without atypia (3/45) but a 21% upgrade rate to DCIS for atypical papillomas (11/52). Of note, in the group without atypia, the two patients with DCIS both had palpable breast masses, and the patient with invasive cancer had a BI-RADS 4c lesion on mammography, so their biopsies were all discordant [11].

Other retrospective studies have reported somewhat higher upgrade rates for benign solitary intraductal papillomas, although upgrade rates for atypical papillomas are consistently high across the literature. For example, a series of 276 patients found an upgrade rate of 9% (8% to DCIS, and 1% to invasive ductal carcinoma) for papillomas without atypia, and among papillomas with associated ADH or atypical lobular hyperplasia (ALH) on core biopsy, 33% were upgraded to DCIS and 5% to invasive ductal carcinoma. In another study of 71 papillary lesions diagnosed on core biopsy, among 47 papillomas without atypia, 4 (9%) were upgraded to carcinoma on excision, and 2 of the 4 malignant lesions diagnosed on excision were found to be arising directly from the papilloma; among 16 atypical papillomas in this series, 7 (44%) were upgraded to malignancy [12].

Overall, the available literature suggests that surgical excision is appropriate for atypical papillomas due to high upgrade rates to malignancy and for palpable papillomas due to clinical-pathologic discordance. However, the management of benign solitary intraductal papillomas is more controversial, as all the existing literature addressing it is retrospective and the reported upgrade rates range from 0% to 9%, making clinical decision-making and patient counseling challenging. Currently, a prospective single-arm trial to address this issue is underway through the Translational Breast Cancer Research Consortium (TBCRC) (TBCRC 034, ClinicalTrials.gov identifier NCT02489617).

Multiple papillomas are defined as a radiographic cluster of at least five papillomas in the same quadrant of the breast [13]. As mentioned above, they are typically located more peripherally compared to solitary papillomas and more often present as clinically palpable masses. Furthermore, multiple papillomas are more frequently associated with atypical hyperplasia, DCIS, and radial scars/complex sclerosing lesions [14], and the reported upgrade rates to a malignant diagnosis range between 20% and 29%, based on small retrospective series [15, 16]. In addition, recurrence risk of multiple papillomas after surgical excision may be as high as 24% [17], although this evidence stems from literature from the 1980s. Currently, surgical excision is advocated for multiple papillomas due to the consistently high upgrade rate to malignancy of up to 29%.

In addition to the risk of missed associated malignancy, patients with intraductal papillomas are also associated with an increased risk of developing future breast cancer. Data from the Mayo Clinic Surgical Index and Pathology Index, which had a median follow-up of 15 years [18], showed that benign solitary intraductal papillomas are associated with a twofold increase in risk, similar to that of other proliferative lesions without atypia, and atypical papillomas are associated with a fivefold increase in risk, similar to that of atypical hyperplasia. Multiple papillomas are associated with a threefold increase in risk, but if atypia is also present, the future risk increases by sevenfold [19]. Overall, neither solitary nor multiple papillomas with or without atypia have been formally evaluated in any chemoprevention trials [20–23], and the actual magnitude of the increase in future breast cancer risk appears to be lower than that of atypical hyperplasias and LCIS. Therefore, chemoprevention is not indicated for these patients.

Radial Scars and Complex Sclerosing Lesions

A radial scar is a benign breast lesion that is usually asymptomatic and is typically discovered via screening mammography or incidentally as part of a biopsy specimen for another indication [24]. In fact, they can be found in up to 16.5% of biopsy or mastectomy specimens [25]. A complex sclerosing lesion (CSL) is generally a larger lesion (>1 cm) with more complex architecture [26].

Radiographically, radial scars may present as stellate densities, spiculated masses, or areas of architectural distortion (Fig. 4.2a), and thus can closely mimic malignancy on imaging, which unfortunately makes concordance especially difficult to establish. Radial scars can also rarely present as isolated microcalcifications. Histologically, a radial scar contains a central zone of sclerosis and elastosis surrounded by radiating ducts and lobules. Obliterated ducts and acini with angulated contours are entrapped within the fibroelastotic stroma (Fig. 4.2b). The radiating ducts and lobules are

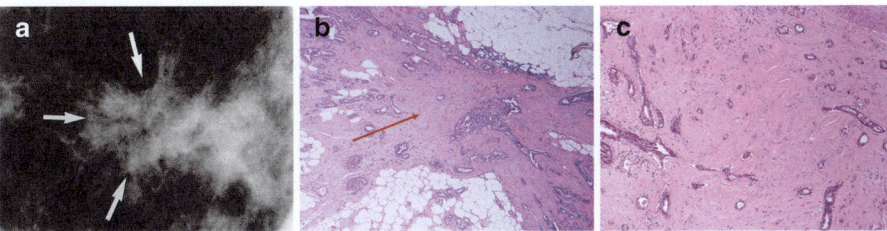

Fig. 4.2 (a) Mammographic appearance of a radial scar presenting as an irregular mass (arrows) with spiculated borders. (b) A radial scar consisting of a central zone of sclerosis and elastosis surrounded by radiating ducts and lobules. (c) Glands entrapped within the fibroelastotic center of a sclerosing lesion may mimic invasive ductal carcinoma. (Courtesy of Dr. B.T. Harrison)

typically involved by a variety of non-proliferative and proliferative changes, including cysts, apocrine metaplasia, sclerosing adenosis, papillomatosis, usual and atypical hyperplasia, and carcinoma in situ. A complex sclerosing lesion is composed of the same elements, but it contains multiple sclerotic areas and a non-radial configuration (Fig. 4.2c). The angulated glands entrapped within the sclerotic stroma may raise consideration for a diagnosis of invasive carcinoma, particularly tubular or well-differentiated ductal types. This is especially true for limited core needle biopsy specimens in which the fibroelastotic core of the lesion is predominantly sampled. In such circumstances, immunohistochemical stains for myoepithelial markers should confirm that the myoepithelial cell layer is retained in the sclerosing lesion or lost in an invasive carcinoma. Of note, multiple markers should be utilized in equivocal cases as the myoepithelial cell layer may be attenuated in the entrapped glands.

Most radial scars with mammographic architectural distortion are excised due to difficulty establishing radiologic-pathologic concordance, while those with associated atypia are also excised primarily due to the presence of atypia. However, radial scars can present solely as mammographic calcifications without either associated atypia or architectural distortion. Brenner et al. evaluated 198 radial scars diagnosed on core biopsy. Seventy patients had a vacuum-assisted device employed for the core biopsy, of whom 68 patients had at least 12 core biopsy specimens removed, and 157 ultimately underwent an excision; among 28 patients in this cohort whose only imaging abnormalities were microcalcifications, there were no upgrades [27]. Another study examined 19 patients with mammographically occult radial scars/CSLs without atypia that were diagnosed on ultrasound with imaging characteristics ranging from BI-RADS 3 to BI-RADS 4b. Eighteen of 19 patients underwent an excision, and 1 patient was followed, with a 0% upgrade rate for all patients [28]. In another cohort of 161 patients with radial scar without an associated proliferative lesion, only 1 patient was upgraded to malignancy on excision, and this was a 2 mm DCIS that was 5 mm away from the core biopsy site. Furthermore, in the upgraded case, there were residual calcifications on post-core biopsy mammogram, suggesting the possibility of insufficient core biopsy sampling [29]. In this study, 3% of biopsies were performed for architectural distortion, and the majority (59%) were performed for calcifications. Finally, in a recent report of 34 excisions for radial scars, 17 of which had concordance and BI-RADS information available, 3 cases (9%) were upgraded. All upgraded cases were discordant with BI-RADS classification of 4b or higher, all presented as mammographic distortions, and one of these three patients had a palpable mass [30].

In some studies without well-specified radiographic indications for the initial core biopsy yielding the diagnosis of pure radial scar, such as BI-RADS classification and concordance, the upgrade rates range between 0% and 10% [31]. The presence of clinical symptoms may be a significant predictor of a higher likelihood of upgrade, as was shown in a cohort of 175 patients with radial scar/CSL diagnosed on core biopsy, 89 of whom presented with clinical symptoms that were not specified. In the clinically symptomatic group, the upgrade rate was 33% vs. a 7% upgrade rate in the clinically asymptomatic group [32]. The presence of clinical symptoms, such as a palpable mass, suggests the possibility of discordance, which was not reported in the study. Better quality data as to whether radial scars/CSLs without mammographic architectural distortion or associated atypia may be safely observed would be helpful to improve patient counseling and management of these patients.

As for future breast cancer risk implications, it is unclear whether radial scars/CSLs are potential precursors to atypical hyperplasia and/or breast carcinoma. One study examined 117 radial scar cases and noted a statistically significant correlation between age and the association of radial scars with atypical lesions and malignancy [33]. Several studies have also shown an increased risk for future malignancy in patients with radial scars. A large case-control study of 1396 women, including 99 patients with radial scars, found that radial scars conferred a 1.8-fold increased risk of breast cancer [34]. This risk increase is similar to that of other proliferative lesions without atypia, though the study also found that among patients with proliferative lesions without atypia, the presence of radial scar further independently increased their risk of cancer from 1.5-fold to 3-fold. Another large retrospective study found a 1.8-fold increased risk of developing a future breast cancer in patients with radial scars [35]. Interestingly, in this study, 92% of patients with radial scars also had atypia (Table 4.1). Similarly to intraductal papillomas, radial scars and CSLs were not formally studied in any of the completed chemoprevention trials [20–23], but the reported small increase in future breast cancer risk associated with radial scars is helpful for patient counseling and reassurance [34–36].

Flat Epithelial Atypia

Flat epithelial atypia (FEA) is a breast lesion found in 5% of percutaneous breast biopsies. Over the years, it has been defined by a variety of other names, including "clinging carcinoma, monomorphic type," "atypical cystic lobules," and "columnar cell change/hyperplasia with atypia" [37]. In 2003, the World Health Organization established FEA as a "presumably neoplastic intraductal alteration characterized by

Table 4.1 Studies of the risk of future breast cancer in patients with radial scar or complex sclerosing lesions

Study	Number of patients with radial scar/CSL	Relative risk of future breast cancer (95% CI)	Comments
Nurses' Health Study (Jacobs et al. 1999) [34]	99	1.8 (1.1–2.9)	Increased risk was found to be independent of presence of other proliferative breast diseases
Vanderbilt (Sanders et al. 2006) [35]	880	1.82 (1.2–2.7)	92% of patients also had other proliferative breast diseases
Mayo Clinic (Berg et al. 2008) [36]	439	1.88 (1.36–2.53)	There was no increase in the risk found in patients with proliferative disease without atypia with or without concurrent radial scar/CSL

CSL complex sclerosing lesion, *CI* confidence interval

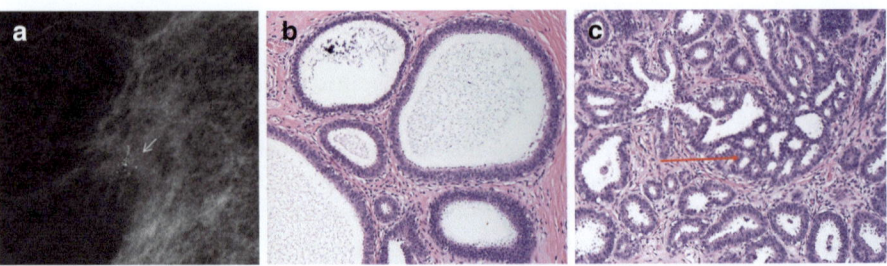

Fig. 4.3 (**a**) Mammographic appearance of a flat epithelial atypia as a cluster of calcifications (arrow). (**b**) Flat epithelia atypia consisting of dilated and rounded acini lined by a multilayered epithelium with low-grade cytologic atypia. (**c**) Atypical ductal hyperplasia with a cribriform growth pattern (red arrow) arising in flat epithelial atypia. (Courtesy of Dr. B.T. Harrison)

the replacement of native epithelial cells by a single layer of three to five layers of mildly atypical cells." [38] FEA is usually asymptomatic and most often presents as breast calcifications on screening mammography (Fig. 4.3a).

Histologically, FEA is usually present within enlarged terminal duct lobular units (TDLUs) containing variably dilated acini and intraluminal calcifications (Fig. 4.3b). The normal luminal epithelium is replaced by one to multiple layers of cuboidal-to-columnar cells with low-grade cytologic atypia of the monomorphic type. FEA often arises in a background of columnar cell change/hyperplasia and appears to serve as a direct precursor to ADH and low-grade DCIS, the spectrum of changes from benign to malignant sometimes coexistent in the same or adjacent TDLUs (Fig. 4.3c). Moreover, it is also commonly identified in close proximity to other entities in the low-grade breast neoplasia pathway, including lobular neoplasia and tubular carcinoma, a finding referred to as the "Rosen triad" [39].

The reported upgrade rates for pure or isolated FEA, i.e., FEA without associated ADH, range from 0% to 21%. One study by Kunju et al. examined 60 core biopsies of pure FEA, pure ADH, or both. They found a 21% upgrade rate to DCIS and/or invasive carcinoma even in the pure FEA group, which was equivalent to that of the overall group [40]. However, another study of 156 cases of FEA diagnosed on core biopsy with or without additional atypical lesions included 36 patients with pure FEA who underwent subsequent surgical excision, and none had malignancy on final surgical pathology [41]. Interestingly, the upgrade rates from more recent studies appear to be generally lower, possibly due to improved sampling with larger core biopsy needles [42]. Prowler et al. reported no upgrades in 24 patients with pure FEA on core biopsy [43], and another study reported a 6.9% (2/29) upgrade rate of pure FEA to in situ carcinoma, but both of the upgraded cases had residual microcalcifications on post-core biopsy mammogram, suggesting inadequate sampling [44]. At this time, for patients with pure FEA on core biopsy, the existing evidence to support either monitoring or surgical excision is insufficient. The TBCRC 034 study discussed previously also has an FEA arm and will be able to provide prospective data to help address this issue.

As is the case with intraductal papillomas, FEA associated with atypical lesions should be excised, as the reported upgrade rates for these are significantly higher. One study of 77 patients, 46 with pure FEA and 31 with FEA plus ADH, ALH, or LCIS, found an upgrade of 2% (1 DCIS) in the pure FEA group but an upgrade rate of 16% (4 DCIS and 1 invasive tubular carcinoma) in the FEA plus atypia group [45]. Another study found similar results, with no upgrades in 20 patients with pure FEA and a 30% upgrade rate in 10 patients with FEA plus ADH (2 DCIS and 1 invasive carcinoma) [46].

There is some molecular evidence that FEA may be a precursor lesion to in situ or invasive ductal carcinoma [47]. FEA lesions often have loss of chromosome 16q, a genetic alteration also commonly found in DCIS [48]. Expression of miR-21, which is associated with invasive breast carcinoma, also increases in frequency from normal breast tissue to FEA to DCIS to invasive ductal carcinoma [49]. There is also pathologic evidence that FEA may be a precursor to atypical lesions, as a study by Said et al. that evaluated surgical excision specimens containing ADH and ALH found that 30–46% of these cases also had FEA present.

However, the actual risk of future breast cancer associated with the diagnosis of FEA is less clear. The same study by Said et al. found that FEA did not confer any additional cancer risk if found in biopsy specimens in conjunction with other proliferative lesions with or without atypia [50]. Another report from the Nurses' Health Study came to similar conclusions: the study found that columnar cell lesions, including FEA, did not significantly increase the risk of future breast cancer after controlling for the presence of proliferative histology and/or atypia, though it did not describe FEA separately from other columnar cell lesions such as columnar hyperplasia or columnar cell change [51]. In the context of these studies, chemoprevention is not currently indicated for patients with FEA.

Summary

Table 4.2 summarizes the upgrade rates and current management recommendations for these lesions. For all lesions, it is critical to first determine concordance of clinical findings, radiologic characteristics, and the histopathologic diagnosis on core biopsy. Patients with discordant lesions should proceed to surgical excision. For concordant lesions, clinicians should consider the upgrade rates associated with

Table 4.2 Summary of upgrade rates and management options for benign breast lesions

Core biopsy diagnosis	Upgrade rate on excision (%)	Management
Intraductal papilloma		
BISP	0–9	Excision vs. observation
Atypical papilloma	21–67	Excision
Palpable papilloma	–	Excision[a]
Multiple papillomas	20–29	Excision
Radial scar/CSL	0–33	Excision[a]
Radial scar/CSL without architectural distortion or atypia	0	Excision vs. observation
FEA	0–21	Excision vs. observation

BISP benign intraductal solitary papilloma, *CSL* central sclerosing lesion, *FEA* flat epithelial atypia
[a]Decision to excise is driven by lack of concordance

each particular pathologic diagnosis. Unfortunately, the literature currently consists almost entirely of retrospective series, and upgrade rates vary from study to study. Two lesions with evidence demonstrating acceptably low upgrade rates are benign solitary intraductal papilloma and pure FEA, and the TBCRC 034 study will be able to add prospective and presumably more definitive data to the existing evidence about the management of these lesions. Radial scars/CSLs that present only as calcifications on mammogram that do not have associated atypia on core biopsy also have low upgrade rates, though prospective data are similarly needed to inform the optimal management of these lesions.

References

1. Mercado CL. BI-RADS update. Radiol Clin N Am. 2014;52(3):481–7.
2. The uniform approach to breast fine needle aspiration biopsy. A synopsis. Acta Cytol 1996;40(6):1120–6; discussion 19.
3. Bassett LW, Mahoney MC, Apple SK. Interventional breast imaging: current procedures and assessing for concordance with pathology. Radiol Clin N Am. 2007;45(5):881–94. vii
4. Neal L, Sandhu NP, Hieken TJ, Glazebrook KN, Mac Bride MB, Dilaveri CA, et al. Diagnosis and management of benign, atypical, and indeterminate breast lesions detected on core needle biopsy. Mayo Clin Proc. 2014;89(4):536–47.
5. Liberman L, Bracero N, Vuolo MA, Dershaw DD, Morris EA, Abramson AF, et al. Percutaneous large-core biopsy of papillary breast lesions. AJR Am J Roentgenol. 1999;172(2):331–7.
6. Shah VI, Flowers CI, Douglas-Jones AG, Dallimore NS, Rashid M. Immunohistochemistry increases the accuracy of diagnosis of benign papillary lesions in breast core needle biopsy specimens. Histopathology. 2006;48(6):683–91.
7. Wen X, Cheng W. Nonmalignant breast papillary lesions at core-needle biopsy: a meta-analysis of underestimation and influencing factors. Ann Surg Oncol. 2013;20(1):94–101.
8. Pareja F, Corben AD, Brennan SB, Murray MP, Bowser ZL, Jakate K, et al. Breast intraductal papillomas without atypia in radiologic-pathologic concordant core-needle biopsies: rate of upgrade to carcinoma at excision. Cancer. 2016;122(18):2819–27.
9. Swapp RE, Glazebrook KN, Jones KN, Brandts HM, Reynolds C, Visscher DW, et al. Management of benign intraductal solitary papilloma diagnosed on core needle biopsy. Ann Surg Oncol. 2013;20(6):1900–5.
10. Sydnor MK, Wilson JD, Hijaz TA, Massey HD. Shaw de Paredes ES. Underestimation of the presence of breast carcinoma in papillary lesions initially diagnosed at core-needle biopsy. Radiology. 2007;242(1):58–62.
11. Nakhlis F, Ahmadiyeh N, Lester S, Raza S, Lotfi P, Golshan M. Papilloma on core biopsy: excision vs. observation. Ann Surg Oncol. 2015;22(5):1479–82.
12. Bernik SF, Troob S, Ying BL, Simpson SA, Axelrod DM, Siegel B, et al. Papillary lesions of the breast diagnosed by core needle biopsy: 71 cases with surgical follow-up. Am J Surg. 2009;197(4):473–8.
13. Azzopardi JG, Ahmed A, Millis RR. Problems in breast pathology. Philadelphia: Saunders; 1979.
14. Muttarak M, Lerttumnongtum P, Chaiwun B, Peh WC. Spectrum of papillary lesions of the breast: clinical, imaging, and pathologic correlation. AJR Am J Roentgenol. 2008;191(3):700–7.
15. Harjit K, Willsher PC, Bennett M, Jackson LR, Metcalf C, Saunders CM. Multiple papillomas of the breast: is current management adequate? Breast. 2006;15(6):777–81.
16. Liberman L, Tornos C, Huzjan R, Bartella L, Morris EA, Dershaw DD. Is surgical excision warranted after benign, concordant diagnosis of papilloma at percutaneous breast biopsy? AJR Am J Roentgenol. 2006;186(5):1328–34.

17. Haagensen CD. Diseases of the breast. 3rd ed. Philadelphia: Saunders; 1986.
18. Hartmann LC, Sellers TA, Frost MH, Lingle WL, Degnim AC, Ghosh K, et al. Benign breast disease and the risk of breast cancer. N Engl J Med. 2005;353(3):229–37.
19. Lewis JT, Hartmann LC, Vierkant RA, Maloney SD, Shane Pankratz V, Allers TM, et al. An analysis of breast cancer risk in women with single, multiple, and atypical papilloma. Am J Surg Pathol. 2006;30(6):665–72.
20. Cuzick J, Sestak I, Forbes JF, Dowsett M, Knox J, Cawthorn S, et al. Anastrozole for prevention of breast cancer in high-risk postmenopausal women (IBIS-II): an international, double-blind, randomised placebo-controlled trial. Lancet. 2014;383(9922):1041–8.
21. Fisher B, Costantino JP, Wickerham DL, Redmond CK, Kavanah M, Cronin WM, et al. Tamoxifen for prevention of breast cancer: report of the National Surgical Adjuvant Breast and Bowel Project P-1 Study. J Natl Cancer Inst. 1998;90(18):1371–88.
22. Goss PE, Ingle JN, Ales-Martinez JE, Cheung AM, Chlebowski RT, Wactawski-Wende J, et al. Exemestane for breast-cancer prevention in postmenopausal women. N Engl J Med. 2011;364(25):2381–91.
23. Vogel VG, Costantino JP, Wickerham DL, Cronin WM, Cecchini RS, Atkins JN, et al. Effects of tamoxifen vs raloxifene on the risk of developing invasive breast cancer and other disease outcomes: the NSABP Study of Tamoxifen and Raloxifene (STAR) P-2 trial. JAMA. 2006;295(23):2727–41.
24. Krishnamurthy S, Bevers T, Kuerer H, Yang WT. Multidisciplinary considerations in the management of high-risk breast lesions. AJR Am J Roentgenol. 2012;198(2):W132–40.
25. Andersen JA, Gram JB. Radial scar in the female breast. A long-term follow-up study of 32 cases. Cancer. 1984;53(11):2557–60.
26. Adler DD, Helvie MA, Oberman HA, Ikeda DM, Bhan AO. Radial sclerosing lesion of the breast: mammographic features. Radiology. 1990;176(3):737–40.
27. Brenner RJ, Jackman RJ, Parker SH, Evans WP 3rd, Philpotts L, Deutch BM, et al. Percutaneous core needle biopsy of radial scars of the breast: when is excision necessary? AJR Am J Roentgenol. 2002;179(5):1179–84.
28. Park VY, Kim EK, Kim MJ, Yoon JH, Moon HJ. Mammographically occult asymptomatic radial scars/complex sclerosing lesions at ultrasonography-guided core needle biopsy: follow-up can be recommended. Ultrasound Med Biol. 2016;42(10):2367–71.
29. Leong RY, Kohli MK, Zeizafoun N, Liang A, Tartter PI. Radial scar at percutaneous breast biopsy that does not require surgery. J Am Coll Surg. 2016;223(5):712–6.
30. Nakhlis F, Lester S, Denison C, Wong SM, Mongiu A, Golshan M. Complex sclerosing lesions and radial sclerosing lesions on core needle biopsy: low risk of carcinoma on excision in cases with clinical and imaging concordance. Breast J. 2017 [Epub ahead of print]. https://doi.org/10.1111/tbj.12859.
31. Hayes BD, O'Doherty A, Quinn CM. Correlation of needle core biopsy with excision histology in screen-detected B3 lesions: the Merrion Breast Screening Unit experience. J Clin Pathol. 2009;62(12):1136–40.
32. Patterson JA, Scott M, Anderson N, Kirk SJ. Radial scar, complex sclerosing lesion and risk of breast cancer. Analysis of 175 cases in Northern Ireland. Eur J Surg Oncol. 2004;30(10):1065–8.
33. Manfrin E, Remo A, Falsirollo F, Reghellin D, Bonetti F. Risk of neoplastic transformation in asymptomatic radial scar. Analysis of 117 cases. Breast Cancer Res Treat. 2008;107(3):371–7.
34. Jacobs TW, Byrne C, Colditz G, Connolly JL, Schnitt SJ. Radial scars in benign breast-biopsy specimens and the risk of breast cancer. N Engl J Med. 1999;340(6):430–6.
35. Sanders ME, Page DL, Simpson JF, Schuyler PA, Dale Plummer W, Dupont WD. Interdependence of radial scar and proliferative disease with respect to invasive breast carcinoma risk in patients with benign breast biopsies. Cancer. 2006;106(7):1453–61.
36. Berg JC, Visscher DW, Vierkant RA, Pankratz VS, Maloney SD, Lewis JT, et al. Breast cancer risk in women with radial scars in benign breast biopsies. Breast Cancer Res Treat. 2008;108(2):167–74.

37. Georgian-Smith D, Lawton TJ. Variations in physician recommendations for surgery after diagnosis of a high-risk lesion on breast core needle biopsy. AJR Am J Roentgenol. 2012;198(2):256–63.
38. Tavassoli FA, Devilee P, International Agency for Research on Cancer, World Health Organization. Pathology and genetics of tumours of the breast and female genital organs. Lyon: IARC Press; 2003.
39. Rosen PP. Columnar cell hyperplasia is associated with lobular carcinoma in situ and tubular carcinoma. Am J Surg Pathol. 1999;23(12):1561.
40. Kunju LP, Kleer CG. Significance of flat epithelial atypia on mammotome core needle biopsy: should it be excised? Hum Pathol. 2007;38(1):35–41.
41. Senetta R, Campanino PP, Mariscotti G, Garberoglio S, Daniele L, Pennecchi F, et al. Columnar cell lesions associated with breast calcifications on vacuum-assisted core biopsies: clinical, radiographic, and histological correlations. Mod Pathol. 2009;22(6):762–9.
42. Racz JM, Carter JM, Degnim AC. Challenging atypical breast lesions including flat epithelial atypia, radial scar, and intraductal papilloma. Ann Surg Oncol. 2017 [Epub ahead of print]. https://doi.org/10.1245/s10434-017-5980-6.
43. Prowler VL, Joh JE, Acs G, Kiluk JV, Laronga C, Khakpour N, et al. Surgical excision of pure flat epithelial atypia identified on core needle breast biopsy. Breast. 2014;23(4):352–6.
44. Dialani V, Venkataraman S, Frieling G, Schnitt SJ, Mehta TS. Does isolated flat epithelial atypia on vacuum-assisted breast core biopsy require surgical excision? Breast J. 2014;20(6):606–14.
45. Acott AA, Mancino AT. Flat epithelial atypia on core needle biopsy, must we surgically excise? Am J Surg. 2016;212(6):1211–3.
46. Piubello Q, Parisi A, Eccher A, Barbazeni G, Franchini Z, Iannucci A. Flat epithelial atypia on core needle biopsy: which is the right management? Am J Surg Pathol. 2009;33(7):1078–84.
47. Bombonati A, Sgroi DC. The molecular pathology of breast cancer progression. J Pathol. 2011;223(2):307–17.
48. Moinfar F, Man YG, Bratthauer GL, Ratschek M, Tavassoli FA. Genetic abnormalities in mammary ductal intraepithelial neoplasia-flat type ("clinging ductal carcinoma in situ"): a simulator of normal mammary epithelium. Cancer. 2000;88(9):2072–81.
49. Qi L, Bart J, Tan LP, Platteel I, Sluis T, Huitema S, et al. Expression of miR-21 and its targets (PTEN, PDCD4, TM1) in flat epithelial atypia of the breast in relation to ductal carcinoma in situ and invasive carcinoma. BMC Cancer. 2009;9:163.
50. Said SM, Visscher DW, Nassar A, Frank RD, Vierkant RA, Frost MH, et al. Flat epithelial atypia and risk of breast cancer: a Mayo cohort study. Cancer. 2015;121(10):1548–55.
51. Aroner SA, Collins LC, Schnitt SJ, Connolly JL, Colditz GA, Tamimi RM. Columnar cell lesions and subsequent breast cancer risk: a nested case-control study. Breast Cancer Res. 2010;12(4):R61.

Diagnostic Management of Fibroepithelial Lesions: When Is Excision Indicated?

Nicholas Manguso and Catherine Dang

Introduction

Fibroepithelial lesions represent a heterogeneous group of breast disease ranging from benign tumors to malignant neoplasms. This group of lesions is characterized by biphasic proliferation of the epithelial and stromal components of breast tissue, and the clinical presentation of both benign and malignant lesions may overlap. Arising from the fibrous stroma, these lesions share a common etiology and entrap fully developed, normal ducts and ductal lobular units. They occur in women of all ages, though fibroadenomas are more commonly found in younger women in the second and third decades of life, whereas phyllodes tumors typically occur beyond the fourth decade [1]. Benign and malignant lesions share similar clinical and imaging characteristics, with pathologic diagnosis through core needle or excisional biopsy often required in order to direct optimal management. Benign lesions, such as fibroadenomas and PASH, can usually be monitored with close follow-up, whereas phyllodes tumors require excision with widely negative margins. Occasionally, core needle biopsy will be insufficient to establish a diagnosis, and an excisional biopsy will be required to obtain a definitive diagnosis. In the following chapter, we will describe the clinical presentation, imaging characteristics, pathologic features, and management of different fibroepithelial lesions, including fibroadenomas, PASH, and phyllodes tumors.

Fibroadenoma

Fibroadenomas are benign, hyperplastic tumors arising from the epithelium and stroma of the breast. The true incidence is difficult to determine as many of these lesions never come to the attention of a medical provider due to their benign nature.

N. Manguso · C. Dang (✉)
Cedars-Sinai Medical Center, Department of Surgery, Los Angeles, CA, USA
e-mail: Nicholas.Manguso@cshs.org; Catherine.Dang@cshs.org

Some studies report an incidence of 7–13% in women examined in a breast clinic [2], whereas incidence in autopsy specimens report fibroadenomas in 10% of patients [2, 3]. Fibroadenomas are the most common benign breast tumors occurring in 25% of asymptomatic women with a peak incidence around 20–30 years of age though they be detected later in life as well [1, 4]. Fibroadenomas represent 50% of all biopsied breast lesions and 75% of all biopsied lesions in women under the age of 20 [5, 6]. These lesions are also more common in African-American women compared to Caucasians [7, 8]. Typically, patients with simple fibroadenomas have no increased risk of breast cancer, although some studies have shown that patients with complex fibroadenomas may have as much as a twofold increased risk of breast cancer [9]. Rarely, DCIS or even invasive cancer may arise within fibroadenomas [10].

Diagnosis

Diagnosis of fibroadenomas and other fibroepithelial lesions relies on the triple test of clinical examination, imaging, and biopsy. Histologic diagnosis may not be necessary if clinical exam and imaging support a benign etiology and the lesion has been demonstrated to be stable over a course of close follow-up.

Clinical Presentation

Patients with fibroadenomas often present with a palpable, well-defined, non-tender, mobile, oval, or lobulated mass on physical examination. Non-palpable masses may also be identified on screening mammogram in older women undergoing regular surveillance. They may be hormone-responsive tumors that can grow in size with pregnancy, the menstrual cycle, or with the use of exogenous hormones in postmenopausal women [11, 12]. These lesions rarely show evidence of skin changes, nipple retraction, or discharge, and the presence of any of these symptoms should prompt thorough investigation and biopsy to rule out a malignant process. Fibroadenomas are typically less than 3 cm in size, though giant fibroadenomas, often larger than 5 cm, occur less commonly. These lesions can arise anywhere in the breast and most are solitary lesions, with only 10–20% of women known to present with multiple fibroadenomas in the same breast [4, 7].

Imaging Findings

Diagnostic breast ultrasound is critical to the evaluation of any palpable breast mass. This is especially true in younger women who typically have denser breast tissue, which lowers the sensitivity of mammography. Benign lesions, such as fibroadenomas, usually appear on ultrasound as an oval or gently lobulated, well-defined

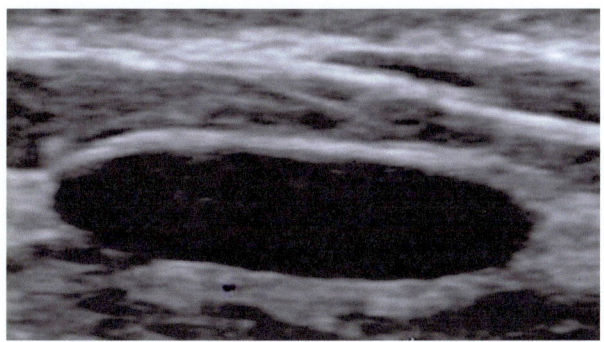

Fig. 5.1 On ultrasound, fibroadenomas typically are described as being well-circumscribed, hypoechoic, wider-than-tall masses and are internally homogeneous

mass [13–15]. Often these lesions have a parallel orientation to the skin and are generally wider than they are tall [16]. Fibroadenomas are generally homogenous internally and have weak acoustic edge shadowing and/or posterior acoustic enhancement [13] (Fig. 5.1). In older women, involuting fibroadenomas may contain course, hyperechoic calcifications [17]. These findings, while typical, are actually only present in 20–30% of cases [17].

Mammogram is commonly used for the evaluation of a breast mass especially in women over the age of 30. In younger, premenopausal women, it may be less useful as younger women typically have radiographically dense breast tissue. Aside from evaluating the palpable compliant, non-palpable masses elsewhere in the breasts and suspicious microcalcifications may help the clinician identify malignancy and determine if the mass was present previously if prior mammograms are available for comparison. On mammography, fibroadenomas are usually well-circumscribed, round, or oval masses. Lobulation may present especially in larger fibroadenomas [14]. Well-delineated borders can indicate a benign histology. Older fibroadenomas and those beginning to involute can have characteristic coarse, "popcorn"-like calcifications [17] that differ from malignant calcifications which are microscopic and pleomorphic.

MRI is not routinely used in the diagnosis of fibroadenomas. However, patients occasionally undergo MRI for other reasons, and fibroadenomas may be incidentally found. The usual appearance of a fibroadenoma on MRI is an oval, enhancing, well-circumscribed mass [18, 19]. Fibroadenomas may have slow or rapid initial enhancement with a persistent late-phase enhancement, which helps differentiate them from breast cancers [19].

Imaging is an important aspect of the workup of a fibroadenoma, specifically to rule out malignancy. In younger women, a mass with characteristics typical of a fibroadenoma can be monitored with serial imaging alone. However, if there are any concerning features on clinical examination or imaging, the mass should be biopsied to confirm the clinical and radiographic impression. Biopsy remains an important diagnostic tool as fibroadenomas frequently have similarities to other fibroepithelial lesions, some of which are best managed by aggressive resection.

Pathologic Findings

Both fine-needle aspiration cytology (FNAC) and core needle biopsy (CNB) can be used in the diagnosis of fibroadenomas. FNAC is used primarily in younger women with a high suspicion for fibroadenoma though it often is less definitive than CNB, which remains the preferred method of histologic examination. Pathologic examination of suspected fibroadenomas should be considered for all masses that do not have typically benign characteristics or for masses that are changing or growing on follow-up imaging and exam.

On gross examination, fibroadenomas are pseudo-encapsulated masses with sharply delineated borders surrounding normal breast tissue [20]. These tumors are typically spherical or ovoid in shape with some being multilobulated. The cut surface will show a tan-white mass through the pseudocapsule [20]. The typical cytologic findings of a fibroadenoma on FNAC are benign epithelial cells with dark-staining myoepithelium and light staining luminal cells [21]. In young women, cytology is often cellular with low false-negative rates. While FNAC may be adequate in young women, CNB is more appropriate for the vast majority of patients. In premenopausal women, CNB often shows a mixture of epithelial cells separated by viable stroma [20, 22] (Fig. 5.2). Typically, there is no increase in stromal cellularity, atypia, or mitotic activity. These features are important in the differentiation between fibroadenomas and phyllodes tumors (Table 5.1). In postmenopausal women, fibroadenomas often show hyalinized stroma and may be associated with coarse calcifications [21]. Fibroadenomas may also be classified as complex if epithelial hyperplasia, apocrine metaplasia, sclerosing adenosis, and cysts with calcifications exist [22].

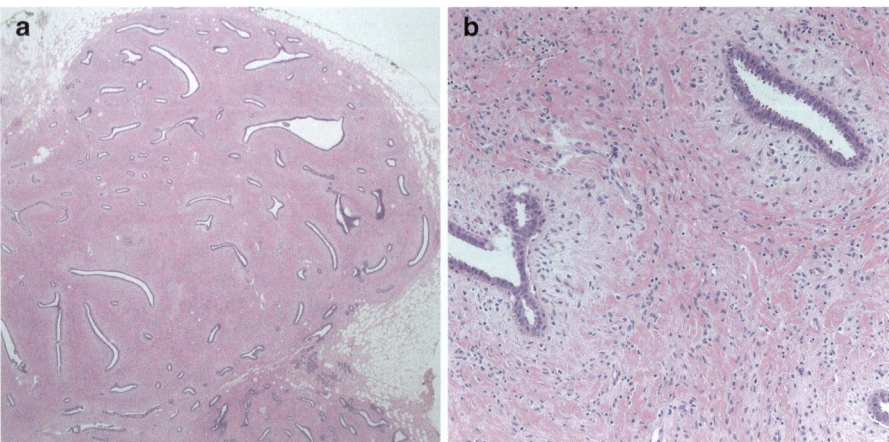

Fig. 5.2 (**a**) Histologic features of fibroadenomas include a pseudocapsule with abundant fibrous stroma (pink) within which are interspersed epithelial cells (purple) which are better seen at higher magnification (**b**)

5 Diagnostic Management of Fibroepithelial Lesions: When Is Excision Indicated?   67

Table 5.1 Features associated with fibroepithelial lesions

Lesion	Clinical exam findings	Imaging findings	Pathologic findings	Management
Fibroadenomas	Slow growing, palpable, mobile, well-defined, oval, changes with pregnancy or menstrual cycle, typically <3 cm, usually solitary, occasionally non-palpable	Oval, well-defined mass, wider than tall, homogenous, "popcorn"-like coarse calcifications weak acoustic echo and posterior acoustic enhancement on US, persistent enhancement on MRI	Pseudocapsule, white-tan color, mixture of epithelial cells separated by stroma, no increased stromal cellularity or mitotic activity, hyalinized stroma and calcifications in older lesions	Simple – close clinical monitoring every 6 months for 2 years, if morphology changes or continues to grow then surgical enucleation
			Complex features: epithelial hyperplasia, apocrine metaplasia, sclerosing adenosis, cysts	Complex – surgical excision for definitive diagnosis
Pseudoangiomatous stromal hyperplasia	Slow growing, well-defined, solitary, firm, oval, mobile	Well-circumscribed, round/oval density without calcifications, hypo- or isoechoic on US, can be heterogeneous or irregular, focal asymmetry on MMG, persistent enhancement on MRI	Round or oval, rubbery, well-circumscribed, unencapsulated mass, gray-white, occasional cyst, complex anastomosing slit-like spaces in hyalinized stroma, no nuclear atypia or mitosis, variable cellularity	Clinical monitoring for changes in size and morphology. Surgical excision with negative margins if rapid enlargement or patients preference
Phyllodes tumor	Palpable, painless mass with continued growth over months, occasional skin changes, rare nipple changes	Well-circumscribed, lobulated mass, hypoechoic, cystic or cleft-like regions on US, lobular with smooth margins and slow persistent enhancement on MRI	Circumscribed or infiltrative border, round or oval mass, multinodular, whorled patter with visible fissures, occasional necrosis, infarcts, leaf-like pattern, increased stromal cellularity and mitotic activity	Wide local excision with margins greater than 1 cm

Management and Prognosis

The typical management of fibroadenomas involves observation and close surveillance. These lesions typically grow to a size no greater than 3 cm and will usually involute slowly over time [23]. When a patient presents with a suspected fibroadenoma, the appropriate workup should be performed to rule out malignancy. After excluding malignancy, patients can be followed clinically every 6 months for at least 2 years, monitoring the lesion for size increase or morphologic changes. If fibroadenomas continue to grow beyond 3 cm during the surveillance period or the patient experiences significant symptoms such as pain or anxiety related to the presence of the mass, surgical resection can be performed. Resection is also indicated if there is discordance between the imaging and clinical impression and the core biopsy results or if atypia, DCIS, LCIS, or invasive carcinoma are identified on CNB [23, 24]. Complex fibroadenomas should be closely monitored as there is data indicating these patients may be at higher risk of developing breast cancer; however, the lesion itself is not at risk for malignant transformation [9]. The operative approach to resection is enucleation of the mass, with shelling out of the fibroadenomas from the surrounding breast tissue as they typically sit in a well-defined pseudocapsule. There is no reason to perform wide excision of these tumors as they carry extremely low malignant potential, and wide excision has never been shown to improve outcomes [5].

Cancer Risk

Fibroadenomas are considered benign hyperplastic tumors, and most studies have not shown any increase in breast cancer risk in patients with simple fibroadenomas [25]. In cases of complex fibroadenomas with atypical features, calcifications, or atypia, studies have shown that patients may be at a 2.2-fold increased risk for breast cancer compared to the normal-risk population [9]. As such, complex fibroadenomas should be surgically resected for complete pathologic analysis, and clinicians should make appropriate surveillance recommendations for these patients.

Pseudoangiomatous Stromal Hyperplasia (PASH)

First described in 1986, PASH is a rare, benign fibroblastic stromal lesion characterized by anastomosing slit-like spaces in a hyalinized stroma [26]. Data about PASH is limited and limited to case reports and small case series. These lesions are thought to be hormonally responsive, typically presenting in pre- and perimenopausal women [27]. Presentation of this benign disease varies from palpable masses and imaging abnormalities to incidental findings on biopsies performed for other reasons. Approximately 50% of these lesions will present on imaging, often appearing similar to fibroadenomas, and about 40% will present with a palpable breast mass

[28, 29]. PASH is believed to be a hormonally responsive lesion with high progesterone receptor expression [30]. These lesions are benign, and there is no evidence to suggest that they have malignant potential, although some studies have shown PASH to be present in biopsies of invasive carcinoma [31, 32].

Clinical Presentation

PASH can either present as a well-defined, homogenous mass or coexist with other breast lesions. It is more commonly seen in premenopausal women but can be seen in older women on hormone replacement therapy. Patients with PASH typically present with a slow-growing mass that is typically solitary, firm, painless, and mobile [33]. Occasionally, patients can experience rapid growth of this mass which often raises suspicion for a malignant tumor [34, 35].

Imaging Findings

Ultrasound and mammogram remain the main imaging modalities used in the evaluation of PASH, as they are often similar on clinical exam to fibroadenomas. Up to 69% of these lesions will not appear on mammogram [32]. For those that do, the mammographic appearance is typically that of a well-circumscribed, round to oval density without calcifications [32, 36]. On mammography, PASH also commonly presents as a focal asymmetry which should prompt further diagnostic imaging to better define the lesion [32, 36]. The sonographic appearance of PASH is that of a well-circumscribed, hypoechoic, or isoechoic oval mass [32, 36]. Occasionally these masses may have poorly defined, irregular margins or heterogeneous echogenicity which results in a BIRADS 4 classification and should prompt biopsy. While not indicated for PASH, MRI can demonstrate divergent findings including progressive enhancement, non-enhancing masses, or even circumscribed mass similar to a fibroadenoma [36]. While the radiologic features of PASH are typically those of other benign lesions, occasionally, PASH may exhibit irregular margins. Radiographically, it may be impossible to distinguish PASH from other benign or even malignant lesions, so patients often undergo a core needle biopsy.

Pathologic Findings

On gross examination, PASH can range from small tumors less than 1 cm in diameter to larger tumors greater than 10 cm in size; however, most are less than 3 cm in size [29, 37, 38]. PASH is usually a round or oval, well-circumscribed, rubbery, nonencapsulated mass [33]. The cut surface shows a homogenous, solid lesion with a gray-white color. Occasionally, cysts may be present [33]. The typical

Fig. 5.3 Histologically, pseudoangiomatous stromal hyperplasia (PASH) appears to have complex, anastomosing, slit-shaped spaces in the intra- and interlobular hyalinized stroma of the breast. Here, anastomosing vessels are seen within the area of PASH

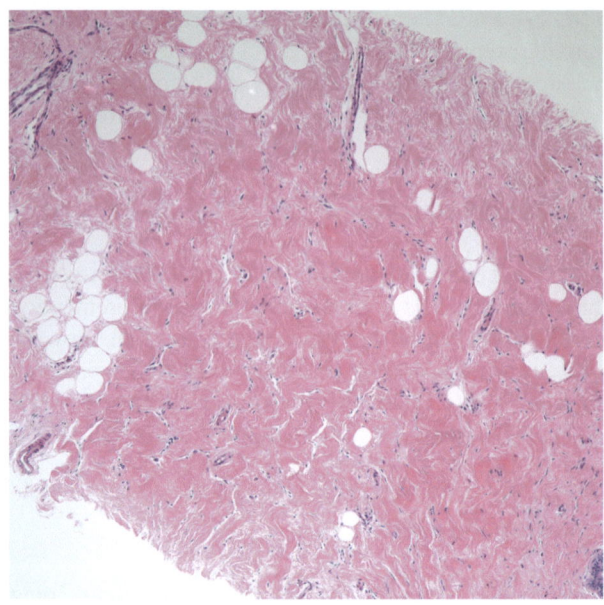

histologic appearance is that of complex, anastomosing, slit-shaped spaces in the intra- and interlobular hyalinized stroma of the breast [33, 39] (Fig. 5.3). Benign spindle fibers are usually present in discontinuous layers surrounding these spaces without nuclear atypia or mitosis [33, 38]. The epithelium of lobules and ducts with PASH lesions can vary from normal to ductal or apocrine hyperplasia [33]. Additionally, PASH shows variable cellularity from increased stromal cellularity to the formation of cellular bundles in a dense collagenous background, but again cytologic atypia is rare [33]. The pathogenesis of PASH is felt to be secondary to an exaggerated, aberrant responsiveness of mammary myofibroblasts to hormonal stimuli. The main hormone providing the stimuli is believed to be progesterone as prior studies have shown intense patchy staining of the progesterone receptor in tumor samples [30].

Management and Prognosis

There are no clear guidelines for the management of PASH, although most data support the notion that these lesions can be followed clinically [27, 40]. PASH can occasionally be present along with malignant lesions, so discordance between imaging and core biopsy results warrants surgical excision. In rare cases, PASH can present as a rapidly enlarging breast mass causing significant breast asymmetry and discomfort, and surgical excision may be performed [34, 35]. When excising PASH, the surgeon should attempt to achieve negative margins to decrease recurrence; however, wide excision is not necessary as these lesions are not malignant. In cases of large tumors or diffuse PASH, patients may even require mastectomy to adequately resect the tumor or achieve an acceptable cosmetic outcome. PASH can recur in up to 22% of cases though recurrence is more likely with incomplete surgical excision of the mass [36, 38, 41]. Recurrences of PASH behave in a benign fashion and can be managed with re-excision. PASH has not been shown to increase breast cancer risk or to be a premalignant marker [32].

Phyllodes Tumor (PT)

Phyllodes tumors are fibroepithelial neoplasms differentiated from fibroadenomas by their leaf-like projections and increased stromal cellularity on histology. These are rare tumors compromising less than 1% of all malignancies of the breast and only 2–3% of fibroepithelial lesions [42–44]. The typical age at presentation is later than that of fibroadenomas with most women presenting in their 40 [45], with one population-based study finding that Latino and Asian women may have a higher risk of developing PTs compared to Caucasians [46]. They are classified as either benign, borderline, or malignant based on histologic features of the tumors. The clinical course varies with the histologic subtype, with malignant PTs having potential for invasion, local recurrence, and even distant metastases. Malignant phyllodes tumors generally behave more like sarcomas, as opposed to invasive breast carcinoma, with respect to recurrence and metastatic spread, which is primarily to the lungs rather than regional lymph nodes. Again, as with other fibroepithelial lesions, diagnosis can be difficult but is critically important as management is dictated by the histologic diagnosis.

Clinical Presentation

Phyllodes tumors usually present as a painless palpable masses in the breast with ongoing growth that often occurs over the course of months and may provide insight to the diagnosis, as fibroadenomas typically don't grow this rapidly. However, growth rate has not been shown to be an indicator of malignancy [47]. Tumors typically grow to a size of 4–7 cm, but size can vary depending on the aggressiveness of the tumor and time from presentation. The rapid growth may lead to visible skin changes and development of varicose veins as the tumor pushes against the skin. In advanced cases, skin ulceration can also be present at diagnosis. This can occur in all categories of PT, so ulceration alone does not indicate malignant PT [47]. Nipple retraction and nipple discharge are uncommon. Diagnosis cannot be made on clinical evaluation alone because these lesions are indistinguishable from fibroadenomas clinically.

Imaging Findings

Phyllodes tumors are often difficult to distinguish from fibroadenomas and PASH on imaging alone. Approximately 20% will be detected on imaging alone [48]. They typically appear as well-circumscribed, lobulated masses on mammography, mimicking fibroadenomas [49–51]. Ultrasound shows a solid hypoechoic, well-circumscribed solid mass, where larger size and cystic or cleft regions should raise suspicion for PT [49, 50, 52]. On MRI, tumors again appear as oval, round, or lobular structures with smooth margins and high signal intensity on T2-weighted images [47]. The lesion often displays a slow initial enhancement with persistent and progressive delayed phase enhancement [47].

Pathologic Findings

The gross appearance of phyllodes tumors is usually that of a circumscribed, round, or oval mass that is often multinodular [53]. The tumor size is variable, ranging from less than 1 cm to as big as 50 cm. Axillary lymph node involvement is rare [53, 54]. Differentiation of the PT from fibroadenomas is only achieved through histologic analysis, usually on CNB, though CNB may be inconclusive and surgical excision may be required. Gross examination reveals a whorled pattern with visible cracks or fissures, and in some cases cystic changes, necrosis, and hemorrhage may be present, especially in larger and malignant PTs [48, 53, 55]. The characteristic leaf-like pattern seen in PTs is the most defining feature on pathologic analysis (Fig. 5.4) and occurs due to the exaggerated intracanalicular stromal proliferation and dilated ducts [20]. Additional features which differentiate PT from fibroadenoma include stromal overgrowth, increased stromal cellularity, and mitotic activity. Phyllodes tumors are categorized by their histologic features as benign, borderline, and malignant tumors, with the benign tumors often appearing very similar to fibroadenomas [56] (Table 5.2). It is important to appropriately categorize these lesions as treatment varies depending on the type of PT. Classification is based

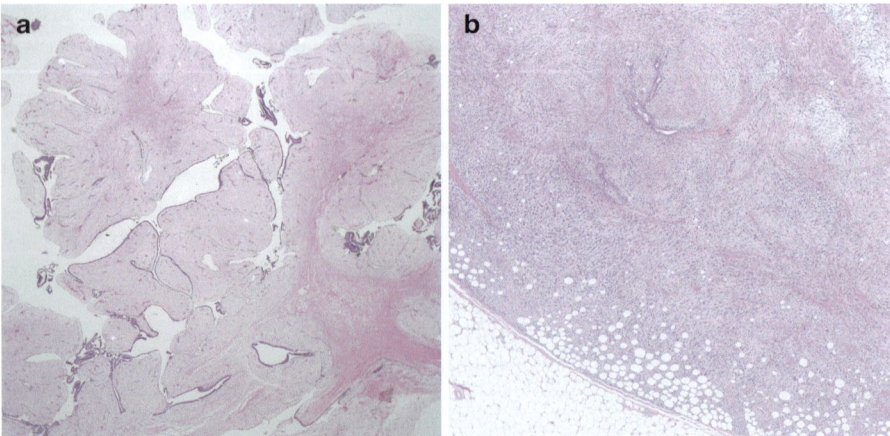

Fig. 5.4 (a) The characteristic leaf-like projections of phyllodes tumors are seen on this low magnification image of a benign phyllodes tumor. (b) Additionally, malignant phyllodes tumors exhibit expanded stroma with excess mitotic activity (>10/HPF) along with significant cellular atypia and may invade into the surrounding fat as shown here

Table 5.2 WHO classification for phyllodes tumors [57]

	Border	Stroma	Mitoses	Malignant elements
Benign	Well-defined	No overgrowth, no atypia, mild hypercellularity, uniform distribution	<5 per 10 HPF	None
Borderline	Well-defined, focally infiltrative	No or focal overgrowth, mild to moderate atypia, moderate cellularity, heterogeneous expansion	5–9 per 10 HPF	Rare
Malignant	Invasive	Marked hypercellularity, marked overgrowth, marked atypia	>10 per HPF	Can be present

Reprinted from Ilvan [57] and Tan et al. [71], with permission from the World Health Organization

on mitotic count, degree of stromal overgrowth, and whether the border is infiltrative or circumscribed.

Benign phyllodes tumors are characterized by having few mitoses per high-power field, no more than mild atypia and no stromal overgrowth [53, 57] (Table 5.2). On gross pathology, they are often well-circumscribed, unencapsulated, lobulated lesions without grossly infiltrative margins. Histologically, they can be difficult to distinguish from fibroadenomas, although PTs have more heterogeneity in stromal cellularity and mitotic activity. The stroma is mildly atypical and typically has euchromatic or hyperchromatic spindle cells with scant cytoplasm [48, 58]. Mitotic figures are often few or absent and localized to periductal areas [48].

Borderline PTs have variable morphologies and characteristics that fall between benign and malignant PTs. They usually have an expanded stromal compartment and pronounced intracanalicular growth pattern compared to benign PTs [57]. Based on the World Health Organization (WHO) classification, borderline PTs have a well-defined border with mild to moderate stromal atypia [56]. They may have focal stromal overgrowth, but this can be absent, and most typically have five to nine mitoses per high-power field [48] (Table 5.2). Additionally, these tumors lack malignant heterologous differentiation such as osteosarcomatous, chondrosarcomatous, and liposarcomatous elements which may be seen in malignant PTs [48, 57].

Malignant PTs have an expanded stroma with excess mitotic activity (>10/HPF) along with significant cellular atypia and invasive borders [57] (Fig. 5.4). These tumors exhibit stromal overgrowth, cellular pleomorphism, and foci of malignant heterologous elements described as sarcomatous in nature (Table 5.2). In some cases, stromal overgrowth may be so marked that the appearance is similar to primary breast sarcoma [57]. In these cases, identification of the aforementioned malignant heterologous features can aid in the appropriate classification as malignant phyllodes tumors [48, 57].

Management and Prognosis

Malignant phyllodes tumors should be managed with wide local excision to negative margins to achieve optimal local control. Per National Comprehensive Cancer Network (NCCN) guidelines, resection margins should be >1 cm, although there is a paucity of data supporting these recommendations as many studies do not show a survival benefit when comparing negative margins and >1 cm margins [59, 60]. Most of these malignant PTs can be excised with breast-conserving therapy; though if the tumor is large or an unacceptable cosmetic outcome is likely, mastectomy may be a better choice. Often, a pseudocapsule of dense normal breast tissue is present, and within this pseudocapsule are microscopic projections of the phyllodes tumor. Consequently, wider resection than might typically be expected needs to be performed in order to achieve the recommended 1 cm margins [61]. With respect to breast-conserving therapy, it may be difficult and impractical to resect these tumors through peri-areolar incisions as tunneling through fibroglandular tissue risks seeding normal breast tissue with tumor cells. It can be helpful to use an elliptical excision and remove the tumor en bloc with a portion of the skin. A previous study from MD Anderson did not show a difference between mastectomy and breast-conserving therapy with respect to local recurrence, indicating breast conservation is reasonable and preferred when tumor and patient characteristics are appropriate [62]. In contrast to invasive breast carcinomas, axillary staging is not recommended for PTs as fewer than 5% will actually have nodal involvement [60, 63, 64]. These tumors tend to behave more like sarcomas with hematogenous rather than lymphatic spread. Adjuvant radiation therapy for primary malignant phyllodes tumors remains a topic of debate but has been utilized increasingly over the years. It may be used in patients with lager tumors and positive margins, although there is no data showing that the use of radiation therapy improves long-term outcomes [65].

Prognosis

As expected, local recurrence rates are highest in malignant PTs (23–30%), followed by borderline (14–25%) and then benign PTs (10–20%) [56, 57, 66, 67]. The median time to recurrence is usually less than 2 years, and most of these tumors recur locally, stressing the importance of widely negative margins [68]. While local recurrence has not been shown to be associated with decreased survival [43], data has shown that tumors are typically more malignant with subsequent recurrences [55, 69]. One study showed that factors predicting recurrence included stromal overgrowth, tumor necrosis, and positive surgical margins [55]. Treatment of PT recurrence is again wide local excision with negative margins [59]. Breast-conserving surgery may again be the preferred method; however, these patients may require mastectomy in order to achieve appropriate 1 cm margins. In addition to re-excision of tumor recurrence, the NCCN guidelines recommend consideration of radiation therapy, but this is based on lower-level evidence (2B) [59]. Distant metastasis can occur through hematogenous spread of tumor with the most common locations including the lung and bone. Patients developing distant metastasis have a poor prognosis with an average survival of 30 months after identification of distant metastasis [70].

> **Conclusion**

Fibroepithelial lesions represent a broad spectrum of breast disease ranging from benign fibroadenomas to malignant phyllodes tumors. They are characterized by biphasic growth of the epithelial and stromal components of the breast tissue. Differentiating between the various types of fibroepithelial lesions can be difficult but is important given that appropriate diagnosis impacts management. Diagnosis should be based on clinical, imaging, and ultimately pathologic findings. While a clear diagnosis of simple fibroadenomas or PASH can often be monitored with close imaging surveillance and serial exams, CNB or even surgical excision should be performed if there is any doubt as to the diagnosis. Once diagnosis is confirmed, the appropriate management is surveillance for fibroadenomas and PASH, while individuals with phyllodes tumors should undergo wide local excision to >1 cm margins. While diagnosis can be difficult, patients often have a good prognosis no matter the histology, especially in comparison to primary invasive carcinoma of the breast.

References

1. Foster ME, Garrahan N, Williams S. Fibroadenoma of the breast: a clinical and pathological study. J R Coll Surg Edinb. 1988;33(1):16–9.
2. Dent D, Hacking E, Wilkie W. Benign breast disease: clinical classification and disease distribution. Br J Clin Pract. 1988;42(Supplemental):69–71.
3. Frantz VK, Pickren JW, Melcher GW, Auchincloss H. Incidence of chronic cystic disease in so-called "normal breasts"; a study based on 225 postmortem examinations. Cancer. 1951;4(4):762–83.
4. El-Wakeel H, Umpleby HC. Systematic review of fibroadenoma as a risk factor for breast cancer. Breast. 2003;12(5):302–7.
5. Greenberg R, Skornick Y, Kaplan O. Management of breast fibroadenomas. J Gen Intern Med. 1998;13(9):640–5.
6. Schuerch C, Rosen PP, Hirota T, Itabashi M, Yamamoto H, Kinne DW, et al. A pathologic study of benign breast diseases in Tokyo and New York. Cancer. 1982;50(9):1899–903.
7. Organ CH, Organ BC. Fibroadenoma of the female breast: a critical clinical assessment. J Natl Med Assoc. 1983;75(7):701–4.
8. Funderburk WW, Rosero E, Leffall LD. Breast lesions in blacks. Surg Gynecol Obstet. 1972;135(1):58–60.
9. Dupont WD, Page DL, Parl FF, Vnencak-Jones CL, Plummer WD, Rados MS, et al. Long-term risk of breast cancer in women with fibroadenoma. N Engl J Med. 1994;331(1):10–5.
10. Dent DM, Cant PJ. Fibroadenoma. World J Surg. 1989;13(6):706–10.
11. Mohs FE. The effect of the sex hormones on the growth of transplanted mammary adenofibroma in rats. Am J Cancer. 1940;38(2):212–6.
12. Geschickter CF, Lewis D, Hartman CG. Tumors of the breast related to the oestrin hormone. Am J Cancer. 1934;21:828–59.
13. Cole-Beuglet C, Soriano RZ, Kurtz AB, Goldberg BB. Fibroadenoma of the breast: sonomammography correlated with pathology in 122 patients. AJR Am J Roentgenol. 1983;140(2):369–75.
14. Harvey JA, Nicholson BT, Lorusso AP, Cohen MA, Bovbjerg VE. Short-term follow-up of palpable breast lesions with benign imaging features: evaluation of 375 lesions in 320 women. AJR Am J Roentgenol. 2009;193(6):1723–30.

15. Jackson VP, Rothschild PA, Kreipke DL, Mail JT, Holden RW. The spectrum of sonographic findings of fibroadenoma of the breast. Investig Radiol. 1986;21(1):34–40.
16. Goel NB, Knight TE, Pandey S, Riddick-Young M, de Paredes ES, Trivedi A. Fibrous lesions of the breast: imaging-pathologic correlation. Radiographics. 2005;25(6):1547–59.
17. Heywang-Köbrunner S, Dershaw D, Schreer I. Benign tumors. In: Thieme S, editor. Diagnostic breast imaging. New York: Thieme; 2001. p. 209–35.
18. Kuhl CK, Klaschik S, Mielcarek P, Gieseke J, Wardelmann E, Schild HH. Do T2-weighted pulse sequences help with the differential diagnosis of enhancing lesions in dynamic breast MRI? J Magn Reson Imaging. 1999;9(2):187–96.
19. Wurdinger S, Herzog AB, Fischer DR, Marx C, Raabe G, Schneider A, et al. Differentiation of phyllodes breast tumors from fibroadenomas on MRI. AJR Am J Roentgenol. 2005;185(5):1317–21.
20. Yang X, Kandil D, Cosar EF, Khan A. Fibroepithelial tumors of the breast: pathologic and immunohistochemical features and molecular mechanisms. Arch Pathol Lab Med. 2014;138(1):25–36.
21. Chinyama C. Fibroepithelial lesions. Benign breast diseases. 2nd ed. Berlin: Springer; 2014. p. 101–26.
22. Collins L, Schnitt S. Pathology of benign breast disorders. Diseases of the breast. 5th edn. Philadelphia: Wolters Kluwer Health; 2014.
23. Carty NJ, Carter C, Rubin C, Ravichandran D, Royle GT, Taylor I. Management of fibroadenoma of the breast. Ann R Coll Surg Engl. 1995;77(2):127–30.
24. Cant PJ, Madden MV, Coleman MG, Dent DM. Non-operative management of breast masses diagnosed as fibroadenoma. Br J Surg. 1995;82(6):792–4.
25. Dixon JM. Cystic disease and fibroadenoma of the breast: natural history and relation to breast cancer risk. Br Med Bull. 1991;47(2):258–71.
26. Vuitch MF, Rosen PP, Erlandson RA. Pseudoangiomatous hyperplasia of mammary stroma. Hum Pathol. 1986;17(2):185–91.
27. Degnim AC, Frost MH, Radisky DC, Anderson SS, Vierkant RA, Boughey JC, et al. Pseudoangiomatous stromal hyperplasia and breast cancer risk. Ann Surg Oncol. 2010;17(12):3269–77.
28. Jones KN, Glazebrook KN, Reynolds C. Pseudoangiomatous stromal hyperplasia: imaging findings with pathologic and clinical correlation. AJR Am J Roentgenol. 2010;195(4):1036–42.
29. Ferreira M, Albarracin CT, Resetkova E. Pseudoangiomatous stromal hyperplasia tumor: a clinical, radiologic and pathologic study of 26 cases. Mod Pathol. 2008;21(2):201–7.
30. Anderson C, Ricci A, Pedersen CA, Cartun RW. Immunocytochemical analysis of estrogen and progesterone receptors in benign stromal lesions of the breast. Evidence for hormonal etiology in pseudoangiomatous hyperplasia of mammary stroma. Am J Surg Pathol. 1991;15(2):145–9.
31. Gresik CM, Godellas C, Aranha GV, Rajan P, Shoup M. Pseudoangiomatous stromal hyperplasia of the breast: a contemporary approach to its clinical and radiologic features and ideal management. Surgery. 2010;148(4):752–7. discussion 7-8
32. Hargaden GC, Yeh ED, Georgian-Smith D, Moore RH, Rafferty EA, Halpern EF, et al. Analysis of the mammographic and sonographic features of pseudoangiomatous stromal hyperplasia. AJR Am J Roentgenol. 2008;191(2):359–63.
33. Virk RK, Khan A. Pseudoangiomatous stromal hyperplasia: an overview. Arch Pathol Lab Med. 2010;134(7):1070–4.
34. Ryu EM, Whang IY, Chang ED. Rapidly growing bilateral pseudoangiomatous stromal hyperplasia of the breast. Korean J Radiol. 2010;11(3):355–8.
35. Shahi KS, Bhandari G, Gupta RK, Sawai M. Pseudoangio-matous stromal hyperplasia: a rare tumor of the breast. J Cancer Res Ther. 2015;11(4):1032.
36. Raj SD, Sahani VG, Adrada BE, Scoggins ME, Albarracin CT, Woodtichartpreecha P, et al. Pseudoangiomatous stromal hyperplasia of the breast: multimodality review with pathologic correlation. Curr Probl Diagn Radiol. 2017;46(2):130–5.
37. Polger MR, Denison CM, Lester S, Meyer JE. Pseudoangiomatous stromal hyperplasia: mammographic and sonographic appearances. AJR Am J Roentgenol. 1996;166(2):349–52.

38. Powell CM, Cranor ML, Rosen PP. Pseudoangiomatous stromal hyperplasia (PASH). A mammary stromal tumor with myofibroblastic differentiation. Am J Surg Pathol. 1995;19(3):270–7.
39. Koerner F. Pseudoangiomatous stromal hyperplasia. Diagnostic problems in breast pathology. 1st ed. Philadelphia: Saunders, Elsevier; 2009. p. 351–8.
40. Wieman SM, Landercasper J, Johnson JM, Ellis RL, Wester SM, Lambert PJ, et al. Tumoral pseudoangiomatous stromal hyperplasia of the breast. Am Surg. 2008;74(12):1211–4.
41. Bowman E, Oprea G, Okoli J, Gundry K, Rizzo M, Gabram-Mendola S, et al. Pseudoangiomatous stromal hyperplasia (PASH) of the breast: a series of 24 patients. Breast J. 2012;18(3):242–7.
42. Vorherr H, Vorherr UF, Kutvirt DM, Key CR. Cystosarcoma phyllodes: epidemiology, pathohistology, pathobiology, diagnosis, therapy, and survival. Arch Gynecol. 1985;236(3):173–81.
43. Parker SJ, Harries SA. Phyllodes tumours. Postgrad Med J. 2001;77(909):428–35.
44. Geisler DP, Boyle MJ, Malnar KF, McGee JM, Nolen MC, Fortner SM, et al. Phyllodes tumors of the breast: a review of 32 cases. Am Surg. 2000;66(4):360–6.
45. Salvadori B, Cusumano F, Del Bo R, Delledonne V, Grassi M, Rovini D, et al. Surgical treatment of phyllodes tumors of the breast. Cancer. 1989;63(12):2532–6.
46. Bernstein L, Deapen D, Ross RK. The descriptive epidemiology of malignant cystosarcoma phyllodes tumors of the breast. Cancer. 1993;71(10):3020–4.
47. Calhoun K, Allison K, Kim J, Rahbar H, Anderson B. Phyllodes tumor. Diseases of the breast. 5th ed. Philadelphia: Wolters Kluwer Health; 2001.
48. Esposito N. Fibroepithelial lesions. In: Dabbs D, editor. Breast pathology. 2nd ed. Philadelphia: Elsevier; 2017.
49. Aydogan F, Tasci Y, Sagara Y. Phyllodes tumors of the breast. Breast disease. 1st ed. Cham: Springer; 2016. p. 421–7.
50. Yilmaz E, Sal S, Lebe B. Differentiation of phyllodes tumors versus fibroadenomas. Acta Radiol. 2002;43(1):34–9.
51. Lifshitz OH, Whitman GJ, Sahin AA, Yang WT. Radiologic-pathologic conferences of the University of Texas M.D. Anderson Cancer Center. Phyllodes tumor of the breast. AJR Am J Roentgenol. 2003;180(2):332.
52. Chao TC, Lo YF, Chen SC, Chen MF. Sonographic features of phyllodes tumors of the breast. Ultrasound Obstet Gynecol. 2002;20(1):64–71.
53. Pinder S, Mulligan AM, O'Malley F. Fibroepithelial lesions, including fibroadenoma and phyllodes tumors. In: O'Malley F, editor. Breast pathology: a volume in the foundations in diagnostic pathology series. 2nd ed. Philadelphia: Saunders, Elsevier; 2011. p. 121–38.
54. Kumar T, Patel MD, Bhargavan R, Kumar P, Patel MH, Kothari K, et al. Largest phyllodes tumor- case report and brief review article. Indian J Surg Oncol. 2011;2(2):141–4.
55. Hawkins RE, Schofield JB, Fisher C, Wiltshaw E, McKinna JA. The clinical and histologic criteria that predict metastases from cystosarcoma phyllodes. Cancer. 1992;69(1):141–7.
56. Tan PH, Ellis IO. Myoepithelial and epithelial-myoepithelial, mesenchymal and fibroepithelial breast lesions: updates from the WHO Classification of Tumours of the Breast 2012. J Clin Pathol. 2013;66(6):465–70.
57. Ilvan S. Fibroepithelial tumors of the breast. In: Aydiner A, Igce A, Soran A, editors. Breast disease. 1st ed. Cham: Springer; 2016. p. 283–8.
58. Koerner F. Phyllodes tumor. Diagnostic problems in breast pathology. 1st ed. Philadelphia: Saunders, Elsevier; 2009. p. 329–41.
59. National Comprehensive Cancer Network. Breast Cancer 2017. Available at: https://www.nccn.org/professionals/physician_gls/pdf/breast.pdf. Accessed 28 Sept 2017.
60. Mangi AA, Smith BL, Gadd MA, Tanabe KK, Ott MJ, Souba WW. Surgical management of phyllodes tumors. Arch Surg. 1999;134(5):487–92; discussion 92–3.
61. August DA, Kearney T. Cystosarcoma phyllodes: mastectomy, lumpectomy, or lumpectomy plus irradiation. Surg Oncol. 2000;9(2):49–52.
62. Chaney AW, Pollack A, McNeese MD, Zagars GK, Pisters PW, Pollock RE, et al. Primary treatment of cystosarcoma phyllodes of the breast. Cancer. 2000;89(7):1502–11.
63. Gullett NP, Rizzo M, Johnstone PA. National surgical patterns of care for primary surgery and axillary staging of phyllodes tumors. Breast J. 2009;15(1):41–4.

64. Meneses A, Mohar A, de la Garza-Salazar J, Ramírez-Ugalde T. Prognostic factors on 45 cases of phyllodes tumors. J Exp Clin Cancer Res. 2000;19(1):69–73.
65. Gnerlich JL, Williams RT, Yao K, Jaskowiak N, Kulkarni SA. Utilization of radiotherapy for malignant phyllodes tumors: analysis of the National Cancer Data Base, 1998–2009. Ann Surg Oncol. 2014;21(4):1222–30.
66. Lenhard MS, Kahlert S, Himsl I, Ditsch N, Untch M, Bauerfeind I. Phyllodes tumour of the breast: clinical follow-up of 33 cases of this rare disease. Eur J Obstet Gynecol Reprod Biol. 2008;138(2):217–21.
67. Selvi R. Phyllodes tumors. Breast diseases. 1st ed. New Delhi: Springer; 2015. p. 181–8.
68. Barrio AV, Clark BD, Goldberg JI, Hoque LW, Bernik SF, Flynn LW, et al. Clinicopathologic features and long-term outcomes of 293 phyllodes tumors of the breast. Ann Surg Oncol. 2007;14(10):2961–70.
69. Tan BY, Acs G, Apple SK, Badve S, Bleiweiss IJ, Brogi E, et al. Phyllodes tumours of the breast: a consensus review. Histopathology. 2016;68(1):5–21.
70. Kessinger A, Foley JF, Lemon HM, Miller DM. Metastatic cystosarcoma phyllodes: a case report and review of the literature. J Surg Oncol. 1972;4(2):131–47.
71. Tan PH, Tse G, Lee A. Fibroepithelial tumors. In: Lakhani SR, Ellis IO, Schnitt SJ, Tan PH, van de Vijver MJ, editors. WHO classification of tumours of the breast. 4th ed. Lyon: IARC Press; 2012. p. 141–7.

Diagnostic Management of the Atypical Hyperplasias: Core Biopsy Alone Versus Excisional Biopsy

6

Emily Siegel and Alice Chung

Atypical ductal hyperplasia (ADH) and atypical lobular hyperplasia (ALH) are two indeterminate lesions diagnosed by breast core needle biopsy (CNB) which have related but separate diagnostic characteristics and natural histories. While the usual pattern of hyperplasia is proliferation, atypical ductal hyperplasias are defined as those having cellular variability, nuclear overlap, and indistinct cell borders diagnosed most often on hematoxylin and eosin stained slides [1]. Those secondary interstitial spaces created by the indistinct borders are irregular and on the periphery [2]. This variability can progress to architecturally complex patterns, including cribriform-like secondary lumens or micropapillary formations [1, 3] (Fig. 6.1). It is important to note that ADH has a considerable morphologic spectrum and can at times be difficult to distinguish from ductal carcinoma in situ (DCIS). Generally, there is less cytological atypia in ADH than in DCIS [4]. DCIS is diagnosed when the atypia in ADH is severe, when two adjacent basement membrane bound spaces are completely replaced by neoplastic cells, and/or when the lesion extends greater than 0.2 cm [2, 4]. The difference between ADH and DCIS is therefore often characterized by the extensiveness of the lesion [3], but variability from pathologist to pathologist can exist.

ALH, in contrast, is characterized by expansion of the acini of a lobular unit and by loss of expression of E-cadherin [5]. In addition, the acini are filled with small, monotonous round or polygonal cells. The combination of expansion of cells, hyperplasia, lack of cohesion, and loss of acinar lumens creates the ALH pattern (Fig. 6.2) [3]. The absence of acinar lumens reflects a cells tendency to spread into adjacent terminal ducts when ALH is present [4]. Analogous to the relationship

---

E. Siegel, M.D. · A. Chung, M.D. (✉)
Cedars-Sinai Medical Center, Los Angeles, CA, USA
e-mail: Emily.Siegel@cshs.org; Alice.Chung@cshs.org

© Springer International Publishing AG, part of Springer Nature 2018
F. Amersi, K. Calhoun (eds.), *Atypical Breast Proliferative Lesions and Benign Breast Disease*, https://doi.org/10.1007/978-3-319-92657-5_6

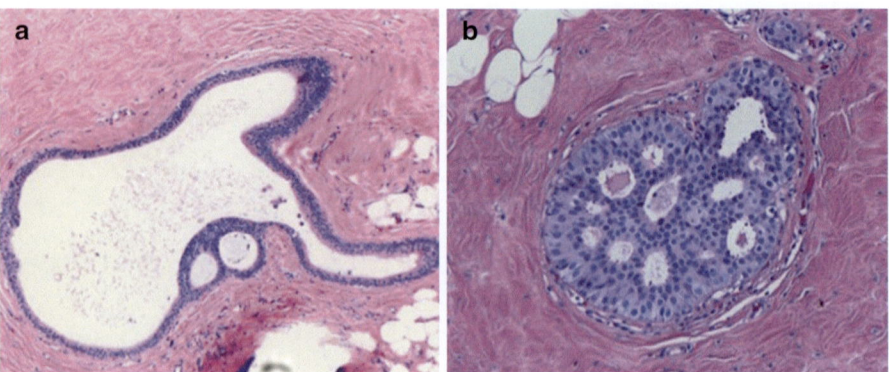

Fig. 6.1 (a) Low-power (10×) view of atypical ductal hyperplasia with proliferation of cells. (b) Higher power (20×) view of atypical ductal hyperplasia with architecturally complex pattern and high cellular variability

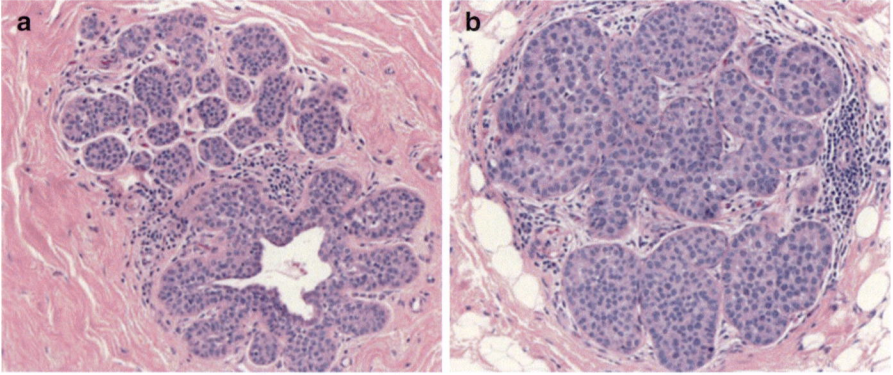

Fig. 6.2 (a) Low-power (10×) view of atypical lobular hyperplasia with expansion of acini. (b) Higher power (20×) view of atypical lobular hyperplasia with expansion and loss of lumens

between ADH and DCIS, ALH can be similar to lobular carcinoma in situ (LCIS) and has a wide spectrum of histological appearances. ALH and LCIS, however, are distinguishable using quantitative criteria; LCIS exists when expansion is greater than 50% of the terminal duct lobular unit, while ALH has expansion to less than 50% [1]. While ADH is usually associated with calcifications on imaging, ALH is less commonly [6], with ALH often diagnosed as an incidental finding on biopsy.

The natural history of ADH and ALH seems to show that the two lesions occupy an intermediate space in the spectrum of benign tissue to carcinoma (Fig. 6.1). Stem cells located within terminal duct lobular units (TLDUs) can give rise to unfolded lobules (ULs). These ULs then develop into ADH using unique molecular pathways which are separate from usual hyperplasia or cystic disease [7]. In contrast, ALH arises directly from normal appearing TLDUs as

Fig. 6.3 Natural history of progression from normal breast parenchyma to atypical lesions and carcinoma

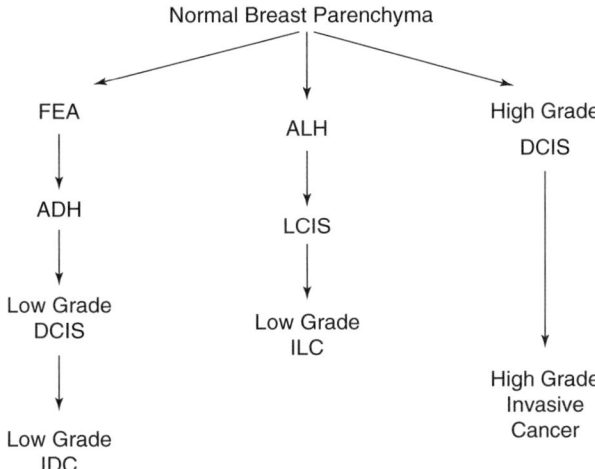

mild atypical epithelial cells. These can, as discussed previously, distend and extend to a large extent at which point they are diagnosed as LCIS [7], just as ADH can extend into DCIS. Based on this behavior, both lesions are often referred to as pre-malignant lesions. It is important to note that there are also separate models for invasive breast cancer which hypothesize that carcinoma arises directly from normal breast parenchyma and that not all breast cancer lesions originate from an ADH or ALH precursor [8] (Fig. 6.3).

ADH is often associated with suspicious calcifications found on mammography. Once identified, these calcifications are then targeted by CNB to determine histology. In one study of 264 stereotactic core biopsies, 105 lesions were initially seen as calcifications on mammography. 20% of these (21/105) were subsequently diagnosed as ADH [9]. ADH may also present as abnormal enhancement on magnetic resonance imaging (MRI). One recent multicenter study examined all biopsies performed by MRI guidance during an 8-year period. Across 4 different institutions, 1655 MRI-guided biopsies showed an incidence of ADH of 3.3–7.1%. The average rate of diagnosis of ADH on MRI biopsy was determined to be 6% [10], while the overall incidence of ADH on biopsy is 8–10% of samples [11].

Patients diagnosed with ADH have an increased risk of breast cancer. A landmark trial by Hartmann et al. studied all patients with ADH from one institution during a 34-year period, with 330 patients with ADH followed for a median of just over 12 years. Fifty-eight of the 330 patients developed either in situ or invasive carcinoma over the follow-up period, and these patients were 2 times more likely to develop a carcinoma on the ipsilateral side as the ADH compared to the contralateral side. DCIS developed in roughly 25% of the 58 patients, with invasive carcinoma found in the remaining 75% [12]. More recently, a single institution review studied all CNB with confirmed ADH across a 4-year period. From the 175 biopsies with ADH, 122 were found to be benign on excisional biopsy. During the median follow-up of 76 months (range 5–180), 14 (11.5%) patients developed DCIS or invasive carcinoma. These were most commonly in the same breast as had previously undergone biopsy (11/14) [13].

The incidence of ALH is lower than ADH, comprising less than 1% of all CNB performed [14]. Although the incidence is low, the risk of subsequent cancer in patients diagnosed previously with ALH is similar to that of ADH. The risk of developing cancer with ALH was first reported in the 1980s and has since been studied extensively. All reports have since suggested a similar fourfold increased relative risk of lifetime cancer despite benign initial excisional biopsy [3].

CNB remains the preferred method of tissue diagnosis for those lesions detected by either palpation or imaging. Early single center studies showed a diagnostic accuracy of greater than 95% for CNB, and the procedure has now been widely adopted and is the optimal method of tissue diagnosis in 88–98% of all breast biopsies [15, 16]. The advantages of CNB include that it is minimally invasive, can be performed under imaging guidance using a wide variety of modalities, and provides timely diagnosis for management planning.

There are, however, some disadvantages to performing CNB. Complications can occur infrequently, including minor wound complications, hematoma formation, and infection. The more frequent problem that can arise is a discordance between pathological and radiographic interpretation of CNB. Elmore et al. studied concordance among pathologists in 2015 using attending pathologists from 8 different states (total of 115 participants). Each pathologist independently reviewed slides from a range of breast diagnoses resulting in 6300 interpretations of 60 slides. Overall, the concordance rate of diagnostic interpretations was only 75.3%. Nonconcordance was higher with biopsies from women with higher breast density and with pathologists whose clinical practices had lower volume or were in nonacademic settings [17]. Another study, the B-Path Study, asked US Pathologists to interpret test slides of CNB from breast patients whose diagnoses ranged from benign to malignant. A subset of this trial analyzed the verification between pathologists when using only one slide for analysis. The authors found that 92.3% of slides could be verified by consensus diagnosis. Over-interpretation occurred in approximately 5% of slides and under-interpretation in 3.2% of slides. Furthermore, as biopsies approached atypia and were not clearly invasive or benign lesions, the rate of verification became less probable: 53.6% of slides were over-interpreted and 8.6% of slides were under-interpreted [18]. In order to specifically examine the atypical diagnoses and rate of pathological concordance, Gomes et al. looked at 610 cases which had been selected for second opinion. While the inter-observer variability for ALH and LCIS were good (Kappa 0.62 and 0.66, respectively), the determination of ADH was much less reproducible (Kappa 0.44) [19]. Therefore, the authors concluded that CNB findings of ADH, and ALH to a lesser extent, are indeterminate diagnoses.

As mentioned previously, ADH and ALH are lesions that may progress to DCIS and LCIS. Within any lesion there may be both ADH and ALH, as well as an area which may have already progressed into DCIS or LCIS and were missed on CNB. Given the variability in diagnosis and possibility of upstaging, excisional biopsy provides a more definitive diagnosis than CNB for atypical lesions. One advantage of excisional biopsy is that the specimen obtained is much larger and therefore is less susceptible to sampling error. In addition, excisional biopsy can be performed on an outpatient basis with minimal complications. There is significantly increased cost with utilization of the operating room, surgeon, and associated hospital operations and surgical excision also creates anxiety and stress for patients. Therefore, it is prudent to use excisional biopsy judiciously and only when appropriate.

Excisional biopsy for ADH has been challenged given the increased expenditure and stress to the patient associated with a surgical procedure. A number of studies have attempted to identify factors which may be predictive of upgrading to malignancy, thereby hoping to allow conservative management if these features are not present. The overall rate of upstaging on excisional biopsy is highly variable among studies, ranging from 0% to 56%. Differences between digital and film-screen mammography have been examined to determine if there is improved upstaging rate with either modality. McLaughlin et al. reviewed 101 cases of ADH in a 10-year period ending in 2011. They showed an upstage rate of 12.3% when ADH was detected by digital mammography and of 13.6% of patients ADH was detected by film-screen mammography (not statistically significant). There were also no differences in upstage rate when comparing biopsies performed with 11- or 8-gauge CNB needles. Furthermore, there was no statistically significant difference in upstage rate if all calcifications were removed during CNB [20]. Similarly, Kohr et al. analyzed 147 consecutive cases of atypia diagnosed via stereotactic vacuum-assisted CNB, with ADH confirmed in 101 cases, and 19.8% ($N = 20$) cases were upstaged on excisional biopsy. They again showed that there is no difference in upstaging rate if calcifications are removed, but they did determine that the upstage rate was significantly higher where CNB showed three or more foci of ADH [21]. Finally, another multicenter trial looked at data from the Breast Cancer Surveillance Consortium, where 685 mammographically detected lesions were diagnosed as ADH, with 420 undergoing surgical excision within 6 months. Of those excised, 26% were upstaged to either DCIS or invasive carcinoma and was associated with being pre-menopausal and/or having a family history of breast cancer [14].

Upstaging rates have also been studied when CNB is performed under MRI guidance. Weinfurtner et al. analyzed data from all MRI-guided biopsies from a single institution over a 6-year time frame. They show an upstage rate of only 7% from CNB diagnosed as ADH. However, when they included lesions with mixed ADH and ALH diagnosed by CNB, the upstaging rate increased to 22%. This result is similar to that in other studies, which have shown that the presence of multiple high risk lesions increases the risk of upstaging [12, 22]. Finally, Weinfurter et al. showed no MRI characteristics associated with higher upstaging rates [23]. In contrast, Khoury et al. reported an upstage rate of 15%, with 80% DCIS (80%) and 20% invasive carcinoma. They showed that the higher the number of cores containing ADH on MRI-guided biopsy, the higher the risk of upstaging [10]. Another study performed by Verheyden et al. examined 72 cases of ADH from 9 different centers. 66 of these patients then underwent excisional biopsy, with an upstaging rate of 25.8%. They showed that the gauge of needle does in fact have an effect on upstaging, and that those who underwent CNB with a 9- or 10-gauge needle had

Table 6.1 Range of upstaging of atypical ductal hyperplasia (ADH) to carcinoma, ductal carcinoma in situ (DCIS), and invasive carcinoma in patients diagnosed with ADH on core needle biopsy [14, 21, 32–34]

Study	N	Carcinoma (%)	DCIS (%)	Invasive CA (%)
Wagoner (2009)	123	22 (18)	22 (18)	0
Kohr (2010)	101	20 (20)	17 (17)	3 (3)
McGhan (2012)	114	20 (18)	15 (13)	5 (5)
Khoury (2015)	203	57 (28)	47 (23)	10 (5)
Menes (2014)	685	123 (18)	101 (15)	22 (3)

significantly higher rates of upgrading to carcinoma compared to those diagnosed with 7- or 8-gauge needles [24].

Ultrasound guided biopsy typically relies on the presence of a mass to target. Given the propensity of ADH to present as calcifications rather than a mass, few studies have examined the upstaging rate with atypia diagnosed by ultrasound-guided biopsy. One study from McGill University reviewed all sonographically performed biopsies over a 7-year period. These ultrasounds were performed for a variety of reasons – to evaluate specific abnormalities discovered on mammography, on MRI, for screening of women with dense breasts, or as part of initial screening. Of 6325 biopsies, only 56 revealed ADH (0.9%), with 28 of the lesions subsequently upstaging on to malignancy excisional biopsy (56%). There were no mammographic or sonographic features associated with malignancy at final diagnosis. However, age less than 50 years old at time of biopsy was found to be independently associated with increased risk of upstaging [25]. Overall, there is a wide range of upstaging rates when ADH is diagnosed on CNB across all imaging modalities (Table 6.1).

Similar to ADH, the rate of upstage to invasive carcinoma or LCIS when discussing CNB versus excisional biopsy for ALH is wide and ranges from 0% to 67% of all lesions with an ALH diagnosis. One recent series from the University of Pittsburgh analyzed CNB performed from 2006 to 2013, with only 339 of 32,000 CNB (1.02%) revealing ALH. 12 of these 339 (3.5%) cases were upstaged to malignancy on excision. The majority of malignancies were DCIS (75%) with a minority of patients diagnosed with invasive carcinomas (25%). Imaging findings showing mammographic fine linear calcifications were significantly more likely to be associated with upstaging on excision [26]. An additional study examined all atypical lesions diagnosed by CNB in a 2-year period ending in 2010 and reported ALH in 28% ($N = 42$) of all atypical specimens. Of these 42 patients, 4 patients upstaged to carcinoma (9.5%). Neither the gauge of the needle used for CNB, nor the number of cores was significantly associated with upstage [27]. An additional study examined all CNB from MD Anderson Cancer Center during a 6-year period ending in 2001. Over 2300 CNB were reviewed, with only 17 showing a diagnosis of ALH. Four of these 17 (24%) patients were upstaged to invasive carcinoma on final excision. All of these specimens were reported as having pagetoid extension on CNB, but this was not analyzed in a regression model to determine predictive value [28].

Table 6.2 Upstaging rates of atypical lobular hyperplasia (ALH) in various publications [28, 29, 35–39]

Study	N	Upstages (%)
Middleton (2003)[a]	17	24
Subhawong (2010)	56	0
Zhao (2012)	163	3
Murray (2013)	30	3
Nakhlis (2016)	49	0
Susnik (2016)	246	3

[a]Study performed prior to using radiologic, clinical, and pathologic concordance

While the rate of upstaging in early studies is quite high, review of clinical and radiological information for pathologic concordance was not performed in many of the earlier studies. Atkins et al. studied CNB diagnosed as ALH from 2000 to 2010. 50 cases were examined to determine if the biopsy findings were concordant or discordant with clinical and imaging information. Of the 43 benign concordant biopsy findings, none were found to upgrade at excisional biopsy after 3 years of follow-up. Of seven discordant biopsy findings, five were upstaged to DCIS at excision. Another analysis from Memorial-Sloan-Kettering Cancer Center studied ALH diagnosed on CNB during a 5-year period ending 2009. Thirty-four cases of ALH were discovered, and 30 of these had concordant pathologic, imaging and clinical findings. Of these 30, only 2 (6.7%) were upstaged at excision and both lesions contained calcifications within the biopsy specimen. In contrast, 50% of the cases with discordant pathologic and imaging findings were upstaged to either IDC or LCIS. While the total number of cases is very low [2], this difference in upstage rate afforded by concordance between imaging and pathologic findings is significant [29]. This finding has been corroborated by more recent studies, and the estimated risk of upstaging after cases of radiologic-pathologic discordance are excluded has been consistently in the range of 2–3%. As such, current practice now requires combined assessment of clinical, imaging and pathologic findings of CNB for ALH. The histologic findings as reported by the pathologist must be interpreted in the context of clinical and imaging findings, with input from both surgeon and radiologist [30] (Table 6.2).

With the low rate of upstaging in patients who have CNB with pathologic findings that are concordant with imaging and clinical information, expectant follow-up has been suggested as a possible management strategy for lobular neoplasia. Middleton et al. investigated 104 patients diagnosed with ALH, ALH/LCIS, or LCIS on CNB. Twenty of the 104 patients underwent immediate excision secondary to discordant pathologic and imaging findings, with an upstage rate for patients whose original CNB revealed ALH of 1.7%. Those with concordant findings were followed for a median of 3.4 years. Of the 84 patients who were followed, only 2 (2.3%) patients originally diagnosed with pure ALH developed DCIS [31]. Such low upstage rates argue that patients with ALH may be appropriate for observation and do not require mandatory excision.

Although surgical excision remains a safe approach in ALH diagnosed by CNB, in the absence of any other high-risk lesions or unassessed suspicious imaging findings, surveillance is a reasonable alternative for patients diagnosed with pure ALH on CNB. Cases with associated non-classic LCIS or ADH should still be excised.

In summary, all CNB pathology results should be correlated with pre-biopsy imaging findings. CNB revealing a diagnosis of ADH currently necessitates surgical consultation for excisional biopsy. Surgical consultation should also be obtained for ALH, and while excisional biopsy is often recommended, in the appropriately selected patient, close interval follow-up appears to be a safe and acceptable alternative. The recommendation for follow-up without surgical excision for ALH requires a team approach with close discussion and collaboration between surgeons, radiologists and pathologists.

References

1. Calhoun BC, Collins LC. Recommendations for excision following core needle biopsy of the breast: a contemporary evaluation of the literature. Histopathology. 2016;68(1):138–51. PMID: 26768035. https://doi.org/10.1111/his.12852.
2. Simpson JF. Update on atypical epithelial hyperplasia and ductal carcinoma in situ. Pathology. 2009;41(1):36–9. PMID: 19089738. https://doi.org/10.1080/00313020802568097.
3. Hartmann LC, Degnim AC, Dupont WD. Atypical hyperplasia of the breast. N Engl J Med. 2015;372(13):1271–2. PMID: 25806929. https://doi.org/10.1056/NEJMc1501046.
4. Neal L, Sandhu NP, Hieken TJ, Glazebrook KN, Mac Bride MB, Dilaveri CA, et al. Diagnosis and management of benign, atypical, and indeterminate breast lesions detected on core needle biopsy. Mayo Clin Proc. 2014;89(4):536–47. PMID: 24684875. https://doi.org/10.1016/j.mayocp.2014.02.004.
5. Jacobs TW, Pliss N, Kouria G, Schnitt SJ. Carcinomas in situ of the breast with indeterminate features: role of E-cadherin staining in categorization. Am J Surg Pathol. 2001;25(2):229–36. PMID: 11176072.
6. Simpson PT, Gale T, Fulford LG, Reis-Filho JS, Lakhani SR. The diagnosis and management of pre-invasive breast disease: pathology of atypical lobular hyperplasia and lobular carcinoma in situ. Breast Cancer Res. 2003;5(5):258–62. PMID: 12927036. https://doi.org/10.1186/bcr624.
7. Allred DC, Mohsin SK, Fuqua SA. Histological and biological evolution of human premalignant breast disease. Endocr Relat Cancer. 2001;8(1):47–61. PMID: 11350726.
8. Bombonati A, Sgroi DC. The molecular pathology of breast cancer progression. J Pathol. 2011;223(2):307–17. PMID: 21125683. https://doi.org/10.1002/path.2808.
9. Liberman L, Cohen MA, Dershaw DD, Abramson AF, Hann LE, Rosen PP. Atypical ductal hyperplasia diagnosed at stereotaxic core biopsy of breast lesions: an indication for surgical biopsy. AJR Am J Roentgenol. 1995;164(5):1111–3. PMID: 7717215. https://doi.org/10.2214/ajr.164.5.7717215.
10. Khoury T, Li Z, Sanati S, Desouki MM, Chen X, Wang D, et al. The risk of upgrade for atypical ductal hyperplasia detected on magnetic resonance imaging-guided biopsy: a study of 100 cases from four academic institutions. Histopathology. 2016;68(5):713–21. PMID: 26291517. https://doi.org/10.1111/his.12811.
11. Pearlman MD, Griffin JL. Benign breast disease. Obstet Gynecol. 2010;116(3):747–58. PMID: 20733462. https://doi.org/10.1097/AOG.0b013e3181ee9fc7.
12. Hartmann LC, Radisky DC, Frost MH, Santen RJ, Vierkant RA, Benetti LL, et al. Understanding the premalignant potential of atypical hyperplasia through its natural history: a longitudinal cohort study. Cancer Prev Res (Phila). 2014;7(2):211–7. PMID: 24480577. https://doi.org/10.1158/1940-6207.CAPR-13-0222.

13. Renshaw AA, Gould EW. Long term clinical follow-up of atypical ductal hyperplasia and lobular carcinoma in situ in breast core needle biopsies. Pathology. 2016;48(1):25–9. PMID: 27020205. https://doi.org/10.1016/j.pathol.2015.11.015.
14. Menes TS, Rosenberg R, Balch S, Jaffer S, Kerlikowske K, Miglioretti DL. Upgrade of high-risk breast lesions detected on mammography in the breast cancer surveillance consortium. Am J Surg. 2014;207(1):24–31. PMID: 24112677. https://doi.org/10.1016/j.amjsurg.2013.05.014.
15. Pettine S, Place R, Babu S, Williard W, Kim D, Carter P. Stereotactic breast biopsy is accurate, minimally invasive, and cost effective. Am J Surg. 1996;171(5):474–6. PMID: 8651388. https://doi.org/10.1016/S0002-9610(96)00007-4.
16. Silverstein MJ, Recht A, Lagios MD, Bleiweiss IJ, Blumencranz PW, Gizienski T, et al. Special report: consensus conference III. Image-detected breast cancer: state-of-the-art diagnosis and treatment. J Am Coll Surg. 2009;209(4):504–20. PMID: 19801324. https://doi.org/10.1016/j.jamcollsurg.2009.07.006.
17. Elmore JG, Longton GM, Carney PA, Geller BM, Onega T, Tosteson AN, et al. Diagnostic concordance among pathologists interpreting breast biopsy specimens. JAMA. 2015;313(11):1122–32. PMID: 25781441. https://doi.org/10.1001/jama.2015.1405.
18. Elmore JG, Nelson HD, Pepe MS, Longton GM, Tosteson AN, Geller B, et al. Variability in Pathologists' interpretations of individual breast biopsy slides: a population perspective. Ann Intern Med. 2016;164(10):649–55. PMID: 26999810. https://doi.org/10.7326/M15-0964.
19. Gomes DS, Porto SS, Balabram D, Gobbi H. Inter-observer variability between general pathologists and a specialist in breast pathology in the diagnosis of lobular neoplasia, columnar cell lesions, atypical ductal hyperplasia and ductal carcinoma in situ of the breast. Diagn Pathol. 2014;9:121. PMID: 24948027. https://doi.org/10.1186/1746-1596-9-121.
20. McLaughlin CT, Neal CH, Helvie MA. Is the upgrade rate of atypical ductal hyperplasia diagnosed by core needle biopsy of calcifications different for digital and film-screen mammography? AJR Am J Roentgenol. 2014;203(4):917–22. PMID: 25247961. https://doi.org/10.2214/AJR.13.11862.
21. Kohr JR, Eby PR, Allison KH, DeMartini WB, Gutierrez RL, Peacock S, et al. Risk of upgrade of atypical ductal hyperplasia after stereotactic breast biopsy: effects of number of foci and complete removal of calcifications. Radiology. 2010;255(3):723–30. PMID: 20173103. https://doi.org/10.1148/radiol.09091406.
22. Polat AK, Kanbour-Shakir A, Andacoglu O, Polat AV, Johnson R, Bonaventura M, et al. Atypical hyperplasia on core biopsy: is further surgery needed? Am J Med Sci. 2012;344(1):28–31. PMID: 22205116. https://doi.org/10.1097/MAJ.0b013e318234cc67.
23. Weinfurtner RJ, Patel B, Laronga C, Lee MC, Falcon SL, Mooney BP, et al. Magnetic resonance imaging-guided core needle breast biopsies resulting in high-risk histopathologic findings: upstage frequency and lesion characteristics. Clin Breast Cancer. 2015;15(3):234–9. PMID: 25579460. https://doi.org/10.1016/j.clbc.2014.12.005.
24. Verheyden C, Pages-Bouic E, Balleyguier C, Cherel P, Lepori D, Laffargue G, et al. Underestimation rate at MR imaging-guided vacuum-assisted breast biopsy: a multi-institutional retrospective study of 1509 breast biopsies. Radiology. 2016;281(3):708–19. PMID: 27355898. https://doi.org/10.1148/radiol.2016151947.
25. Mesurolle B, Perez JC, Azzumea F, Lemercier E, Xie X, Aldis A, et al. Atypical ductal hyperplasia diagnosed at sonographically guided core needle biopsy: frequency, final surgical outcome, and factors associated with underestimation. AJR Am J Roentgenol. 2014;202(6):1389–94. PMID: 24848840. https://doi.org/10.2214/AJR.13.10864.
26. Sen LQ, Berg WA, Hooley RJ, Carter GJ, Desouki MM, Sumkin JH. Core breast biopsies showing lobular carcinoma in situ should be excised and surveillance is reasonable for atypical lobular hyperplasia. AJR Am J Roentgenol. 2016;207(5):1132–45. PMID: 27532153. https://doi.org/10.2214/AJR.15.15425.
27. Linsk A, Mehta TS, Dialani V, Brook A, Chadashvili T, Houlihan MJ, et al. Surgical upgrade rate of breast atypia to malignancy: an academic center's experience and validation of a predictive model. Breast J. 2017 PMID: 28833923. https://doi.org/10.1111/tbj.12885.

28. Middleton LP, Grant S, Stephens T, Stelling CB, Sneige N, Sahin AA. Lobular carcinoma in situ diagnosed by core needle biopsy: when should it be excised? Mod Pathol. 2003;16(2):120–9. PMID: 12591964. https://doi.org/10.1097/01.MP.0000051930.68104.92.
29. Murray MP, Luedtke C, Liberman L, Nehhozina T, Akram M, Brogi E. Classic lobular carcinoma in situ and atypical lobular hyperplasia at percutaneous breast core biopsy: outcomes of prospective excision. Cancer. 2013;119(5):1073–9. PMID: 23132235. https://doi.org/10.1002/cncr.27841.
30. Degnim AC, King TA. Surgical management of high-risk breast lesions. Surg Clin North Am. 2013;93(2):329–40. PMID: 23464689. https://doi.org/10.1016/j.suc.2012.12.005.
31. Middleton LP, Sneige N, Coyne R, Shen Y, Dong W, Dempsey P, et al. Most lobular carcinoma in situ and atypical lobular hyperplasia diagnosed on core needle biopsy can be managed clinically with radiologic follow-up in a multidisciplinary setting. Cancer Med. 2014;3(3):492–9. PMID: 24639339. https://doi.org/10.1002/cam4.223.
32. Wagoner MJ, Laronga C, Acs G. Extent and histologic pattern of atypical ductal hyperplasia present on core needle biopsy specimens of the breast can predict ductal carcinoma in situ in subsequent excision. Am J Clin Pathol. 2009;131(1):112–21. PMID: 19095574. https://doi.org/10.1309/AJCPGHEJ2R8UYFGP.
33. McGhan LJ, Pockaj BA, Wasif N, Giurescu ME, McCullough AE, Gray RJ. Atypical ductal hyperplasia on core biopsy: an automatic trigger for excisional biopsy? Ann Surg Oncol. 2012;19(10):3264–9. PMID: 22878619. https://doi.org/10.1245/s10434-012-2575-0.
34. Khoury T, Chen X, Wang D, Kumar P, Qin M, Liu S, et al. Nomogram to predict the likelihood of upgrade of atypical ductal hyperplasia diagnosed on a core needle biopsy in mammographically detected lesions. Histopathology. 2015;67(1):106–20. PMID: 25529860. https://doi.org/10.1111/his.12635.
35. Subhawong AP, Subhawong TK, Khouri N, Tsangaris T, Nassar H. Incidental minimal atypical lobular hyperplasia on core needle biopsy: correlation with findings on follow-up excision. Am J Surg Pathol. 2010;34(6):822–8. PMID: 20431477. https://doi.org/10.1097/PAS.0b013e3181dd8516.
36. Zhao C, Desouki MM, Florea A, Mohammed K, Li X, Dabbs D. Pathologic findings of follow-up surgical excision for lobular neoplasia on breast core biopsy performed for calcification. Am J Clin Pathol. 2012;138(1):72–8. PMID: 22706860. https://doi.org/10.1309/AJCPYG48TUTFIBMR.
37. Chaudhary S, Lawrence L, McGinty G, Kostroff K, Bhuiya T. Classic lobular neoplasia on core biopsy: a clinical and radio-pathologic correlation study with follow-up excision biopsy. Mod Pathol. 2013;26(6):762–71. PMID: 23307062. https://doi.org/10.1038/modpathol.2012.221.
38. Nakhlis F, Gilmore L, Gelman R, Bedrosian I, Ludwig K, Hwang ES, et al. Incidence of adjacent synchronous invasive carcinoma and/or ductal carcinoma in-situ in patients with lobular Neoplasia on Core biopsy: results from a prospective multi-institutional registry (TBCRC 020). Ann Surg Oncol. 2016;23(3):722–8. PMID: 26542585. https://doi.org/10.1245/s10434-015-4922-4.
39. Susnik B, Day D, Abeln E, Bowman T, Krueger J, Swenson KK, et al. Surgical outcomes of lobular neoplasia diagnosed in core biopsy: prospective study of 316 cases. Clin Breast Cancer. 2016;16(6):507–13. PMID: 27425222. https://doi.org/10.1016/j.clbc.2016.06.003.

Diagnostic Management of LCIS: Core Biopsy Alone Versus Core Biopsy plus Excision for Classic Versus Pleomorphic LCIS

Batul Al-zubeidy and Nora Hansen

Introduction

Lobular carcinoma in situ (LCIS) was first introduced as a precancerous lesion by Ewing in 1919 and later was described as "rare form of mammary carcinoma" with "peculiar and somewhat obscure" features by Foote and Stewart in 1941 [1–3]. LCIS is considered to be relatively uncommon breast lesion typically found in breast biopsies targeting other lesions. Despite its increased incidence from 2 in 100,000 to 2.5–4 in 100,000 with increasing mammographic screening, it remains an infrequent pathology [4, 5]. The increase in the incidence of LCIS has been more apparent in postmenopausal women compared with premenopausal women [6].

Since its initial recognition as a potential malignant lesion, its peculiar classification, associated risk, and appropriate management continue to raise debate within the scientific community. The World Health Organization (WHO) classifies lobular neoplastic breast lesions (which LCIS belongs to) as those originating from the terminal ductal-lobular unit and "characterized by small, non-cohesive cells" [7]. Initially, LCIS was considered as a precursor toward invasive lobular breast cancer, and thus excision of the lesion was considered essential as part of the surgical management. Nonetheless, studies showed that the majority of women who did not undergo surgical treatment of LCIS did not develop invasive breast cancer. Furthermore, while LCIS patients have higher incidence of breast cancer, their subsequent invasive lesions develop at different locations of the ipsilateral breast or even on the opposite the breast. This gave rise to the notion that LCIS is a marker of high risk of breast cancer development rather than an obligate precursor.

Based on the results at Memorial Hospital between 1952 and 1965, LCIS was treated with mastectomy with contralateral breast biopsy [8]. If the biopsy showed LCIS, a contralateral mastectomy was then performed. Given the higher risk of

B. Al-zubeidy · N. Hansen (✉)
Lynn Sage Comprehensive Breast Center, Chicago, IL, USA
e-mail: batul.al-zubeidy@northwestern.edu; nhansen@nm.org

© Springer International Publishing AG, part of Springer Nature 2018
F. Amersi, K. Calhoun (eds.), *Atypical Breast Proliferative Lesions and Benign Breast Disease*, https://doi.org/10.1007/978-3-319-92657-5_7

invasive breast cancer associated with LCIS, many patients opted for bilateral mastectomy as a prophylactic measure to reduce their chance of future breast cancer development. In fact, during the 1980s, bilateral mastectomies were chosen by (13%) of women with LCIS. Nonetheless, several studies, including Haagensen et al., showed that subsequent breast cancer risk was about 1% per year in LCIS patients, much lower than expected from direct precursor [9]. Furthermore, these data show that both breasts were at increased risk, rather than the ipsilateral breast.

Since Haagensen, there were various population-based studies over the past few decades, which revealed that patients diagnosed with LCIS had subsequently higher ipsilateral vs contralateral invasive breast cancer. Furthermore, they had slightly higher rate of invasive lobular carcinoma compared with the overall population based on population studies [10]. Modern genetics and molecular analysis have demonstrated similar clonal genes between the initial LCIS lesions and subsequent IBC [11]. These findings have re-demonstrated a strong link between the initial LCIS lesion and future tumorigenic abilities. Lobular carcinoma in situ should more accurately be viewed as both a marker of high-risk cancer development and nonobligatory precursor toward invasive lesions within the breast.

The evolution of our understanding of this rather rare lesion within the breast has challenged our dogmatic surgical and medical management. The traditional approach of excision of LCIS lesion clearly challenges the idea of LCIS as a marker, given that the remaining breast continue to be at high risk of future cancer. Similarly, a nonsurgical treatment approach questions the theory of LCIS as precursor toward IBC. Hence, it is not surprising that no clear treatment guidelines exist for the management of LCIS.

A major area of debate regarding the management of LCIS is the associated upgrade rate to ductal carcinoma in situ (DCIS) or invasive breast cancer (IBC) with excisional biopsy. Some studies have shown that excisional biopsy of LCIS was associated with an upgrade rate of 10–20% of synchronous malignant or invasive lesions (DCIS or IBC) [12]. However, these studies were underpowered and failed to demonstrate clear association between the subtypes of LCIS and subsequent IBC risks. In order to determine the true upgrade rate of LCIS lesion and thus provide optimal treatment, it is crucial to distinguish the histological LCIS subtypes. As will be argued below, different LCIS histology (pleomorphic and florid) is associated with greater occult invasive and noninvasive cancer compared with classic LCIS (LCIS). Thus, management of these different entities should be tailored differently.

Molecular and Histological Subtypes

Histological Analysis

Classic LCIS (CLIS)
This subtype of LCIS refers to a unique discohesive population of cells compromising at least one-half of the acini (Figs. 7.1 and 7.2). These cells, known as type A, have scant cytoplasm with monomorphic round nuclei and usually lack nucleoli [13]. On the other hand, type B cells have abundant cytoplasm with slight

Fig. 7.1 LCIS

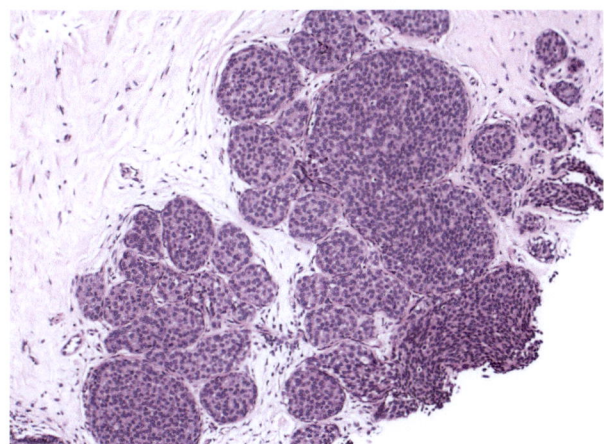

Fig. 7.2 Higher magnification revealing the filling of lobules with monotonous cells

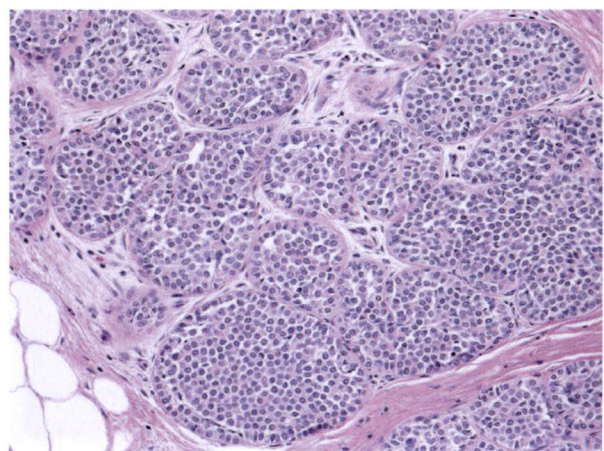

pleomorphism, larger nuclei, and more apparent nucleoli [9, 14]. Furthermore, LCIS cells may demonstrate signet ring morphology due to intracytoplasmic mucin inclusions. As demonstrated in Table 7.1, classic LCIS rarely presents with calcifications on imaging and tends to be an incidental finding on core needle biopsies or surgical specimens for other targeted lesions.

The majority of LCIS cells tend to lose the E-cadherin transmembrane protein that mediates cell-to-cell adhesion. Normally, the intracytoplasmic component of the E-cadherin protein binds to the actin filament via catenin proteins (p120, β-catenin, α-catenin, and δ-catenin). In lobular carcinoma in situ, various disruptions to the E-cadherin and β-catenin result in loss of cell-to-cell adhesion and disjointed cell populations. Hence, immunohistochemical staining for the E-cadherin and p120 can aid in the differentiation of LCIS and DCIS, as well as IDC and ILC (Figs. 7.3 and 7.4). Over three-quarters of lobular neoplastic lesions tend to lack E-cadherin staining, but retain p120 cytoplasmic (rather than membranous) staining [15].

Table 7.1 Histological and clinical features of classic and pleomorphic lobular carcinoma in situ

	CLCIS	PLCIS
Age of patients	40–50 years old	50–60 years old
Histology	Large, loosely cohesive cells	Large, loosely cohesive
Presence of calcifications	Occasional	Common
Presence of necrosis	Absent to rare	Common
Nuclear pleomorphism	Absent to rare	Common with high mitotic figures

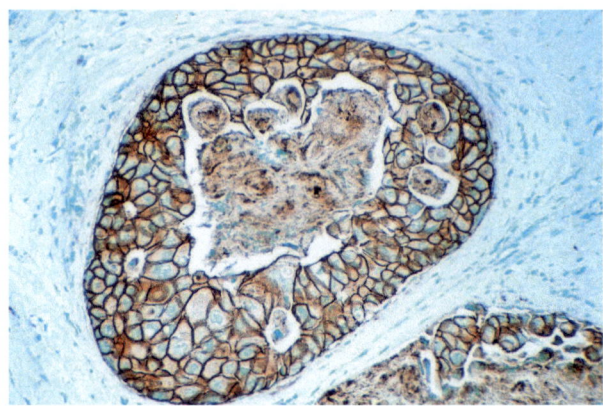

Fig. 7.3 E-cadherin staining demonstrating the ductal structure

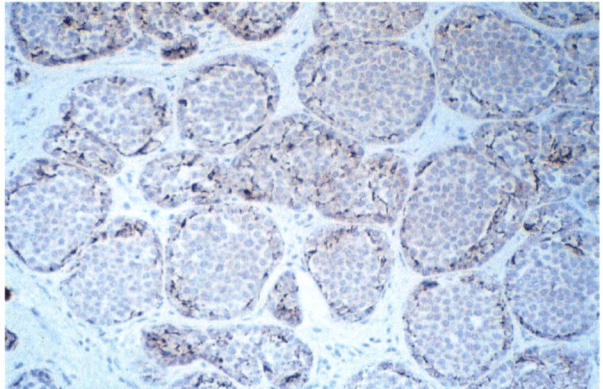

Fig. 7.4 E-cadherin staining demonstrating the lobular structure

Pleomorphic LCIS (PLCIS)

Pleomorphic lobular carcinoma in situ (PLCIS) is a rare distinct histological subtype of LCIS first described in 1982 by Dixon et al. [15]. With an incidence of 2.7–4.4% of all lobular neoplasia, PLCIS can represent a challenging diagnosis that requires experience and possibly additional reviews by other pathologists [16, 17]. Similar to classic LCIS, it lacks E-cadherin staining and high cytoplasmic P120 catenin staining. However, subsequent studies showed that PLCIS has similar aggressive histological features as infiltrating ductal carcinoma [18]. It is of paramount importance to distinguish LCIS from DCIS, as they associated with different cancer risks and thus dictate different management.

Pleomorphic LCIS is characterized by discohesive large pleomorphic cells with eosinophilic cytoplasm [19]. These cells harbor pleomorphic nucleoli with high degree of variability. PLCIS reported to have higher rates of comedo necrosis and calcifications and demonstrate florid growth patterns (cells extending to fill the lobule and the duct). This has traditionally made it difficult to differentiate it from high-grade DCIS [20]. Unlike classic LCIS, PLCIS cells demonstrated greater binucleated and multinucleated appearance [21]. Similarly, PLCIS is reported to be associated with higher proliferation activity (45%) and higher multifocal and extensive lesions [19].

Florid

This rare form of LCIS describes the solid architectural growth pattern of cells along the ducts, similar to that of DCIS. Florid LCIS has been occasionally described as LCIS with comedo necrosis, or macroacinar lobular intraepithelial neoplasia. This chapter will not discuss florid LCIS in any further detail.

Hormonal Receptors Expression in LCIS

Classic LCIS tends to have significantly higher estrogen and progesterone receptors expression compared with pleomorphic LCIS. Similarly, classic LCIS has lower HER2 expression, as shown in Table 7.1 [22]. This has significant impact in terms of progression of the lesion, treatment, and impact on survival. Chen et al. have reported that pleomorphic LCIS lesions were associated with 44% ER negative, 48% PR negative, and 13% HER2 overexpression [23]. Florid LCIS has been observed to have ER expression similar to CLCIS, but unlike CLCIS, it has higher HER2+ overexpression [24].

Molecular Analysis

Through the use of genomic hybridization analyses, we came to recognize the various genetic alterations and molecular changes that distinguish LCIS from other breasts pathologies. Various molecular studies have demonstrated that LCIS lesions have loss of heterozygosity that characterizes their genetic makeups. Classic LCIS is notably known for loss of 16q and gain of 1q, both of which have been recognized in well-differentiated tumors, such as tubular carcinoma, ADH, and low-grade DCIS [14, 25, 26]. It also has been shown that LCIS lesions lose their E-cadherin expression due to premature truncation of the CDH1 gene (the cell-to-cell adhesion receptor gene E-cadherin) [27]. The loss of molecular expression of this gene is a result of promotor methylation, various missense mutations, and allelic loss [27].

Advances in molecular and genetic analysis have allowed scientists to investigate the molecular relationships between LCIS lesions and invasive cancers. These studies have demonstrated that certain somatic genetic mutations were found in both

LCIS and ILC, which suggest clonal similarities between the two. One such study from Memorial Sloan Kettering showed that the most frequently mutated genes in LCIS and ILC are CDH1 (56% and 66%, respectively), PIK3CA (41% vs 52%, respectively), and CBFB (12% and 19% respectively) [28]. Analysis of microarray gene expression of healthy LCIS and ILC patients have revealed over 150 potential genes involved in the progression from LCIS to ILC [29]. While these findings suggest a potential nonobligatory precursor pathway between some LCIS and ILC lesions, further molecular analytical and population-based studies are required.

Similar to classic LCIS, the majority of pleomorphic LCIS has shown to have loss of 16q and 17p and gain of 1q. However, there are key histological and molecular differences between the two lesions. Comparative genomic hybridization analysis by Chen et al. showed that PLCIS had higher Ki67 index, lower estrogen and progesterone receptor expression, and higher incidence of HER2 gene amplification [23]. Similarly, apocrine PLCIS showed more genomic alterations than non-apocrine PLCIS. Moreover, PLCIS have been linked to various mutations with known cancer genes, such as *p53, MEN1, ATM, RB, CCND1, and CCNF* [14]. Similar to PLCIS, florid LCIS showed HER2 overexpression and CCND1 gene alterations, among others. These important clinical, histological, immunophenotypic, and molecular differences between PLCIS and CLCIS point to more aggressive tumors.

Upgrade Rates

Various studies have attempted to determine the true upgrade rates of LCIS lesions to DCIS or invasive cancers upon surgical excisions. However, the majority of these studies are retrospective and do not differentiate between ALH, classic LCIS, or PLCIS. For those who attempt to differentiate between the different subtypes of lobular neoplastic lesions, the PLCIS cohorts are usually small and thus tend to be underpowered.

Classic LCIS has been reported to have an upgrade rate of 3.5% but 26.7% for variable LN (representing mostly pleomorphic) [28]. Chaudhary et al. have reported their experience with an upgrade rate of classic LCIS with concordant radiographic-pathological finding to be 1.7% [19]. Similarly, Hwang et al. reported a 1% upgrade rate when excluding non-CLCIS and discordant radio-pathologic results (shown in Table 7.2) [34].

Nonetheless, the strongest factor associated with high upgrade rate was PLCIS on core needle biopsy, with or without synchronous lesion. As Table 7.2 demonstrates, PLCIS lesions have an upgrade rate of 25–65% range. A meta-analysis of five studies with 42 patients with PLCIS on core biopsies revealed an upgrade rate of 36% [41]. Similarly, a review of 21 patients with PLCIS from the University of Washington Medical Center between 2000 and 2014 revealed an upgrade rate to invasive cancer of 33.3% and to DCIS 17.4% upon surgical excision [33]. Rendi et al. showed that their overall upgrade rate of 31% in LCIS patients undergoing surgical excision was much higher with PLCIS compared with CLCIS [38].

Table 7.2 Upgrade rate following surgical excision for a core biopsy

Series	N	Upgrade rate on excision
Pleomorphic LCIS		
Carder et al. (2010) [30]	10	30%
Chivukula et al. (2008) [31]	12	25%
Fasola et al. (2012) [32]	34 (13 pure, 21 mixed w/DCIS or IDC)	62%
Flanagan et al. (2015) [33]	21	52% (33.3% IBC and 19% DCIS)
Hwang et al. (2008) [34]	13	46%
Morris et al. (2013) [35]	17 (3 pure, 7 with DCIS, 7 with IC)	65%
Niell et al. (2012) [36]	5	62%
Sullivan et al. (2010) [16]	17	18%; 36% upgrade rate when LCIS with necrosis
Classic LCIS (or unclassified LCIS)		
King et al. (2015) [5]	1060	
Hussain et al. (2011) [37]	241	32%
Rendi et al. (2012) [38]	23	5%
Elsheikh et al. (2005) [43]	13	31%
Choudhry et al. (2013) [19]	87	3.4%
Hwang et al. (2008) [34]	26	11%; but 1% when excluding radiology-pathology discordance
Lewis et al. (2012) [39]	99	19%
Karabakhtsian et al. (2007) [40]	19	21%; 19% when excluding mass lesions
Middleton et al. (2003) [55]	9	22%; both patients had mass lesions

Sullivan et al.'s review of 28 patients with pleomorphic and LCIS with necrosis revealed an upgrade rate of 18% and 36%, respectively [16].

In addition to pleomorphic histological finding within LCIS lesions, many studies attempted to investigate key factors that point toward higher correlation between classic LCIS on core biopsy and invasive breast lesions on excisional biopsy. One such study demonstrated that a high upgrade rate was associated with discordant imaging-pathological findings in lobular neoplasia compared with concordant results (38% vs 3%, respectively) [42]. Hence, discordant pathological-imaging finding warrants a surgical excision or close monitoring.

Moreover, patients with concurrent pathological finding in addition to the LCIS lesion have higher upgrade rates compared with those who do not. Patients with simultaneous ADH and LCIS were shown to have 29% upgrade rate compared with 5% in LCIS alone [38]. Similarly, a mixed DCIS and LCIS lesion detected on core needle biopsies were found to be associated with 60% upgrade rate toward invasive carcinoma. Also, a greater risk of occult malignancy was reported in patients found to have a mass on physical exam or imaging but who subsequently had LCIS only lesions on core biopsy [39, 43]. These lesions were found to correlate with higher rate of occult malignancy requiring excision (21.4% vs 3.3%).

Furthermore, the volume and extent of LCIS on core needle biopsy have been linked in some studies, but not all, to high upgrade rate. While this factor has not been reproducible in multiple studies, it can be considered as potential risk for an occult malignancy [38]. Extensive LCIS, >4 foci, was associated with high upgrade rate compared with focal lesion, <4 foci. Chaudhary et al.'s analysis of classic lobular neoplasia on core biopsies did not find a number of cores and lobules involved, pagetoid duct extension, or presence of microcalcification important in the upgrade rates to DICS or invasive cancer [19].

Management

Patients who are diagnosed with LCIS should be counseled regarding their increased risk (8–11-fold increase) of breast cancer compared with the general population. These patients have a probability of developing breast cancer equivalent of 1–2% per year. Furthermore, patients with LCIS appear to have this increased risk persist over their lifetime and thus should remain vigilant about surveillance for the disease.

Surveillance

The NCCN and ACS have issued recommendations regarding surveillance in this high-risk group. It recommends biannual or annual breast exam with annual mammography, with possible consideration of MRI [44]. However, the ACS has refrained from supporting or discouraging MRI screening pointing to high false-positive rate. The utilization of MRI as a mode of surveillance has not shown improved cancer detections or overall survival in this group. A large study from Memorial Sloan Kettering of 776 patients with LCIS, of which 59% were undergoing MRI screening with conventional modalities compared with conventional screening alone in the remaining cohort. The study failed to show any difference in cancer detection rate between the two groups [45]. Similar studies have not demonstrated earlier cancer stages detected in the LCIS patients undergoing MRI [46]. The lack of survival benefits and/or improved detection rates, as well as high biopsy rates, makes MRI less optimal as a routine screening modality in this group of patients.

Chemoprevention

It has been shown in large randomized controlled trials that patients with high-risk lesions, such as LCIS, benefit from chemoprevention with selective estrogen receptor blocker and aromatase inhibitors. The NSABP P-1 trial demonstrated 56% risk reduction of breast cancer development in women with LCIS with 5 years of tamoxifen administration (8 breast cancers in the chemoprevention group vs 18 in the placebo group). Also, it showed more dramatic reduction, 86% risk reduction, in the over 1196 women with atypical hyperplasia lesions with the same period of tamoxifen [47].

Various other studies showed similar risk reduction rates with chemoprevention in LCIS cohorts. The Memorial Sloan Kettering cohort of 1032 patients who underwent surveillance reported 12% incidence of breast cancer at 10 years in patients electing tamoxifen compared with 21% in those who did not [5]. Similarly, Coopey et al. showed a breast cancer incidence rate of 10.3% in LCIS patients taking tamoxifen, raloxifene, or exemestane at 10 years vs 32.4% in those who did not [48]. These studies have changed practice guidelines in terms of treatment of LCIS. The American Society of Clinical Oncology has endorsed the use of estrogen receptor blockers and aromatase inhibitors as chemopreventive options in high-risk patients, such as LCIS [49].

While the benefits of tamoxifen in LCIS patients were observed in all age groups, the greatest benefits were seen during the premenopausal period [5]. Women who are 45 years of age and older undergoing chemoprevention did not show the same significant risk reduction rates observed in those under the age of 45 [5].

Despite the reported benefits from tamoxifen in risk reduction of subsequent breast cancer development in patients with LCIS, a minority of patients choose this route of management. It has been reported that 4–20% of LCIS patients offered chemoprevention actually take it for the specified duration period [48, 50]. A meta-analysis of patient decisions about breast cancer chemoprevention showed a real uptake of 14.8% compared with 24.7% reported hypothetical uptake [50]. This is likely a result of several factors. First, despite its documented reduction in breast cancer incidence rates, chemoprevention has not demonstrated clear long-term breast cancer-specific mortality within this patient population group [51].

Second, various chemoprevention drugs have been associated with long-term side effects with potential lifelong complications. The NSABP P-1 trial reported a statistically significant increased risk of invasive endometrial cancer in women who took tamoxifen with RR = 3.28, 95% CI = 1.87–6.03, with greatest risk being in postmenopausal women (4.68 vs 15.64 in 1000 in the placebo and tamoxifen groups, respectively) [47]. Similarly, tamoxifen has been shown to increase the incidence of thromboembolic events, particularly pulmonary emboli among women aged 50 and over (RR = 2.16, 95% CI = 1.02–4.89) [47].

The risk-benefit ratio of chemoprevention in LCIS patients should be thoroughly assessed in patient prior to initiation of the treatment. Certainly, history of thromboembolic disorders, interfering comorbidities, and menopausal status should be part of an individualized treatment plan of affected patients.

Surgical Intervention

Many patients opt for surgical excision (mastectomy) of LCIS rather than observation with surveillance and chemoprevention. Given the higher risk of breast cancer in both breasts with incidence rates of 1–2% per year, many patients elect bilateral mastectomy. Approximately 5–10% of LCIS patients elect to undergo prophylactic bilateral mastectomies and are more likely to be of younger age, denser breast, and has stronger family history of breast cancer compared with those electing surveillance [5]. Analysis of the National Cancer Institute's Surveillance, Epidemiology, and End Results (SEER) database demonstrated a reduction in prophylactic bilateral mastectomy in LCIS patients from 58.8% in 1983 to 10.3% in 2013 ($p < 0.001$) [52].

As has been demonstrated above, the risk of synchronous malignant lesion and the risk of breast cancer development in patients with LCIS will dictate the most optimal treatment plan. The appropriate management of LCIS should be based on histological subtypes, concordant radiological and pathological findings, and patient's clinical presentation. Review of the SEER database demonstrated that surveillance without surgical intervention of LCIS lesions was not reported until 1988 [52]. This resembled the point of recognizing LCIS as a marker rather than obligate precursor toward invasive breast cancer and thus did not dictate surgical excision.

Pleomorphic LCIS

Following histological and clinical recognition of PLCIS as a unique form of LCIS with high risk of upgrade rate to DCIS and invasive breast cancers (ILC or IDC), many clinicians agree that the most optimal treatment of PLCIS is surgical excision. However, given the extensive nature of PLCIS in breast tissue, positive margins are reported to be high in patients who undergo breast conservation therapy. Khoury et al. reported a positive margin of 21% within their 46 patients with PLCIS, while Flanagan et al. reported 35% within their 21 patients [17, 33]. Similarly, close margins, <0.1 mm, were shown to be between 20% and 50%. This multicentric and diffuse nature of PLCIS makes it difficult to be surgically removed with aesthetically acceptable results. With approximately 50% of PLCIS being extensive and multifocal lesions, re-excisions for positive margins is common [33]. While it varies across institutions, the rate of re-excision and/or mastectomy has been reported to be as high as 85% in pursuit of negative surgical margin [33]. Hence, many clinicians find it more cosmetically appropriate to treat with mastectomy [53].

Incidence of Subsequent Breast Cancer

The Memorial Sloan Kettering patient population with LCIS had a median follow-up of 81 months, which revealed 14% incidence of breast cancer over the 29-year period in patients who chose surveillance with or without chemoprevention. In this large single-institution study, the risk of invasive breast cancer was found to be 1–2% per year, with a risk of 26% at 15 years. To determine whether any particular factors predicted progression toward future breast cancer, King et al. reported the ratio of LCIS lesions on reviewed slides (0.5) associated with higher subsequent breast cancer incidence rate. While family history, age of LCIS detection, and menopausal status were examined, none were found to be a statistically significant contributor.

The presence of LCIS in surgical margins has not been associated with higher breast cancer recurrence rates. The presence of incidental LCIS on the margin specimen of invasive cancer or ductal carcinoma in situ does not statistically influence future cancer occurrence. Ciocca et al. showed that the 5-year actuarial rates of local recurrences in 290 patients with LCIS and 2604 without LCIS were 2% in both groups [54]. Approximately 29% of the LCIS cohort had positive margin (LCIS on ink), with reported 5-year recurrence rate of 6% compared with 1% in the "negative" margin. However, the difference between the two was not statistically significant. This study points to factors other than LCIS on margin, such as age, menopause, and adjuvant therapy, as important predictors of breast cancer recurrence [54]. Furthermore, Downs-Kelly et al.'s study of 26 patients with PLCIS reported 1 patient with PLCIS at the margin who subsequently developed recurrence (3.8%) [53]. In the same study, 5 other patients with PLCIS at the margin and 11 patients within 2 mm of the margin had no recurrence at a mean follow-up of 46 months. These patients had received chemoprevention.

For patients who elect breast conservation therapy, the margin status is an important factor that should be investigated. To determine whether the margin status of excised PLCIS lesions is important in breast cancer recurrences, it is important to have long-term follow-ups. The current studies are small and underpowered, and most lack long-term follow-ups. As mentioned earlier, Downs-Kelly et al. report of one BC recurrence (3.8%) in a patient with PLCIS margin, while Khoury et al. reported six BC recurrences (19.4%) in four patients who had positive surgical margin [17]. To have a greater understanding of the role of margin status in excised PLCIS specimen, a multi-institutional cooperative study with long follow-up is required. The current NCCN guidelines do not make a specific recommendation regarding the margin status with PLCIS, but rather leave them to the discretion of clinician.

Our understanding of the diagnosis and treatment of LCIS has evolved since its initial description over seven decades ago. Due to greater understanding of its pathological presentation and improved diagnostic tools, we are diagnosing LCIS more frequently (higher incidence) and are able to subclassify it. As shown earlier, PLCIS carries a greater risk of harboring invasive ductal or lobular cancer and DCIS compared with CLCIS. Hence, it is of high importance to determine the histopathologic subtype in order to formulate the most optimal management. Currently, we are lacking large randomized controlled trials with sufficient numbers to delineate the most optimal management. However, based on the current literature, CLCIS continues to be a marker of high risk toward breast cancer, as well as nonobligatory precursor. Patients with CLCIS should be managed with chemoprevention and close surveillance. On the other hand, PLCIS should be managed similar to DCIS, with surgical excision with or without radiation.

References

1. Ewing J. Neoplastic diseases: a textbook on tumors. Philadelphia: W.B. Saunders; 1919.
2. Foote FW, Stewart FW. Lobular carcinoma in situ: a rare form of mammary cancer. Am J Pathol. 1941;17(4):491–6.
3. King TA, Reis-Filho J. Lobular carcinoma in situ: biology and management. In: Harris JR, Lippman ME, Morrow M, Osborn CK, editors. Diseases of the breast. 5th ed. Philadelphia: Lippincott Williams & Wilkins; 2014.
4. Portschy PR, Marmor S, Nzara R, et al. Trends in incidence and management of lobular carcinoma in situ: a population-based analysis. Ann Surg Oncol. 2013;20:3240–6.
5. King TA, Pilewskie M, Muhsen S, et al. Lobular carcinoma in situ: a 29-year longitudinal experience evaluating clinicopathologic features and breast cancer risk. J Clinic Oncol. 2015;33(33):3945–52.
6. Ci L, Anderson BO, Porter P, et al. Changing incidence rate of invasive lobular breast carcinoma among older women. Cancer. 2000;88(11):2561–9.
7. Lakhani SR, Ellis IO, Schnitt SJ, et al. WHO classification of tumours of the breast, vol. 4. Lyon: IARC Press; 2012.
8. Rosen PP, Kosloff C, Lieberman PH, et al. Lobular carcinoma in situ of the breast. Detailed analysis of 99 patients with average follow up of 24 years. Am J Surg Pathol. 1978;2(3):225–51.
9. Haagensen CD, Lane N, Lattes R, et al. Lobular neoplasia (so-called lobular carcinoma in situ) of the breast. Cancer. 1978;42(2):737–69.
10. Middleton LP, Sneige N, Coyne R, et al. Most lobular carcinoma in situ and atypical lobular hyperplasia diagnosed on core needle biopsy can be managed with radiologic follow-up in a multidisciplinary setting. Cancer Med. 2014;3(3):492–9.
11. Shah V, Nowinski S, Levi D, et al. PIK3CA mutations are common in lobular carcinoma in situ, but are not a biomarker of progression. Breast Cancer Res. 2017;19(1):7.
12. Aripno G, Allred DC, Mohsin SK, et al. Lobular neoplasia on core-needle biopsy: clinical significance. Cancer. 2004;101:242–50.
13. Reis-Filho JS, Pinder SE. Non-operative breast pathology: lobular neoplasia. J Clin Pathol. 2007;60(12):1321–7.
14. Ginter P, D'Alfonos T. Current concepts in diagnosis, molecular features, and management of lobular carcinoma in situ of the breast with a discussion of morphologic variants. Arch Pathol Lab Med. 2017;141(12)1668–78.
15. Dixon JM, Anderson TJ, Page DL, et al. Infiltrating lobular carcinoma of the breast. Histopathology. 1982;6:149–61.
16. Sullivan ME, Khan SA, Sullu Y, et al. Lobular carcinoma in situ variants in breast cores: potential for misdiagnosis, upgrade rates at surgical excisions, and practical implications. Arch Pathol Lab Med. 2010;134(7):1024–8.
17. Khoury T, Karabakhtsian RG, Mattson D, et al. Pleomorphic lobular carcinoma in situ of the breast: clinicopathological review of 47 cases. Histopathology. 2014;64(70):981–93.
18. Eusebi V, Magalhaes F, Azzopardi JG. Pleomorphic lobular carcinoma of the breast: an aggressive tumor showing apocrine differentiation. Hum Pathol. 1992;23:655–62.
19. Chaudhary S, Lawrence L, McGinty G, et al. Classic lobular neoplasia on core biopsy: a clinical and radio-pathologic correlation study with follow-up excision biopsy. Mod Pathol. 2013;26:762–71.
20. Sapino A, Frigerio A, Peterse JL, et al. Mammographically detected in situ lobular carcinomas of the breast. Virchows Arch. 2000;436:421–30.
21. Blanco LZ, Thurow TA, Mahajan A, et al. Multinucleation is an objective feature useful in the diagnosis of pleomorphic lobular carcinoma in situ. Am J Clin Pathol. 2015;144(5):772–26.
22. Brogi E, Corhen A, Murray M. Morphologic precursor of mammary carcinoma and their mimics. Difficult diagnoses in breast pathology. Palazio JP. 2011. Demos Med. New York.
23. Chen YY, Hwang ES, Roy R, et al. Genetic and phenotypic characteristics of pleomorphic lobular carcinoma in situ of the breast. Am J Surg Pathol. 2009;33(11):1683–94.

24. Shin S, Lal A, De Vries S, et al. Florid lobular carcinoma in situ: molecular profiling and comparison to classic lobular carcinoma in situ and pleomorphic lobular carcinoma in situ. Hum Pathol. 2012;44:1198–2009.
25. Mohsin SK, O'Connell PR, Allred DC, Libby AL. Biomarker profile and genetic abnormalities in lobular carcinoma in situ. Breast Cancer Res Treat. 2005;90(3):249–56.
26. Green AR, Krivinskas S, Young P, et al. Loss of expression of chromosome 16q genes DPEP1 and CTCF in lobular carcinoma in situ of the breast. Breast Cancer Res Treat. 2009;113(1):59–66.
27. Droufakou S, Deshmane V, Roylance R, et al. Multiple ways of silencing E cadherin gene expression in lobular carcinoma of the breast. Int J Cancer. 2001;92(3):404–8.
28. Sakr RA, Schiza M, Carniello JV, et al. Targeted capture massively parallel sequencing analysis of LCIS and invasive lobular cancer: repertoire of somatic genetic alterations and clonal relationships. Mol Oncol. 2016;10(2):360–70.
29. Andrade VP, Morrogh M, Qin LX, et al. Gene expression profiling of lobular carcinoma in situ reveals candidate precursor genes for invasion. Mol Oncol. 2015;9(4):772–82.
30. Carder PJ, Shaaban A, Alizadeh Y, Kumarasuwamy V, Liston JC, Sharma N. Screen-detected pleomorphic lobular carcinoma in situ (PLCIS): risk of concurrent invasive malignancy following a core biopsy diagnosis. Histopathology. 2010;57:472–8.
31. Chivukula M, Haynik DM, Brufsky A, et al. Pleomorphic lobular carcinoma in situ (PLCIS) on breast core needle biopsies: clinical significance and immune profile. Am J Surg Pathol. 2008;32:1721–6.
32. Fasola CE, Jensen KC, Horst KC. Local regional recurrence among patients with pleomorphic lobular carcinoma in situ: is there a role for radiation therapy? Int J Radiat Oncol Biol Phys. 2012;1:S238.
33. Flanagan MR, Rendi MH, Calhoun KE, et al. Pleomorphic lobular carcinoma in situ: radiologic-pathologic features and clinical management. Ann Surg Oncol. 2015;22(13):4263–9.
34. Hwang H, Barke LD, Mendelson EB, et al. Atypical lobular hyperplasia and classic lobular carcinoma in situ in core biopsy specimens: routine excision is not necessary. Mod Pathol. 2008;21:1208–16.
35. Morris K, Howe M, Kirwan C, et al. Clinical and phenotypic characteristics of core biopsy diagnosed pleomorphic lobular carcinoma-in-situ in a UK population (PLCIS). Eur J Surg Oncol. 2013;39:484.
36. Niell B, Specht M, Gerade B, Rafferty E. Is excisional biopsy required after a breast core biopsy yields lobular neoplasia? AJR Am J Roentgenol. 2012;199:929–35.
37. Hussain M, Cunnick GH. Management of Lobular carcinoma in-situ and atypical lobular hyperplasia of the breast –a review. Eur J Surg Oncol. 2011;37(4):279–89.
38. Rendi MH, Dintzis SM, Lehman CD, et al. Lobular in-situ neoplasia on breast core needle biopsy: imaging indication and pathologic extent can identify which patients require excisional biopsy. Ann Surg Oncol. 2012;19(3):914–21.
39. Lewis JL, Lee DY, Tartter PI. The significance of lobular carcinoma in situ and atypical lobular hyperplasia of the breast. Ann Surg Oncol. 2012;19(13):4124–8.
40. Karabakhtsian RG, Johnson R, Sumkin J, et al. The clinical significance of lobular neoplasia on breast core biopsy. Am J Surg Pathol. 2007;31(5):717–23.
41. Pieri A, Harvey J, Bundred N. Pleomorphic lobular carcinoma in situ of the breast: can the evidence guide practice? World J Clin Oncol. 2014;4(3):546–53.
42. Murray M, Brogi E. Lobular carcinoma in situ, classical type and unusual variants. Surg Pathol Clin. 2009;2:273–99.
43. Elsheikh TM, Silverman JF. Follow-up surgical excision is indicated when breast core needle biopsies show atypical lobular hyperplasia or lobular carcinoma in situ: a correlative study of 33 patients with review of the literature. Am J Surg Pathol. 2005;29(4):534–43.
44. Bevers TB, Anderson BO, Bonaccio E, et al. Breast cancer screening and diagnosis. J Nat Compr Netw. 2006;4(5):480–508.
45. Port ER, Park A. Borgen pi, et al. results of MRI screening for breast cancer in high-risk patients with LCIS and atypical hyperplasia. Ann Surg Oncol. 2007;14(3):1051–7.

46. King TA, Muhsen S, Patil S, et al. Is there a role for routine screening MRI in women with LCIS? Breast Cancer Res Treat. 2013;142(2):445–53.
47. Fisher B, Costantino JP, Wickerham DL, et al. Effects of tamoxifen vs raloxifene on the risk of developing invasive breast cancer and other disease outcomes: the NSABP study of tamoxifen and raloxifene (STAR) P-2 trial. JAMA. 2006;295(23):2727–41.
48. Coopey SB, Mazzola E, Buckley JM, et al. The role of chemoprevention in modifying the risk of breast cancer in women with atypical breast lesions. Breast Cancer Res Treat. 2012;136:627–33.
49. Visvanathan K, Hurely P, Bantug E, et al. Use of pharmacologic interventions for breast cancer risk reduction: American Society of Clinical Oncology clinical practice guideline. J Clin Oncol. 2013;31:2942–62.
50. Ropka ME, Keim J, Philbrik JT. Patient decisions about breast cancer chemoprevention: a systematic review and meta-analysis. J Clin Oncol. 2009;28(18):3090–5.
51. Cuzick J, Sestak I, Cawathorn S, Hamed H, Holli K, Howell A, et al. Tamoxifen for prevention of breast cancer: extended long-term follow-up of the IBIS0I breast cancer prevention trial. Lancet Oncol. 2015;16:67–75.
52. Wong S, King TA, Boileau JF, et al. Population-based analysis of breast cancer incidence and survival outcomes in women diagnosed with lobular carcinoma in situ. Ann Surg Oncol. 2017 Sep;24(9):2509–17.
53. Downs-Kelly E, Bell D, Sneige N, et al. Management of pleomorphic lobular carcinoma in situ (supplement 1): Abstract no. 119:29A. Modern Pathology 2008; 97th Annual Meeting of United States and Canadian Academy of Pathology, March 1–7, Denver.
54. Ciocca RM, Li T, Freedman GM, et al. Presence of lobular carcinoma in situ does not increase local recurrence in patients treated with breast-conservation therapy. Ann Surg Oncol. 2008;15(8):2263–71.
55. Middleton LP, Grant S, et al. Lobular Carcinoma In Situ Diagnosed By Core Needle Biopsy: When Should It Be Excised? Modern Pathology 2003;16(2):120–129.

Breast Cancer Risk Prediction in Women with Atypical Breast Lesions

8

Suzanne B. Coopey and Kevin S. Hughes

Introduction

There are several atypical breast lesions which are known to significantly increase a woman's risk of developing breast cancer. These include lobular carcinoma in situ, atypical ductal hyperplasia, and atypical lobular hyperplasia. Data suggest that long-term cancer risk for women diagnosed with these lesions is greater than 20%, which puts them into a high-risk category, even in the absence of family history. This chapter provides an in-depth review of the breast cancer risks associated with these high-risk lesions, methods for estimating a woman's cancer risk, and data on medication for risk reduction.

Part I. Lobular Carcinoma In Situ

Lobular carcinoma in situ (LCIS) was initially described by Foote and Stewart in 1941 [1]. They hypothesized that LCIS was a direct precursor to invasive lobular carcinoma and recommended simple mastectomy for treatment [1]. This practice continued until the 1970s when subsequent studies led to reclassification of LCIS as a risk factor for breast cancer, since the risk was found to be equal in both breasts [2–4]. Currently, there is renewed interest in the concept of LCIS as a direct, but non-obligate, precursor to invasive lobular carcinoma, as when LCIS and invasive lobular carcinoma co-exist, they are phenotypically and cytologically similar [5]. Plus, invasive lobular carcinoma (ILC) occurs two to three times more frequently in women with LCIS than in women in the general population [4, 6–8]. In the United States in 2009, the incidence of LCIS was approximately 2.75/100,000 women [9].

S. B. Coopey (✉) · K. S. Hughes
Division of Surgical Oncology, Massachusetts General Hospital, Boston, MA, USA
e-mail: scoopey@mgh.harvard.edu; kshughes@partners.org

Relative Risk of Breast Cancer

Studies have shown that the risk of invasive breast cancer in women with LCIS is seven- to ninefold greater than the risk in the general population [2, 3]. Haagensen and colleagues followed 209 patients with LCIS between 1930 and 1972, of whom 35 developed invasive breast cancer with 14-year mean follow-up [2]. The number of women afflicted with breast cancer was seven times the expected number for women of similar ages living in the same geographic region [2]. Rosen et al. followed 77 women who were diagnosed with LCIS between 1940 and 1950. With 24-year median follow-up, 28 developed breast cancer, 9-fold higher than the number of cases expected ($p < 0.001$) [3].

Cumulative Risk of Breast Cancer

There are several studies which have estimated long-term cancer risks with LCIS (Table 8.1). Some of the studies included cases of invasive cancer only, and others included both ductal carcinoma in situ (DCIS) and invasive cancer. The study by Bodian and colleagues has the longest follow-up at 35 years; their results suggest that a woman's lifetime risk is steady at approximately 1% per year after a diagnosis of LCIS [6]. A more recent study by King et al. suggests that the risk may be higher at 2% per year for at least the first 6 years after diagnosis, which is corroborated by Coopey and colleagues [7, 8].

Table 8.1 Risk of breast cancer with lobular carcinoma in situ

Author, year	# Patients	5-year risk (%)	10-year risk (%)	15-year risk (%)	20-year risk (%)	35-year risk (%)	% ILC
McDivitt (1967)[a] [10]	50	8	15	27	35	–	–
Ottesen (1993) [11]	88[b]	17	–	–	–	–	37
Bodian (1996) [6]	236	–	13	–	26	35	27
Levi (2005)[a] [12]	88	–	–	–	28	–	23
Chuba (2005)[a] [4]	4853	4	7	11	–	–	23
Coopey (2012) [8]	568	10	24	–	–	–	31
King (2015) [7]	831	7	21	26	–	–	27

ILC invasive lobular carcinoma
[a]Included invasive cancers only
[b]Included LCIS and mixed ductal and lobular carcinoma in situ

Risk Based on Age

Data regarding the impact of patient age on breast cancer risk in women with LCIS is variable. In Bodian's review of 236 patients with LCIS and a median follow-up of 18 years, she and her co-authors found that age at LCIS diagnosis was a significant risk factor for the development of breast cancer [6]. Specifically, patients under 40 years of age at LCIS diagnosis had the highest relative risk (RR = 10.5), and patients diagnosed after age 55 had the lowest relative risk (RR = 3.2), although the number of patients in each age subgroup was small [6]. In contrast, when Chuba and colleagues reviewed the SEER database of 4853 women with LCIS, they found that the cumulative incidence of breast cancer increased with increasing age similar to what occurs in the general population [4]. In King's multivariable analysis of 831 women with LCIS, she and her colleagues also found no association between age at diagnosis and breast cancer risk with nearly 7-year median follow-up [7].

Risk Based on Family History

Once a woman has been diagnosed with LCIS, having a family history of breast cancer (defined as one or more first-degree relative or two or more second-degree relatives) does not seem to further increase breast cancer risk [7].

Risk Based on Extent of Disease

There is evidence that the volume of LCIS may impact the risk of breast cancer [7, 11]. When Ottesen and colleagues reviewed 88 cases of LCIS and mixed ductal and lobular carcinoma in situ, they found that the presence of ≥10 lobules with LCIS was significantly associated with breast cancer risk, 24% cancer with ≥10 lobules versus 8% cancer with <10 lobules with just over 5-year median follow-up ($p = 0.028$) [11]. In a nested case-controlled analysis, King et al. found that a higher proportion of slides containing LCIS increased the risk of breast cancer, with a ratio of 0.5–1 having the highest risk [7].

Chemoprevention for Lobular Carcinoma In Situ

In the National Surgical Adjuvant Breast and Bowel Project (NSABP) P-1 trial, which randomized high-risk women to 5 years of tamoxifen versus 5 years of placebo, tamoxifen reduced the number of invasive breast cancers by 49% compared with placebo through 69 months of follow-up [13]. When participants were broken down into subgroups, 826 women with a history of LCIS who took tamoxifen reduced their breast cancer risk even further, by 56% [13]. When Coopey and colleagues reviewed the outcomes of 568 women with LCIS, they found that the 10-year risk of breast cancer (invasive and DCIS) was significantly reduced from 32% to 10% with the use of chemoprevention medications [8]. Women who took chemoprevention in King's study also had a significant reduction in 10-year cumulative cancer rates from 21% to 7% [7]. Current guidelines from the American Society of Clinical Oncology and the National Comprehensive Cancer Network (NCCN) endorse chemoprevention for high-risk women with LCIS [14, 15]. Note that in the NSABP P-1 trial, women with a history of LCIS could start tamoxifen at any time after diagnosis. This suggests that breast cancer risk and chemoprevention benefits persist long after diagnosis. Thus, women may be offered chemoprevention even many years after their LCIS diagnosis.

Risk Models and Lobular Carcinoma In Situ

Only the Bodian and Tyrer-Cuzick breast cancer risk models include women with LCIS [16]. The Bodian model is based on a cohort of 236 patients with LCIS followed for a median of 18 years [6]. This model includes age, first-degree relatives with breast cancer, parity and age of first birth, extent of LCIS, number of times diagnosed with LCIS, and the presence of additional benign breast disease [6]. Validation of this model is limited; one study found it to be most accurate compared to the Gail model, Claus model, and BRCAPRO for predicting risk in women with LCIS [17], though, these other risk models do not account for the presence of LCIS [16].

The Tyrer-Cuzick model is very comprehensive and includes age and body mass index; age at menarche, age at first live birth, parity, age at menopause, and use of hormone replacement therapy; breast biopsies, presence of hyperplasia, atypical hyperplasia (ductal or lobular), or LCIS; and hereditary information including first- and second-degree relatives with breast cancer and/or ovarian cancer, incorporating age of onset, and the presence of bilateral breast cancers [16, 18]. LCIS calculations are based on an assigned eightfold increased risk if present based on the work of Page et al. which studied 39 women with lobular neoplasia over 18 years [19]. However, the Tyrer-Cuzick model has not been formally validated in patients with LCIS. Until the models are better validated for this cohort, it may be best to talk to women about their cumulative risk based on the data presented in Table 8.1 rather than a calculated risk.

Pleomorphic Lobular Carcinoma In Situ

Pleomorphic LCIS was initially described by Frost in 1996 [20]. Compared to classical LCIS, pleomorphic LCIS is characterized by large, pleomorphic nuclei and massively distended acini with large, discohesive cells with abundant cytoplasm [21]. Because of its rarity, the long-term cancer risk of pure pleomorphic LCIS is largely unknown (Table 8.2). Interestingly, when Ottesen and colleagues reviewed 88 cases of LCIS and mixed ductal and lobular carcinoma in situ in 1993, they

Table 8.2 Risk of breast cancer with pleomorphic lobular carcinoma in situ

Author, year	# Patients	Treatment	Length of follow-up	Breast cancers (%)
Sneige (2002) [22]	5	5 excision alone	17 months	0
Downs-Kelly (2011) [23]	26	10 excision alone	46 months	1 (3.8%)
		6 excision + CP		
		4 excision + RT		
		6 excision + RT +CP		
Khoury (2014) [24]	31	17 excision alone	56 months	4 (12.9%)
		11 excision + CP		
		3 excision + RT		
Flanagan (2015) [25]	12	5 excision alone	4.1 years	0
		5 excision + CP		
		2 excision + RT		
De Brot (2017) [26]	7	6 excision alone	67 months	4 (57.1%)
		1 excision + CP		

CP chemoprevention, *RT* radiation

found that large nuclear size significantly increased the risk of cancer with median follow-up of 5 years, 31% risk of cancer with large nuclei versus 11% risk of cancer with small nuclei size ($p = 0.032$) [11]. In a recent review by De Brot of 7 patients with pure pleomorphic LCIS, 57% developed ipsilateral breast cancer at a median follow-up of 67 months [26]. Therefore, most suggest treating pleomorphic LCIS with wide excision to obtain negative margins in addition to chemoprevention [21, 23, 26].

Part II. Atypical Hyperplasia

One to two million women per year in the Unites States undergo a benign breast biopsy; of these, 10% are diagnosed with atypical hyperplasia [27]. There are two types of atypical hyperplasia – atypical lobular hyperplasia (ALH) and atypical ductal hyperplasia (ADH). The term atypical lobular hyperplasia was coined by Ackerman in 1977 in a paper which stressed the importance of differentiating a pathologic diagnosis of LCIS from that of ALH based on the degree of involvement and distention of the lobules [28]. The pathologic criteria used today for diagnosing a breast lesion as ALH or ADH come from Page and colleagues from the Nashville study published in 1985 [29].

Relative Risk of Breast Cancer

In 1985, Dupont and Page reported that the risk of invasive breast cancer in women with atypical hyperplasia (ADH and ALH) was four to five times the risk of women of similar ages in the general population [30]. Their study included 3303 women with benign breast biopsies, of which 311 had atypical hyperplasia; their median follow-up was 17 years [30]. In 2005, Hartmann and colleagues from the Mayo Clinic reported similar findings from their cohort of 9087 women with benign breast disease [31]. With a median follow-up of 15 years, patients with atypical hyperplasia ($n = 336$) were 4.24 times more likely to develop cancer than the general population [31].

Relative Risk Based on Type of Atypical Hyperplasia

Dupont and Page found similar risks of invasive breast cancer with ADH and ALH; specifically ADH increased the risk by 4.1-fold and ALH increased the risk by 4.5-fold [30]. In contrast, in a case-control study of 856 women from the Nurses' Health Study with benign breast biopsies, Marshall and colleagues found that the odds of breast cancer (invasive and DCIS) in women with ALH was 5.3 times higher than women with non-proliferative breast lesions, while the odds of breast cancer with ADH was lower at 2.4 [32]. This study included 70 women with ADH and 49 women with ALH, and the difference between these odds ratios was of borderline significance ($p = 0.05$) [32]. In a meta-analysis of 5 case-control studies, Zhou determined that the odds of breast cancer in women with ADH was 2.93 times that of women with non-proliferative breast disease, while the odds with ALH was higher at 5.14 [33]. In a more recent update from the Mayo Clinic investigators, the risk was found to be similar for women with ADH or ALH; the standardized incidence ratio (SIR) comparing observed number of breast cancer events to those expected based on Iowa Surveillance, Epidemiology, and End Results (SEER) data was 3.93 for ADH and 4.76 with ALH [34].

Cumulative Risk of Breast Cancer

Few studies have assessed the long-term cancer risks with atypical hyperplasia (Table 8.3). Hartmann and colleagues reported a 29% 25-year risk of breast cancer in patients with atypical hyperplasia (ADH and ALH combined) [34]. Updated, but unpublished, results from the Nashville Breast Cohort were similar with a 25-year risk of in situ or invasive disease of 27.5% [38]. In a larger, more modern, cohort of 2370 patients with ADH, ALH, and severe ADH, Mazzola and colleagues recently reported that the 15-year risk of in situ or invasive disease was 40.1% [36].

Risk Based on Age

The Mayo Cohort study found that the relative risk of breast cancer is higher in women diagnosed with atypical hyperplasia at a younger age; the SIR was 3.54 for women diagnosed over age 55, 5.43 for women diagnosed between ages 45 and 55, and 5.45 for women diagnosed under the age of 45 [34]. In contrast, in a recent publication by Mazzola and colleagues which included 2370 patients with atypical

Table 8.3 Risk of breast cancer with atypical hyperplasia

Author, year	# Patients	5-year risk (%)	10-year risk (%)	15-year risk (%)	20-year risk (%)	25-year risk (%)
Atypical hyperplasia (ADH and ADH)						
Degnim (2007) [35]	331	–	–	–	21	29
Hartmann (2014) [34]	698	–	–	–	–	29
Mazzola (2017)[a] [36]	2370	7.6	25.1	40.1		
ADH						
Coopey (2012) [8]	1198	4.5	17.3	–	–	–
ALH						
McLaren (2006)[b] [37]	252	–	–	19	–	–
Coopey (2012) [8]	827	10.9	20.7	–	–	–

[a]Included 345 cases of severe ADH (bordering on DCIS)
[b]Included invasive cancers only

hyperplasia, their data suggested that for women between the ages of 35 and 75, there was no significant difference in cumulative breast cancer risk up to 15 years' post-diagnosis [36].

Risk Based on Family History

In Dupont and Page's landmark paper, they found that women with atypical ductal or lobular hyperplasia and a family history of breast cancer nearly doubled their risk of invasive breast cancer, RR of 4.4 with atypical hyperplasia and no family history compared to RR of 8.4 with atypical hyperplasia and family history [30]. In contrast, in a cohort of 331 women with atypical hyperplasia, Degnim et al. found no significant difference in breast cancer risk based on family history (RR 3.59 with strong family history, RR 5.59 with weak family history, RR 3.81 with no family history) [35]. Similarly, Hartmann and colleagues found that family history did not significantly alter breast cancer risk in 698 women with atypical hyperplasia (her cohort included Degnim's patients plus patients accrued over an additional 10 years) [34]. In addition, Zhou's meta-analysis found that having a family history did not increase breast cancer risk in women with atypical hyperplasia [33].

Risk Based on Extent of Disease

More foci of atypical hyperplasia present on excision and less age-related regression (involution) of background lobular units have been associated with increased breast cancer risk [34]. Hartmann and colleagues found that the SIR was 3.19 with

1 focus of atypical hyperplasia, 5.53 with 2 foci, and 7.61 with 3 or more foci [34]. They also found that the SIR was 1.91 with complete lobular involution ($\geq$75% of lobules being atrophic), 4.63 with partial lobular involution (1–74% of lobules being atrophic), and 7.66 with no lobular involution [34]. Interestingly, a recent publication by the Mayo Clinic detected no association between mammographic density and breast cancer risk in women with atypical hyperplasia [39].

Chemoprevention for Atypical Hyperplasia

In the NSABP P-1 study, a subgroup of women with atypical hyperplasia who were randomized to 5 years of tamoxifen at any time since diagnosis had a reduction in the number of invasive breast cancers by 85% compared to women randomized to placebo through 69 months of follow-up [13]. In the clinical setting, Coopey and colleagues found that chemoprevention reduced the probability of cancer at 10 years from 20% to 8.5% in 1198 women with ADH and from 19% to 8.5% in 827 women with ALH [8]. NCCN guidelines strongly recommend risk reduction medication for women with atypical hyperplasia [15]. While historic rates of chemoprevention uptake by high-risk women have been low, a recent study of 382 women with atypical breast lesions who underwent individualized education and counseling sessions found that 52% of women were willing to initiate chemoprevention after an informed discussion and approximately 55% of women on treatment would complete 5 years [40].

Risk Models and Atypical Hyperplasia

There are two widely used risk assessment models which include atypical hyperplasia as a variable in their calculations, the Gail model and the Tyrer-Cuzick model [18, 41]. Unfortunately, neither has proven reliable in women with atypical hyperplasia. The Gail model tends to underestimate risk, while the Tyrer-Cuzick model tends to overestimate risk [42, 43]. In a study of 331 women with atypical hyperplasia, 1.66 times more women developed breast cancer than predicted by the Gail model [42]. In a separate study of the same 331 women, the Tyrer-Cuzick model overestimated the number of breast cancers to develop within 10 years by nearly a factor of 2 [43]. Until a more accurate risk prediction model for women with atypical hyperplasia is developed, it may be prudent to use the cumulative risks of breast cancer when counseling patients with atypical hyperplasia. Using the Mayo Clinic data, it is reasonable to advise women with atypical hyperplasia that their 25-year risk of breast cancer approaches 30% [34].

Severe ADH Bordering on Ductal Carcinoma In Situ

Infrequently, a breast lesion may be too atypical to call ADH but not quite meet criteria for DCIS. These lesions are often described as "severe ADH" or "borderline DCIS" or "markedly atypical ductal hyperplasia bordering on DCIS." Little is known about the long-term cancer risk with these lesions. In a review by Tozbikian and colleagues of 105 patients with severe ADH bordering on DCIS, 3.8% developed ipsilateral invasive breast cancer or DCIS at a median follow-up of 37 months [44]. Of note, 13% of patients received chemoprevention [44]. In Coopey et al.'s study of 161 patients with severe ADH bordering on DCIS, investigators estimated that the 5-year risk of invasive cancer or DCIS was 9.7% and 10-year risk was 26.0% without the use of chemoprevention [8].

Flat Epithelial Atypia

Flat epithelial atypia (FEA) is a benign proliferative lesion of the breast characterized by columnar cell changes and cytologic atypia but without the architectural changes required for a diagnosis of atypical hyperplasia [45]. There is limited data regarding the risk of breast cancer with FEA. In a cohort of 152 patients with FEA and a median follow-up of 16.8 years, Said et al. found no increased risk of breast cancer in women with FEA compared to women with proliferative breast disease without atypia (SIR = 2.04 with FEA versus SIR = 1.90 without FEA, $p = 0.76$) [45].

Conclusion

Lobular carcinoma in situ, atypical ductal hyperplasia, and atypical lobular hyperplasia significantly increase a woman's risk of breast cancer. In the absence of accurate risk prediction models for women with these high-risk lesions, cumulative cancer estimations should be used when counseling about risk. Chemoprevention medications should be offered to women with atypical breast lesions, as multiple studies have demonstrated what a significant impact they have in reducing breast cancer risk.

References

1. Foote FW, Stewart FW. Lobular carcinoma in situ. A rare form of mammary cancer. Am J Pathol. 1941;17:491–5.
2. Haagensen CD, Lane N, Lattes R, Bodian C. Lobular neoplasia (so-called lobular carcinoma in situ) of the breast. Cancer. 1978;42:737–69.
3. Rosen PP, Lieberman PH, Braun DW, Kosloff C, Adair F. Lobular carcinoma in situ of the breast: detailed analysis of 99 patients with average follow-up of 24 years. Am J Surg Pathol. 1978;2(3):225–51.
4. Chuba PJ, Hamre MR, Yap J, et al. Bilateral risk for subsequent breast cancer after lobular carcinoma-in-situ: analysis of surveillance, epidemiology, and end results data. J Clin Oncol. 2005;23:5534–41.
5. Murray M, Brogi E. Lobular carcinoma in situ, classical type and unusual variants. Surg Pathol Clin. 2009;2:273–99.
6. Bodian CA, Perzin KH, Lattes R. Lobular neoplasia: long-term risk of breast cancer and relation to other factors. Cancer. 1996;78:1024–34.
7. King TA, Pilewskie M, Muhsen S, et al. Lobular carcinoma in situ: a 29-year longitudinal experience evaluating clinicopathologic features and breast cancer risk. J Clin Oncol. 2015;33:3945–52.

8. Coopey SB, Mazzola EM, Buckley JM, et al. The role of chemoprevention in modifying the risk of breast cancer in women with atypical breast lesions. Breast Cancer Res Treat. 2012;136:627–33.
9. Portschy PR, Marmor S, Nzara R, Virnig BA, Tuttle TM. Trends in incidence and management of lobular carcinoma in situ: a population-based analysis. Ann Surg Oncol. 2013;20:3240–6.
10. McDivitt RW, Hutter RVP, Foote FW, Stewart FW. In situ lobular carcinoma: a prospective follow-up study indicating cumulative patient risks. JAMA. 1967;201(2):82–6.
11. Ottesen GL, Graverson HP, Blichert-Toft M, Zedeler K, Andersen JA, on behalf of the Danish Breast Cancer Cooperative Group. Lobular carcinoma in situ of the female breast: short-term results of a prospective nationwide study. Am J Surg Pathol. 1993;17(1):14–21.
12. Levi F, Randimbison L, Te V, LaVecchio C. Invasive breast cancer following ductal and lobular carcinoma in situ of the breast. Int J Cancer. 2005;116:820–3.
13. Fisher B, Constantino JP, Wickerham L, et al. Tamoxifen for prevention of breast cancer: report of the national surgical adjuvant breast and bowel project P-1 study. J Natl Cancer Inst. 1998;90:1371–88.
14. Visvanathan K, Hurley P, Bantug E, et al. Use of pharmacologic interventions for breast cancer risk reduction: American Society of Clinical Oncology clinical practice guideline. J Clin Oncol. 2013;31:2942–62.
15. NCCN Clinical Practice Guidelines. Breast cancer risk reduction, v1.2016. NCCN.org.
16. Cintolo-Gonzalez JA, Braun D, Blackford AL, et al. Breast cancer risk models: a comprehensive overview of existing models, validation, and clinical applications. Breast Cancer Res Treat. 2017;164:263–84.
17. Euhus DM, Leitch M, Huth JF, Peters GN. Limitations of the gail model in the specialized breast cancer risk assessment clinic. Breast J. 2002;8(1):23–7.
18. Tyrer J, Duffy SW, Cuzick J. A breast cancer prediction model incorporating familial and personal risk factors. Stat Med. 2004;23:1111–30.
19. Page DL, Kidd TE, Dupont WD, Simpson JF, Rogers LW. Lobular neoplasia of the breast: higher risk for subsequent invasive cancer predicted by more extensive disease. Hum Pathol. 1991;22(12):1232–9.
20. Frost AR, Tsangaris TN, Silverberg SG. Pleomorphic lobular carcinoma in situ. Pathol Case Rev. 1996;1(1):27–31.
21. Masannat YA, Bains SK, Pinder SE, Purushotham AD. Challenges in the management of pleomorphic lobular carcinoma in situ of the breast. Breast. 2013;22:194–6.
22. Sneige N, Wang J, Baker BA, Krishnamurthy S, Middleton LP. Clinical, histopathologic, and biologic features of pleomorphic lobular (ductal-lobular) carcinoma in situ of the breast: a report of 24 cases. Mod Pathol. 2002;15(10):1044–50.
23. Downs-Kelly E, Bell D, Perkins GH, Sneige N, Middleton LP. Clinical implications of margin involvement by pleomorphic lobular carcinoma in situ. Arch Pathol Lab Med. 2011;135:737–43.
24. Khoury T, Karabakhtsian RG, Mattson D, et al. Pleomorphic lobular carcinoma in situ of the breast: clinicopathological review of 47 cases. Histopathology. 2014;64:981–93.
25. Flanagan MR, Rendi MH, Calhoun KE, Anderson BO, Javid SH. Pleomorphic lobular carcinoma in situ: radiologic–pathologic features and clinical management. Ann Surg Oncol. 2015;22:4263–9.
26. De Brot M, Koslow Mautner S, Muhsen S, et al. Pleomorphic lobular carcinoma in situ of the breast: a single institution experience with clinical follow-up and centralized pathology review. Breast Cancer Res Treat. 2017;165:411–20.
27. Visscher DW, Frank RD, Carter JM, et al. Breast cancer risk and progressive histology in serial benign biopsies. JNCI J Natl Cancer Inst. 2017;109(10):djx035.
28. Ackerman LV, Katzenstein AL. The concept of minimal breast cancer and the pathologist's role in the diagnosis of "Early Carcinoma". Cancer. 1977;39:2755–63.
29. Page DL, Dupont WD, Rogers LW, Rados MS. Atypical hyperplastic lesions of the female breast: a long-term follow-up study. Cancer. 1985;55:2698–708.

30. Dupont WD, Page DL. Risk factors for breast cancer in women with proliferative breast disease. N Engl J Med. 1985;312(3):146–51.
31. Hartmann LC, Sellers TA, Frost MH, et al. Benign breast disease and the risk of breast cancer. N Engl J Med. 2005;353:229–37.
32. Marshall LM, Hunter DJ, Connolly JL, et al. Risk of breast cancer associated with atypical hyperplasia of lobular and ductal types. Cancer Epidemiol Biomark Prev. 1997;6:297–301.
33. Zhou WB, Xue DQ, Liu XA, Ding Q, Wang S. The influence of family history and histological stratification on breast cancer risk in women with benign breast disease: a meta-analysis. J Cancer Res Clin Oncol. 2011;137:1053–60.
34. Hartmann LC, Radisky DC, Frost MH, et al. Understanding the premalignant potential of atypical hyperplasia through its natural history: a longitudinal cohort study. Cancer Prev Res. 2014;7(2):211–7.
35. Degnim AC, Visscher DW, Herman HK, et al. Stratification of breast cancer risk in women with atypia: a Mayo cohort study. J Clin Oncol. 2007;25:2671–7.
36. Mazzola E, Coopey SB, Griffin M, et al. Reassessing risk models for atypical hyperplasia: age may not matter. Breast Cancer Res Treat. 2017;165:285–91.
37. McLaren BK, Schuyler PA, Sanders ME, et al. Excellent survival, cancer type, and Nottingham grade after atypical lobular hyperplasia on initial breast biopsy. Cancer. 2006;107:1227–33.
38. Hartmann LC, Degnim AC, Santen RJ, Dupont WD, Ghosh K. Atypical hyperplasia of the breast — risk assessment and management options. N Engl J Med. 2015;372(1):78–89.
39. Vierkant RA, Degnim AC, Radisky DC, et al. Mammographic breast density and risk of breast cancer in women with atypical hyperplasia: an observational cohort study from the Mayo Clinic Benign Breast Disease (BBD) cohort. BMC Cancer. 2017;17:84.
40. Roche CA, Tang R, Coopey SB, Hughes KS. Chemoprevention acceptance and adherence in women with high risk breast lesions. Breast J. https://doi.org/10.1111/tbj.13064. EPub 2018 May 21.
41. Gail MH, Brinton LA, Byar DP, et al. Projecting individualized probabilities of developing breast cancer for white females who are being examined annually. J Natl Cancer Inst. 1989;81(24):1879–86.
42. Pankratz VS, Hartmann LC, Degnim AC, et al. Assessment of the accuracy of the gail model in women with atypical hyperplasia. J Clin Oncol. 2008;26(33):5374–9.
43. Boughey JC, Hartmann LC, Andersen SS, et al. Evaluation of the Tyrer-Cuzick (International Breast Cancer Intervention Study) model for breast cancer risk prediction in women with atypical hyperplasia. J Clin Oncol. 2010;28(22):3591–6.
44. Tozbikian G, Brogi E, Vallejo CE, et al. Atypical ductal hyperplasia bordering on ductal carcinoma in situ: interobserver variability and outcomes in 105 cases. Int J Surg Pathol. 2017;25(2):100–7.
45. Said SM, Visscher DW, Nassar A, et al. Flat epithelial atypia and risk of breast cancer: a Mayo cohort study. Cancer. 2015;121:1548–55.

Advanced Screening Options and Surveillance in Women with Atypical Breast Lesions

Erin Crane, Nicole Sondel Lewis, Erini Makariou, Janice Jeon, Judy Song, and Charlotte Dillis

Introduction

Understanding appropriate and evidence-based breast cancer screening recommendations is important in guiding management recommendations for those women who are at increased risk for developing breast cancer. The goal of a screening test is to detect disease in asymptomatic individuals at the earliest stages, when treatment may be more effective, less invasive, and/or less expensive. While screening mammography decreases mortality associated with breast cancer, it has limitations. Women with an elevated lifetime risk of developing breast cancer, including those with a history of atypia, may benefit from additional and adjunct screening modalities which have higher sensitivity and may detect mammographically occult breast cancers.

Screening Recommendations and Risk

In women of average risk, breast cancer screening with mammography or digital breast tomosynthesis (DBT) is recommended by the American Cancer Society (ACS) [1], National Comprehensive Cancer Network (NCCN) [2], Society of Breast Imaging (SBI) [3], American College of Radiology (ACR) [4], and the American College of Obstetricians and Gynecologists (ACOG) [5]. Recommendations for additional/adjunct screening vary according to the patient's risk stratification.

Although women with biopsy-proven atypia are at increased risk for developing breast cancer, this increased risk may not be appropriately reflected using some of

E. Crane (✉) · N. S. Lewis · E. Makariou · J. Jeon · J. Song · C. Dillis
Department of Radiology, Medstar Georgetown University Hospital, Washington, DC, USA
e-mail: erin.p.crane@gunet.georgetown.edu; makariev@gunet.georgetown.edu; Janice.l.jeon@gunet.georgetown.edu; judy.h.song@gunet.georgetown.edu

the available computer-based risk assessment models. Many of the highly utilized risk assessment models generate results based primarily on family history. Thus, if current models are utilized, women with history of atypia but with no family history may not generate a high enough cumulative risk to qualify for supplementary breast cancer screening. The ACR defines "high risk" as a greater than or equal to 20% calculated lifetime risk of developing breast cancer, history of BRCA gene mutation or untested first degree relatives, and women with a history of chest irradiation between 10 and 30 years of age [4]. The ACS and NCCN have similar guidelines which also include recommendations for adjunct screening in women with a calculated lifetime breast cancer risk of 20–25% or greater. However, the clinician must remember that these lifetime risk calculations are largely based on family history and may be misleading in patients with no family history of breast cancer, but with a personal history of atypia, for example.

Women with a personal history of atypia without additional risk factors are currently placed into the "intermediate-risk" category by the ACR. For these women, adjunct screening recommendations are not clearly defined and remain a subject of debate. Intermediate risk is defined as those with a history of atypical ductal hyperplasia (ADH) and lobular neoplasia (ALH and LCIS), personal history of breast cancer, or a calculated 15–20% lifetime risk of breast cancer. In these patients, additional screening "may be appropriate" [4]. ACS similarly considers there to be "insufficient evidence for or against" additional screening in women in this risk category [6]. NCCN guidelines specifically address women with a history of LCIS or ADH/ALH, noting that additional screening should be considered [2].

Recent data suggests that available models may underestimate risk estimates for women with atypia. Atypia, including atypical ductal and lobular hyperplasia, confers an approximate fourfold increase in relative risk of future breast cancer [7–9] (Fig. 9.1). Recent absolute risk analysis performed analyzing the Nashville Breast Cohort and Mayo Clinic confirms that the cumulative increased risk of breast cancer approaches 30% in long-term follow-up studies [10, 11].

Currently, this cumulative risk is not widely recognized, and atypia is not included in many commonly used risk assessment models. Thus atypia is not accounted for in many high-risk guidelines [10]. Family history is included in lifetime risk assessment using available computer models such as Claus, BRCAPro, Breast and Ovarian Analysis of Disease Incidence and Carrier Estimation Algorithm (BOADICEA), and Tyrer-Cuzick. In a prospective comparison of risk assessment models, Tyrer-Cuzick model was the most consistently accurate in calculating a woman's breast cancer risk [12, 13]. It utilizes a comprehensive set of factors including personal risk factors, reproductive risk factors and genetic risk factors (including BRCA gene mutation carrier status). It also takes into account a history of prior biopsies/atypical hyperplasia/LCIS [14].

Additional prospective trials are needed. Meanwhile, given the recently published data citing increased cumulative risk, reevaluation of the available risk assessment models and guidelines should be considered.

Mammography

Mammography is the only method of breast cancer screening that has been shown to decrease mortality. In fact, breast cancer mortality in the era of screening has decreased by 20–38% from 1989 to 2014 [15]. Presumably, this is due to earlier diagnosis of treatable, small, node-negative breast cancers. However, mammography is limited by high false-positive rates as well as decreased sensitivity in women with dense breasts. The sensitivity of mammography ranges from 87% in women

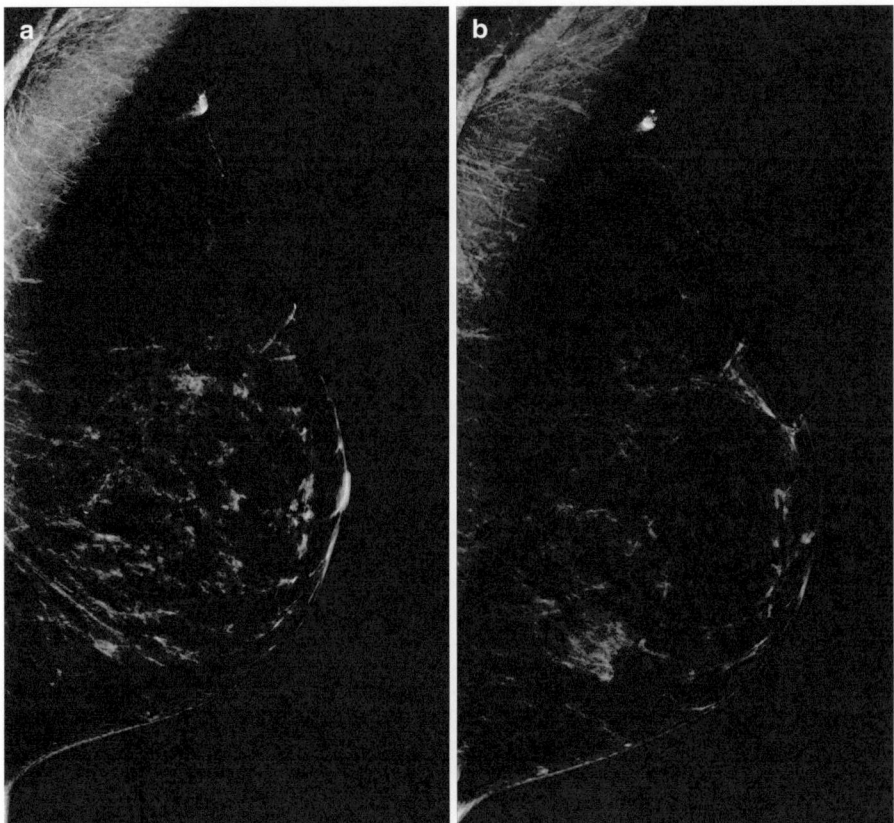

Fig. 9.1 A 63-year-old female with increased risk of breast cancer given history of remote LCIS underwent annual screening mammography with negative results (**a**). She did not undergo adjunct screening MRI. Three years later, she presented with a palpable mass (**b**, triangular marker). Subsequent MIP (**c**) images from her contrast-enhanced MRI demonstrated two irregular heterogeneously enhancing masses in her left breast (**d**). Biopsy revealed invasive lobular carcinoma with negative sentinel nodes. Patient proceeded to mastectomy

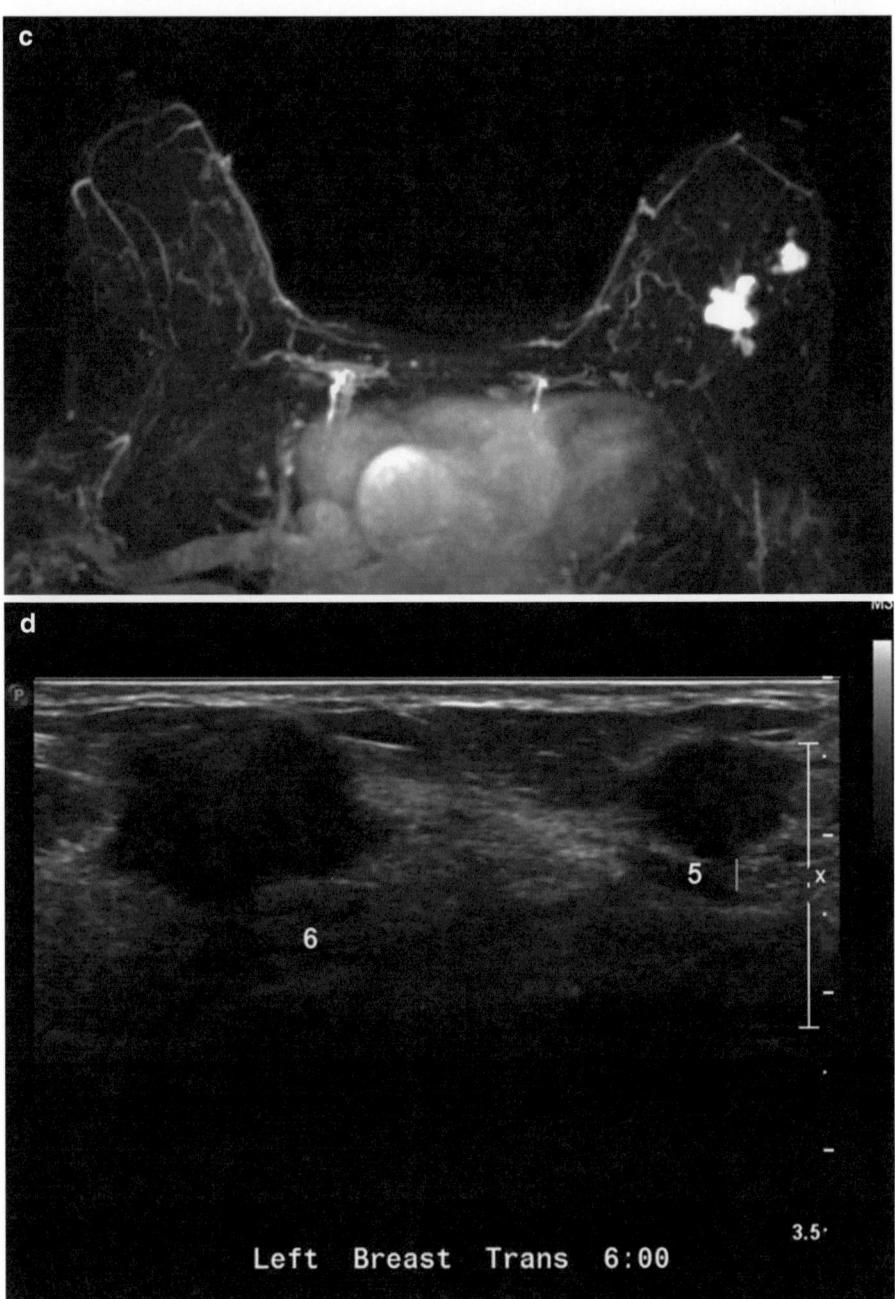

Fig. 9.1 (continued)

with almost entirely fatty tissue to 63% in women with extremely dense breasts, with additional studies demonstrating sensitivity as low as 30% in dense breasts [16, 17]. The lowered sensitivity in dense breasts results from masking effect, or obscuration of masses by overlying tissues. In addition, conventional (2D) mammography is limited by superimposed normal tissue creating summation density and pseudolesions. This leads to an increase in false positives and callbacks for additional evaluation; often cited as a "risk" of mammography as it contributes to heightened anxiety, further imaging and biopsies.

These cited risks of mammography have fueled controversy regarding ages and intervals at which women of average risk should be screened leading to confusion among physicians and patients. Patients with history of previous biopsies demonstrating atypia, and thus at increased risk for breast cancer, should be counseled that the general recommendations apply only to the population of women of average risk. For women with biopsy-proven lobular neoplasia, ADH, or DCIS, for example, annual mammography is recommended per ACR guidelines starting at age 30 [4].

Digital Breast Tomosynthesis (DBT)

Digital breast tomosynthesis (DBT) produces thin-section reconstructed mammographic images of the breast. Projection images are acquired in 0.5–1 mm increments at different angles in an arc around the compressed breast by a rotating X-ray tube. A 3D data set of the breast is created by stacking multiple 2D slices. The radiologist can scroll through the constructed data set on a dedicated workstation. Abnormalities identified can be further scrutinized and triangulated. By scrolling through images, radiologists can resolve superimposed normal tissue which would have otherwise resulted in a false-positive callback on conventional (2D) mammography. Similarly, cancers that may have been obscured by surrounding dense tissue on 2D mammography are more easily detected using tomosynthesis 3D technology (Fig. 9.2). Finally, DBT allows better characterization of benign lesions (such as intramammary lymph nodes) also contributing to decreased false positives. In fact, compared to 2D mammography, DBT has shown a decrease in relative "recall rates" ranging from 14% to as much as 63% [18].

Multiple studies of varying design have been performed comparing DBT to conventional mammography. These have confirmed an increase in cancer detection rate (CDR). The CDR for standard digital mammography is approximately 4–6 per 1000 patients. Adding 3D increases the absolute CDR by 1–3 per 1000 screening mammograms for a total of 5–9 per 1000 patients. This corresponds to a 27–53% increase in cancer detection [18–22].

Despite improvements in technology and addition of tomosynthesis, mammography remains an imperfect anatomic screening test, particularly in younger women and those with dense breasts. Therefore, supplemental screening is recommended in certain patients with increased risk.

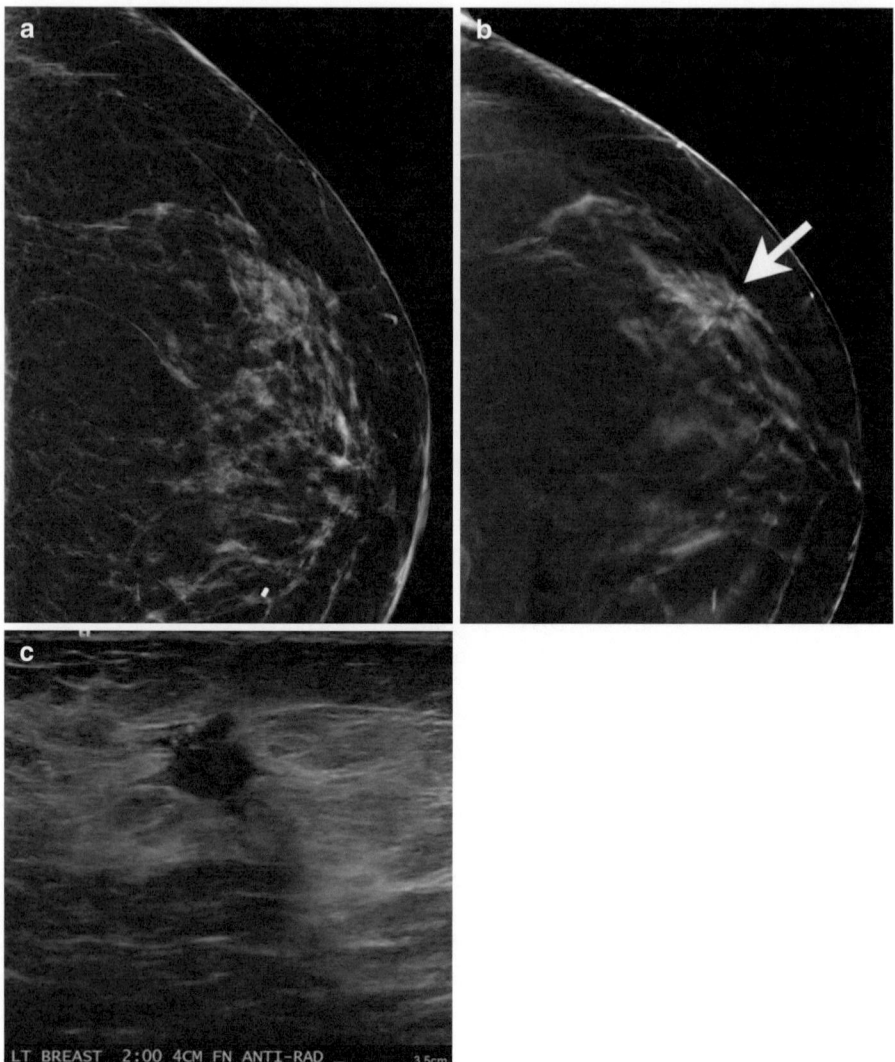

Fig. 9.2 Full-field digital mammogram (FFDM) CC view of the left breast (**a**) demonstrating no obvious abnormality. Corresponding digital breast tomosynthesis (DBT) slice (**b**, arrow) demonstrating distortion not readily apparent on 2D mammography. Targeted ultrasound demonstrates a suspicious hypoechoic mass with irregular margins and architectural distortion (**c**), biopsy-proven invasive ductal adenocarcinoma

Contrast-Enhanced Digital Mammography (CEDM) and Tomosynthesis (CET)

Contrast-enhanced digital mammography (CEDM) and contrast-enhanced tomosynthesis (CET) aim to improve the sensitivity of both 2D and DBT. As in contrast-enhanced MRI, CEDM and CET aim to detect angiogenesis and neovascularity associated with cancers. The protocol typically involves a power injection of iodinated contrast with images acquired following a 90 second delay. Standard mediolateral oblique (MLO) and craniocaudal (CC) views of each breast are obtained. Images are acquired in a dual energy projection, at low energy similar to a conventional mammogram and at high energy to optimally detect iodine. Contrast-enhanced subtraction images are produced for radiologist interpretation.

CEDM has been shown to be more sensitive for cancer detection than conventional mammography with no loss in specificity. This benefit is best appreciated in women with dense breasts [23, 24]. Data from a small study in the screening population has shown similar results [25]. The sensitivity of CEDM has been shown to be similar to MRI [26, 27]. In a small study of 49 participants, patient experience with CEDM was also preferable to MRI, with quicker scan times and less claustrophobia [28].

While promising, this modality is limited given that it is not currently widely available. CEDM, like contrast-enhanced CT, is limited by the risk of contrast reactions, and caution/premedication is advised in patients with known contrast allergy. Less than 1% of patients experience allergic or physiologic reactions and a much smaller percentage, 0.04%, can experience a severe reaction [29]. In addition to screening for allergies, patients should also be screened for renal dysfunction prior to CEDM.

Magnetic Resonance Imaging

Magnetic resonance imaging (MRI) is effective in breast cancer screening with additional cancer detection over mammography alone (Fig. 9.3). Recent literature lends support to the use of supplemental MRI screening in those with history of LCIS [30] as well as dense breasts with a history of atypia [31]; however, additional studies are needed. Screening with MRI is an adjunct tool and does not replace annual screening mammography. High-risk women should receive both annual mammograms and annual MRI. Often, these exams are staggered at 6 month intervals.

MRI is acquired with the patient in prone position utilizing a breast-specific coil. Multiphase, multisequence images of the breast are acquired, including pre- and post-contrast T1-weighted and T2-weighted images with or without diffusion-weighted imaging. The initial MR images are acquired after contrast injection, and serial post-contrast images are subsequently acquired in order to analyze enhancement kinetics. Examinations involve the intravenous injection of gadolinium-based contrast.

MRI is highly sensitive for the detection of breast cancer as it provides information about morphology as well as physiology of breast abnormalities without mammographic limitation of breast density. With the addition of MRI to mammography, incremental cancer detection rate has been reported at 14.7 per 1000 [32].

Although MRI is highly sensitive compared to mammography, it demonstrates a lower specificity [33, 34]. False-positive biopsies as well as short-term follow-up examinations add to financial considerations as well as patient anxiety. With

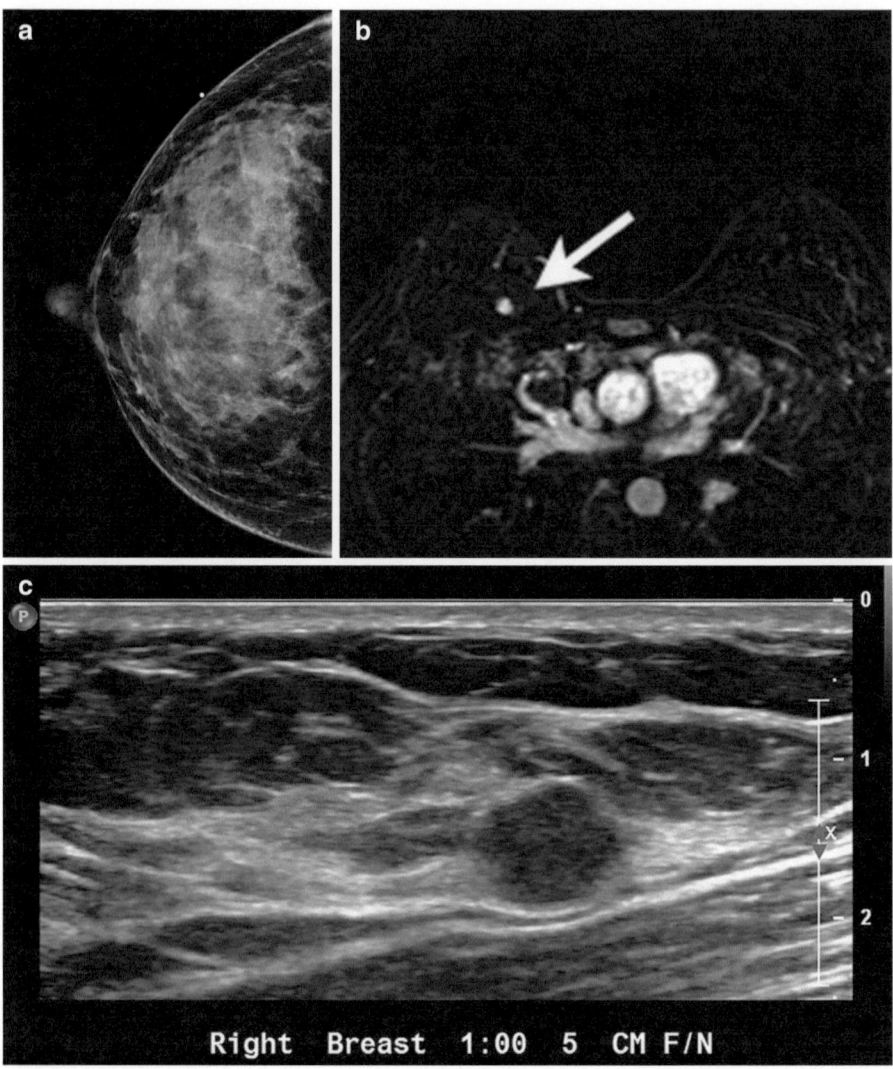

Fig. 9.3 A 38-year-old female with heterogeneously dense breasts and a history of BRCA1 mutation. Patient had a negative mammogram and diagnostic workup for palpable abnormality at the 10 o'clock position (**a**). Approximately 6 months later, the patient had a screening contrast-enhanced breast MRI, and an enhancing mass was seen at the 1 o'clock position of the right breast (arrow, **b**). Subsequent targeted ultrasound demonstrated a suspicious hypoechoic mass at 1 o'clock, biopsy-proven carcinoma (**c**)

improvements in MRI technique and interpreter experience, false-positive rates have improved over those quoted in the early literature. False-positive exams are more frequent with initial MRI exams [35] and tend to decrease once a baseline is established.

In addition to cost and false positives, there are other barriers to screening with MRI. Current breast MRI protocols rely on blood flow to identify and characterize lesions, requiring intravenous gadolinium-based contrast agents. Although these agents are generally considered safe, severe, acute, allergic-like reactions can occur. Fortunately, these are only one third as frequent as with iodine-based agents used in other radiology procedures [29]. Nephrogenic systemic fibrosis (NSF), a serious complication causing fibrosis of skin as well as internal organs, has decreased with the use of newer agents and avoidance of any gadolinium-based agents in patients with severe renal failure. More recent studies describe gadolinium deposition in brain tissue, of unknown clinical significance [36]. Additionally, severe claustrophobia, patient body habitus, and implanted devices may be relative or absolute contraindications to breast MRI in some patients.

Abbreviated Breast MRI (FAST)

A standard breast MRI examination occupies the scanner for up to 40 min and generates several hundred images. A 2014 study by Kuhl et al. describes an abbreviated screening protocol called "FAST," with an MRI acquisition time of 3 min and an expert radiologist reading time of under 1 min. In Kuhl's study of women at mild to moderate increased risk, an additional cancer detection rate of 18.2 per 1000 was achieved after negative mammograms [37]. The negative predictive value was 99.8%. Although these findings have yet to be validated by a multicenter controlled study, results are promising, and the procedure has been adopted by some radiology practices. The abbreviated scan times and shorter interpretation times would improve access to screening breast MRI and reduce costs. The reduced cost would be particularly desirable for women of intermediate risk, for whom insurance may not cover the supplemental screening study. Additional research focuses on developing breast MR imaging protocols that do not require intravenous contrast.

Breast Ultrasound

Ultrasound utilizes sound waves to create images of the breast tissue. Ultrasound is often used as a problem-solving tool in breast imaging. It can further characterize masses and other mammography findings, serve as an adjunct to mammography in the evaluation of palpable findings (Fig. 9.4), and guide biopsies and other interventional procedures. Ultrasound does not utilize radiation and is particularly useful in young and pregnant patients. Recent studies have also evaluated its utility as an adjunct screening modality.

Both handheld ultrasound and automated whole breast ultrasound (ABUS) have been evaluated in the screening population. Both modalities are time intensive, with the average time for hand held ultrasound ranging from 15 to 19 min [32] and automated breast ultrasound averaging 15 min with 9 min for interpretation [38]. Handheld ultrasound requires an adept ultrasound technologist or physician.

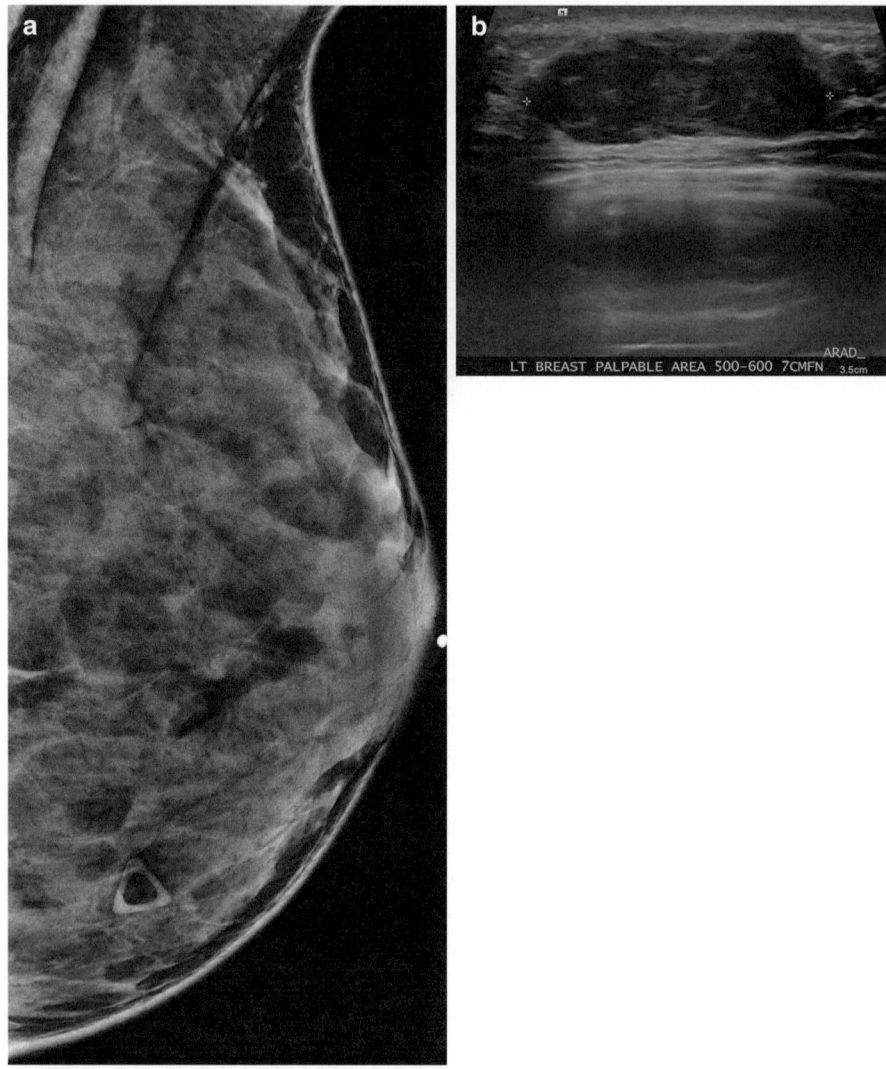

Fig. 9.4 Left MLO mammogram demonstrates extremely dense breast tissue. Triangular marker notes site of palpable concern, without obvious underlying mammogramphic abnormality (**a**). Left breast ultrasound shows a hypoechoic mass at 5–6 o'clock, biopsy-proven invasive ductal carcinoma, which was obscured by surrounding dense fibroglandular tissue on mammogram (**b**)

The ACRIN 6666 trial evaluated cancer detection rates with addition of ultrasound following a negative mammogram. This trial demonstrated additional cancer detection rate of 3.7 cancers per 1000 in women with elevated risk. Positive predictive values however were significantly lower for mammography plus ultrasound than mammography alone, and a larger number of biopsies were noted with incidence screening ultrasound, averaging 5.0% [32]. The positive predictive value

(PPV) of malignancy among women with positive ultrasound screening test who subsequently underwent biopsy was lower than mammography, ranging from 9% to 11.7%, whereas mammography alone was much higher (29–38.1%) [32].

In the high-risk population, screening with ultrasound should be considered if the patient cannot undergo MRI. If MRI and mammography are preformed, there is no additional benefit in cancer detection rate when ultrasound is added, and there is the drawback of added high false-positive rates [32].

Molecular Imaging

Molecular breast imaging (MBI) is a nuclear medicine imaging test that provides high resolution, functional images of the breast. The two commonly utilized radiotracers are 99mTc-sestamibi (gamma emitting) and 18-F-fluorodeoxyglucose (18F-FDG), which relies on positron emission. Radiation doses have generally been considered prohibitive for adopting these as large-scale serial screening examinations. Molecular studies result in radiation to multiple organs throughout the body, in addition to the breast. These studies are also limited by longer imaging times.

Breast-Specific Gamma Imaging (BSGI)

Breast-specific gamma imaging (BSGI) has shown promise as a physiologic molecular imaging modality and adjunct for screening; however, no large population studies of MBI for screening have been performed. The radiotracer 99mTc-sestamibi is injected intravenously, and the breast is imaged for approximately 40 min under mild compression, generating MLO and CC views. A gamma camera is used to detect gamma rays preferentially within carcinoma, and a high-resolution functional image is produced. Studies evaluating BSGI in asymptomatic women at increased risk of breast cancer with a recent negative mammogram, demonstrated a cancer detection rate of 7.5–8.8/1000 [39, 40] and more recently 16.5/1000 [41]. Comparatively, MRI performance in high-risk patients ranges from 9.5 to 14.7/1000 [32, 34]. False-positive rates are lower than that of screening breast ultrasound. Incremental cancer detection rate with BSGI was most pronounced in women with dense tissue. The main disadvantage of this modality as a serial screening method is the associated radiation dose to both the breast and whole body. Dose reduction has been implemented and produces similar diagnostic results; however, continued research is needed.

Positron Emission Mammography (PEM)

Positron emission tomography or mammography (PET or PEM) acquires images created from positron-emitting 18-F-fluorodeoxyglucose (18F-FDG). Following a 4–6 h fast, the patient is injected intravenously and imaged after a 1 h uptake interval. While with PET, the patient's whole body is imaged, using PEM, CC and MLO views (similar to mammography) are acquired with the breast stabilized between two detectors. PEM has been shown to have greater sensitivity than whole-body PET for breast cancer detection [42]. Large-scale screening studies have yet to be performed.

Other Imaging Modalities

There is currently insufficient evidence to support the use of other modalities such as thermography or optical imaging for breast cancer screening in women of any risk category.

Summary

Women with a history of atypia are at an elevated risk for breast cancer and, at the very least, should undergo annual screening mammography. A complete risk assessment should also be performed to quantify a woman's lifetime risk. In patients with a lifetime risk of 20% or greater, supplemental screening with MRI is recommended. Currently, for the subset of women with an increased lifetime risk relative to the general population who do not meet the 20% lifetime risk threshold, there is no universally accepted supplemental screening recommendation. Ideally, each woman at intermediate or high risk would benefit from personalized education and counseling to access the risks, benefits, and additional financial costs of adjunct screening. Due to its superior sensitivity, MRI is the preferred modality for supplemental screening. Ultrasound may be considered for those unable to undergo MRI. Current research is aimed at abbreviated MRI protocols and contrast-enhanced mammography as well as developing additional modalities including molecular breast imaging.

References

1. Oeffinger KC, Fontham ET, Etzioni R, Herzig A, Michaelson JS, Shih YC, et al. Breast cancer screening for women at average risk: 2015 guideline update from the American Cancer Society. JAMA. 2015;314(15):1599–614.
2. Bevers TB, Harris RE, Parker CC, Helvie M, Heerdt AS, Pearlman M, et al. Breast cancer screening and diagnosis. NCCN Clinical Practice Guidelines in Oncology (NCCN Guidelines) [Internet]. June 2, 2017; Version I.2017. Available from: NCCN.org
3. ACR and SBI continue to recommend regular mammography starting at age 40 [press release]. https://www.sbi-online.org/Portals/0/ACR-SBI%20press%20release%20ACS%20FINAL%20for%20web.pdf. October 20, 2015.
4. Mainiero MB, Moy L, Baron P, Didwania AD, diFlorio-Alexander RM, Green ED, et al. ACR appropriateness criteria® breast cancer screening. Available from: https://acsearch.acr.org/docs/70910/Narrative/. American College of Radiology. Accessed 31 Oct 2017.
5. Practice Bulletin Number 179. Breast cancer risk assessment and screening in average-risk women. Obstet Gynecol. 2017;130(1):e1–e16.

6. Saslow D, Boetes C, Burke W, Harms S, Leach MO, Lehman CD, et al. American Cancer Society guidelines for breast screening with MRI as an adjunct to mammography. CA Cancer J Clin. 2007;57(2):75–89.
7. Page DL, Dupont WD, Rogers LW, Rados MS. Atypical hyperplastic lesions of the female breast. A long-term follow-up study. Cancer. 1985;55(11):2698–708.
8. Degnim AC, Visscher DW, Berman HK, Frost MH, Sellers TA, Vierkant RA, et al. Stratification of breast cancer risk in women with atypia: a Mayo cohort study. J Clin Oncol Off J Am Soc Clin Oncol. 2007;25(19):2671–7.
9. Hartmann LC, Sellers TA, Frost MH, Lingle WL, Degnim AC, Ghosh K, et al. Benign breast disease and the risk of breast cancer. N Engl J Med. 2005;353(3):229–37.
10. Hartmann LC, Degnim AC, Santen RJ, Dupont WD, Ghosh K. Atypical hyperplasia of the breast – risk assessment and management options. N Engl J Med. 2015;372(1):78–89.
11. Degnim AC, Dupont WD, Radisky DC, Vierkant RA, Frank RD, Frost MH, et al. Extent of atypical hyperplasia stratifies breast cancer risk in 2 independent cohorts of women. Cancer. 2016;122(19):2971–8.
12. Amir E, Freedman OC, Seruga B, Evans DG. Assessing women at high risk of breast cancer: a review of risk assessment models. J Natl Cancer Inst. 2010;102(10):680–91.
13. Amir E, Evans DG, Shenton A, Lalloo F, Moran A, Boggis C, et al. Evaluation of breast cancer risk assessment packages in the family history evaluation and screening programme. J Med Genet. 2003;40(11):807–14.
14. Tyrer J, Duffy SW, Cuzick J. A breast cancer prediction model incorporating familial and personal risk factors. Stat Med. 2004;23(7):1111–30.
15. Siegel RL, Miller KD, Jemal A. Cancer statistics, 2017. CA Cancer J Clin. 2017;67(1):7–30.
16. Carney PA, Miglioretti DL, Yankaskas BC, Kerlikowske K, Rosenberg R, Rutter CM, et al. Individual and combined effects of age, breast density, and hormone replacement therapy use on the accuracy of screening mammography. Ann Intern Med. 2003;138(3):168–75.
17. Mandelson MT, Oestreicher N, Porter PL, White D, Finder CA, Taplin SH, et al. Breast density as a predictor of mammographic detection: comparison of interval- and screen-detected cancers. J Natl Cancer Inst. 2000;92(13):1081–7.
18. Skaane P. Breast cancer screening with digital breast tomosynthesis. Breast Cancer (Tokyo, Japan). 2017;24(1):32–41.
19. Ciatto S, Houssami N, Bernardi D, Caumo F, Pellegrini M, Brunelli S, et al. Integration of 3D digital mammography with tomosynthesis for population breast-cancer screening (STORM): a prospective comparison study. Lancet Oncol. 2013;14(7):583–9.
20. Skaane P, Bandos AI, Gullien R, Eben EB, Ekseth U, Haakenaasen U, et al. Comparison of digital mammography alone and digital mammography plus tomosynthesis in a population-based screening program. Radiology. 2013;267(1):47–56.
21. Lång K, Andersson I, Rosso A, Tingberg A, Timberg P, Zackrisson S. Performance of one-view breast tomosynthesis as a stand-alone breast cancer screening modality: results from the Malmö Breast Tomosynthesis Screening Trial, a population-based study. Eur Radiol. 2016;26(1):184–90.
22. Friedewald SM, Rafferty EA, Rose SL, Durand MA, Plecha DM, Greenberg JS, et al. Breast cancer screening using tomosynthesis in combination with digital mammography. JAMA. 2014;311(24):2499–507.
23. Cheung YC, Lin YC, Wan YL, Yeow KM, Huang PC, Lo YF, et al. Diagnostic performance of dual-energy contrast-enhanced subtracted mammography in dense breasts compared to mammography alone: interobserver blind-reading analysis. Eur Radiol. 2014;24(10):2394–403.
24. Dromain C, Thibault F, Muller S, Rimareix F, Delaloge S, Tardivon A, et al. Dual-energy contrast-enhanced digital mammography: initial clinical results. Eur Radiol. 2011;21(3):565–74.
25. Lobbes MB, Lalji U, Houwers J, Nijssen EC, Nelemans PJ, van Roozendaal L, et al. Contrast-enhanced spectral mammography in patients referred from the breast cancer screening programme. Eur Radiol. 2014;24(7):1668–76.
26. Fallenberg EM, Dromain C, Diekmann F, Engelken F, Krohn M, Singh JM, et al. Contrast-enhanced spectral mammography versus MRI: initial results in the detection of breast cancer and assessment of tumour size. Eur Radiol. 2014;24(1):256–64.

27. Chou CP, Lewin JM, Chiang CL, Hung BH, Yang TL, Huang JS, et al. Clinical evaluation of contrast-enhanced digital mammography and contrast enhanced tomosynthesis – comparison to contrast-enhanced breast MRI. Eur J Radiol. 2015;84(12):25018.
28. Hobbs MM, Taylor DB, Buzynski S, Peake RE. Contrast-enhanced spectral mammography (CESM) and contrast enhanced MRI (CEMRI): patient preferences and tolerance. J Med Imaging Radiat Oncol. 2015;59(3):300–5.
29. ACR manual on contrast media version 10.3. ACR committee on drugs and contrast media. Available from: https://www.acr.org/~/media/37D84428BF1D4E1B9A3A2918DA9E27A3.pdf. American College of Radiology. Accessed on 31 Oct 2017.
30. Port ER, Park A, Borgen PI, Morris E, Montgomery LL. Results of MRI screening for breast cancer in high-risk patients with LCIS and atypical hyperplasia. Ann Surg Oncol. 2007;14(3):1051–7.
31. Nadler M, Al-Attar H, Warner E, Martel AL, Balasingham S, Zhang L, et al. MRI surveillance for women with dense breasts and a previous breast cancer and/or high risk lesion. Breast (Edinburgh, Scotland). 2017;34:77–82.
32. Berg WA, Zhang Z, Lehrer D, Jong RA, Pisano ED, Barr RG, et al. Detection of breast cancer with addition of annual screening ultrasound or a single screening MRI to mammography in women with elevated breast cancer risk. JAMA. 2012;307(13):1394–404.
33. Lord SJ, Lei W, Craft P, Cawson JN, Morris I, Walleser S, et al. A systematic review of the effectiveness of magnetic resonance imaging (MRI) as an addition to mammography and ultrasound in screening young women at high risk of breast cancer. Eur J Cancer (Oxford, England: 1990). 2007;43(13):1905–17.
34. Kriege M, Brekelmans CT, Boetes C, Besnard PE, Zonderland HM, Obdeijn IM, et al. Efficacy of MRI and mammography for breast-cancer screening in women with a familial or genetic predisposition. N Engl J Med. 2004;351(5):427–37.
35. Abramovici G, Mainiero MB. Screening breast MR imaging: comparison of interpretation of baseline and annual follow-up studies. Radiology. 2011;259(1):85–91.
36. Gulani V, Calamante F, Shellock FG, Kanal E, Reeder SB. Gadolinium deposition in the brain: summary of evidence and recommendations. Lancet Neurol. 2017;16(7):564–70.
37. Kuhl CK, Schrading S, Strobel K, Schild HH, Hilgers R-D, Bieling HB. Abbreviated breast magnetic resonance imaging (MRI): first postcontrast subtracted images and maximum-intensity projection—a novel approach to breast cancer screening with MRI. J Clin Oncol. 2014;32(22):2304–10.
38. Skaane P, Gullien R, Eben EB, Sandhaug M, Schulz-Wendtland R, Stoeblen F. Interpretation of automated breast ultrasound (ABUS) with and without knowledge of mammography: a reader performance study. Acta Radiol (Stockholm, Sweden: 1987). 2015;56(4):404–12.
39. Rhodes DJ, Hruska CB, Phillips SW, Whaley DH, O'Connor MK. Dedicated dual-head gamma imaging for breast cancer screening in women with mammographically dense breasts. Radiology. 2011;258(1):106–18.
40. Rhodes DJ, Hruska CB, Conners AL, Tortorelli CL, Maxwell RW, Jones KN, et al. Journal club: molecular breast imaging at reduced radiation dose for supplemental screening in mammographically dense breasts. Am J Roentgenol. 2015;204(2):241–51.
41. Brem RF, Ruda RC, Yang JL, Coffey CM, Rapelyea JA. Breast-specific gamma-imaging for the detection of mammographically occult breast cancer in women at increased risk. J Nucl Med Off Publ Soc Nucl Med. 2016;57(5):678–84.
42. Kalinyak JE, Berg WA, Schilling K, Madsen KS, Narayanan D, Tartar M. Breast cancer detection using high-resolution breast PET compared to whole-body PET or PET/CT. Eur J Nucl Med Mol Imaging. 2014;41(2):260–75.

The Role of Chemoprevention in the Prevention of Breast Cancer

10

Jinny Gunn, E. Alexa Elder, and Sarah McLaughlin

Introduction

It is estimated that nearly 15% of women in the United States (USA) between 35 and 70 years of age are at high risk for breast cancer and are therefore eligible candidates for breast cancer prevention medications [1]. The US Food and Drug Administration (FDA) have approved Tamoxifen and Raloxifene for breast cancer prevention for women with a Gail model 5-year breast cancer risk estimate of 1.67% or higher [1]. The US Preventive Services Task Force (USPSTF) found prevention medications to have more net benefit than harm caused in women with a 3% or greater 5-year breast cancer risk [2]. Also, women with atypical ductal or lobular hyperplasia (AH) and lobular carcinoma in situ (LCIS) have been shown to have greater benefit from prevention medications than women with elevated risk based on family history alone [3–6].

Atypia

Over the past three decades, the role of screening mammography has gained increasing importance as data demonstrates early detection of breast cancer is critical to decreasing mortality [7]. Approximately 10% of women undergoing screening mammography are recalled for additional imaging, and 8–10% of these women will require a core needle biopsy (CNB) [8, 9]. Among those undergoing CNB, atypical

---

J. Gunn · E. Alexa Elder
Department of Surgery, Mayo Clinic, Jacksonville, FL, USA
e-mail: Gunn.Jinny@mayo.edu; Elder.Erin1@mayo.edu

S. McLaughlin (✉)
Department of Surgery, Mayo Clinic, Jacksonville, FL, USA

Section of Surgical Oncology, Jacksonville, FL, USA
e-mail: Mclaughlin.Sarah@mayo.edu

ductal hyperplasia (ADH) or atypical lobular hyperplasia (ALH) will account for approximately 10% of biopsy results.

For years, researchers have studies atypical lesions focusing on their influence on risk for future invasive disease. While most women diagnosed with ADH or ALH do not develop breast carcinoma, both ADH and ALH are associated with a substantially increased absolute risk of breast cancer approaching 30% at 25 years with an overall relative risk of approximately four- to fivefold [10–19]. However, not all atypical lesions are equal. Sub-studies of ADH identify features such as multiple foci of atypia and presence of calcifications that are associated with "very high risk" status conferring a >50% risk at 20 years [11]. These risk estimates remain controversial and are under study at multiple institutions. Identification of other features of atypical lesions that may confer risk remains the focus of ongoing research and future stratification will likely include molecular and biological characterization.

Chemoprevention History

Discoveries within the last century have pivoted clinicians to specifically focus on personalized medicine in all treatment realms including prevention strategies. As early as the 1920s, physicians understood "estrogen" to be produced by the ovaries and linked estrogen to breast cancer in mice in 1933. Subsequently, scientists first proposed the idea of an estrogen receptor (ER) in 1962. Soon researchers discovered this short-lived protein resided in the nuclei of cells, and the estrogen receptor quickly became the target of interest in the search for a breast cancer cure [20]. As the benefits of estrogen blockade for the treatment of breast cancer were recognized, discussion regarding the use of estrogen blockade for prevention soon followed. In fact, multiple compounds have been investigated as breast cancer chemoprevention agents and extend beyond blockade of the ER and include nonsteroidal anti-inflammatory drugs, bisphosphonates, aromatase inhibitors, selective estrogen receptor modulators, statins, insulin-stimulating agents, vitamins, and synthetic hormones [21]. While historically these medications have been commonly called breast cancer chemoprevention drugs, contemporary clinicians are moving away from the term "chemoprevention" referring to them only as prevention medications. The word "chemoprevention" is felt by many to be associated with a negative connotation or cancer treatment and may be dissuading patients from taking these drugs for prevention purposes.

Selective Estrogen Receptor Modulators

Historically, the premise of using selective estrogen receptor modulators (SERM) for breast cancer prevention rests on the hypothesis that if estrogen leads to breast cancer then antiestrogen drugs will be effective in treating and potentially preventing breast cancer. In study of the estrogen receptor, scientists also realized the ER was present in normal uterine and bone tissue. Researchers feared blocking this receptor had the potential to also result in osteoporosis and/or uterine cancer. Animal studies conducted in the 1980s paradoxically demonstrated that these ER modulating drugs had an antiestrogen effect in some tissues (breast) while simultaneously having a pro-estrogenic effect in others (uterus and bone) [22]. This remained perplexing until researchers discovered that the ER consists of two subunits: ERα and ERβ. ERα is a ubiquitinated protein and is not as simple as an "on/off" switch but rather undergoes conformational changes depending on the ligand binding to it [23]. This results in SERMs being useful as antiestrogen medications in the breast (cancer prevention) while also offering bone protection against osteoporosis and fractures. The side effect of uterine cancer remains associated with some of the SERMs, but not all.

Tamoxifen

Interestingly, Tamoxifen (a triphenylethylene), the first antiestrogen medication proposed for use in prevention of breast cancer, was originally developed as a contraceptive [24]. Tamoxifen is a long-acting nonsteroidal antiestrogen ER modulator with an active metabolite. Professor Trevor Powles unearthed the failed contraceptive drug Tamoxifen to utilize its potential as an anticancer drug in his 1985 pilot toxicology study. This double-blinded clinical trial of Tamoxifen versus placebo was conducted at the Royal Marsden Hospital utilizing a population of 200 women deemed to be at high risk for breast cancer, as indicated by having one or two first-degree relatives with breast cancer. The results of this study demonstrated that Tamoxifen had estrogenic antagonistic properties in certain tissues while showing evidence of estrogenic agonistic effects in others. Additionally, they proved Tamoxifen had an acceptable side effect profile. Not surprisingly, women in the Tamoxifen group had a statistically significant increase in the incidence of hot flashes, though these were generally rated as mild. The trial researchers noted no statistically significant difference in compliance or cessation between the two groups. As a result, Tamoxifen was deemed "an ideal agent" for use as a prevention agent for breast cancer [25]. The results of this study prompted further investigation and in 1986 the Royal Marsden Clinic started enrolling healthy women for a much larger placebo-controlled, double-blinded, randomized clinical trial. Ultimately, the final results of this study with a median follow-up of 13 years were published in 2007 and showed a statistically significant posttreatment reduction in ER-positive breast cancer among women assigned to the Tamoxifen group when compared to placebo (HR = 0.48, 95% CI = 0.29–0.79; $p = 0.004$) [26].

In 1998, the National Surgical Adjuvant Breast and Bowel Project (NSABP) published their results of their NSABP P-1 randomized controlled study that compared Tamoxifen and placebo for the prevention of breast cancer. Tamoxifen was found to reduce the risk of breast cancer by 49% in the total study population [3]. Patients with a history of atypical lesions were found to have a greater benefit from Tamoxifen as the incidence of breast cancer in 1000 women with atypical hyperplasia was 10.1 in the placebo group compared to 1.4 in the Tamoxifen group

Table 10.1 Relative risk of Tamoxifen side effects according to age

Relative risks of serious side effects with Tamoxifen by age			
Side effect/risk	Age >50	Age <50	All women
Uterine cancer	4.01	1.21	2.53
Stroke	1.75	0.76	1.59
Pulmonary embolism	3.19	2.03	3.01
DVT	1.71	1.39	1.60

(relative risk 0.14, 95% CI 0.03–0.47). Tamoxifen decreased invasive breast cancer risk by 56% in women with a history of LCIS and 86% with a history of atypical hyperplasia [3]. The risk of noninvasive breast cancer was reduced by 50% [3]. A 2005 update of the trial after its unblinding demonstrated similar treatment effects with Tamoxifen reducing the rate of both invasive and noninvasive breast cancers [27].

The International Breast Intervention Study I (IBIS-I) trial of Tamoxifen and placebo was completed in over 7000 patients. Recently reported results following an extended follow-up (median 16 years) period found extended protection after cessation of Tamoxifen [28]. The risk of developing breast cancer in the first 10 years was 6.3% in the placebo group and 4.6% in the Tamoxifen group, while the risk after 10 years was 3.8% in the placebo group and 2.6% in the Tamoxifen group [28]. Only 8% of the participants in the study were enrolled based on the presence of a high-risk lesion at biopsy [28]. They determined the number needed to treat to prevent one breast cancer in the next 20 years was 22 patients [28]. They also noted less benefit from Tamoxifen in women who had taken postmenopausal hormone replacement therapy [28].

One of the concerns regarding Tamoxifen is the risk of endometrial cancer in women retaining their uterus. Most studies show a two to threefold increased relative risk when compared to the age-matched population. This has been attributed to the estrogenic agonistic effect of Tamoxifen on endometrial tissues. In the updated analysis of the NSABP trials, endometrial cancer occurrence was significantly increased in woman aged 50 years and older (RR = 5.33, 95% CI = 2.47–13.17). The same was not true for women aged 49 years and under (RR = 1.42, 95% CI = 0.55–3.81) [3, 27]. In addition to endometrial cancers, Tamoxifen users were found to have an increased incidence of deep vein thrombosis (DVT), pulmonary embolism, and cataracts (Table 10.1) [3, 27]. The standard dosing for Tamoxifen as a prevention medication is 20 mg daily for 5 years [2, 29].

Raloxifene

The increased risk of endometrial cancer and other adverse events associated with Tamoxifen encouraged researchers to identify a SERM that would offer the same or better breast cancer prevention while having a more acceptable side effect profile. Raloxifene hydrochloride (keoxifene) is a very short-acting, second-generation benzothiophene derivative. Similar to Tamoxifen, Raloxifene exhibits antiestrogen effects on breast tissue. Unlike Tamoxifen though, it also exhibits antiestrogen effects on endometrial tissue [20].

The Multiple Outcomes of Raloxifene Evaluation (MORE) trial was an international, multicenter, randomized, double-blinded trial comparing Raloxifene to placebo. The results of this study showed that Raloxifene reduced the risk of ER+ breast cancers in postmenopausal women by 90%. While there was no statistical difference in incidence of endometrial cancers ($p = 0.67$), women in the treatment arm did have a statistically significant increase in hot flashes and thromboembolic disease ($p = <0.001$ and 0.002, respectively). Similar to Tamoxifen, Raloxifene use was associated with an increase in subjective hot flashes ($p < 0.001$) [30]. A follow-up study with 4-year results published in 2001 again concluded that Raloxifene significantly reduced the risk of ER+ breast cancer by 84% [31]. As more of the molecular basis for these pharmaceuticals was discovered, it was shown that the difference lies in conformational changes at the ER level based on the binding ligand. Tamoxifen acts as an estrogen agonist in endometrial cells, resulting in recruitment of coactivators. Raloxifene, on the other hand, binds without recruitment of these coactivators, resulting in a neutral effect [32].

The National Surgical Adjuvant Breast and Bowel Project P-2 study of Tamoxifen and Raloxifene (STAR) directly compared Tamoxifen and Raloxifene in postmenopausal women [6, 33]. The STAR trial initially found that Raloxifene was as effective as Tamoxifen in reducing invasive breast cancer risk while having a lower risk of endometrial cancer, thromboembolic events, and cataracts [33]. Fewer cases of noninvasive breast cancer were found in the Tamoxifen group [33]. A long-term analysis of the STAR data extended the initial 47 month median follow-up to a median of 81 months. This updated report found a greater difference between the two agents with Raloxifene only 76–78% as effective as Tamoxifen in reducing breast cancer risk for those patients with the diagnosis of an atypical lesion [6].

In 1998 the FDA approved Raloxifene for the treatment and prevention of osteoporosis. This was followed in 2007 by extended approval for use as a breast cancer reduction medication.

Currently, Raloxifene is only approved for use in postmenopausal women. The side effect profile of Tamoxifen makes Raloxifene an attractive alternative even though it has been shown to be less effective (Table 10.2). The typical dosage of Raloxifene is 60 mg daily for 5 years [2, 29].

Contraindications for use of Tamoxifen or Raloxifene include a history of deep venous thromboembolism, pulmonary embolism, thrombotic stroke, transient ischemic attack (TIA), known inherited hypercoagulable disorder, and pregnancy.

Other SERMS

Other notable SERMs that have been shown to be efficacious in the prevention of breast cancer include Lasofoxifene and Arzoxifene. These pharmaceuticals were developed with the pharmacokinetics in mind as a method to enhance drug delivery to target tissues. Lasofoxifene is a third-generation SERM that is a naphthalene

Table 10.2 Comparison of adverse side effects between selective estrogen receptor modulators (SERM) and aromatase inhibitors (AI)

Comparing SERM and AI risk			
Adverse effects	Tamoxifen	Raloxifene	Exemestane
Uterine cancer	↑[a]	No	No
DVT/PE	↑↑[a]	↑	No
Bone loss/fracture	↓	↓	↑
Stroke	↑	↑	No
Cataracts	↑↑	↑	No
Hot flashes	↑↑	↑	↑
Arthralgia	No	No	↑
Vaginal atrophy	↑	↑	↑↑
Vaginal bleeding	↑	No	No

SERM selective estrogen receptor modulator, *AI* aromatase inhibitor
[a]Excess risk predominantly in postmenopausal women

derivative with a nonpolar tetrahydronaphthalene structure [34]. This structure results in extensive metabolism and improved bioavailability. In fact, the clinical dose of this novel SERM is a mere 1/100th that of Raloxifene. Additionally, the ERα binding affinity for Lasofoxifene is ten times greater than that of Raloxifene or Tamoxifen. The Postmenopausal Evaluation and Risk-Reduction with Lasofoxifene (PEARL) trial was a randomized, double-blinded, placebo-controlled trial of two different Lasofoxifene doses to evaluate the safety and efficacy of this novel SERM in a population of postmenopausal women with osteoporosis. Though underpowered, the results of this study showed a statistically significant reduction in all breast cancer (76%) and an even greater reduction (83%) of ER+ breast cancer among those patients receiving the higher, 0.5 mg, dose of Lasofoxifene when compared to placebo or the lower, 0.25 mg, dose of Lasofoxifene. Furthermore, the higher 0.5 mg dose group also had statistically significantly lower incidences of vertebral and non-vertebral fractures (42% and 24%, respectively). The toxic events experienced were similar to those seen in Tamoxifen and Raloxifene, namely, thromboembolism and vasomotor symptoms (hot flashes). There was no increase in endometrial cancer among either Lasofoxifene groups although there was an increase in benign endometrial thickening. Quite interestingly though this group also had statistically significant reductions in major coronary events and stroke (32% and 36%, respectively). Elevated baseline estradiol levels were associated with increased effect [35].

Another novel SERM is Arzoxifene. This drug was created by chemists seeking to increase the efficacy of Raloxifene without diminishing the desired tissue-specific modulation of previous SERMs. Arzoxifene is a benzothiophene derivative, like Raloxifene, which is rapidly metabolized and has an active metabolite, desmethyl-arzoxifene. Arzoxifene was shown to be exceedingly more active than Raloxifene for breast cancer prevention in animal models and also lowered serum cholesterol, maintained bone density, and was less susceptible to drug resistance [36]. These favorable findings sparked an international, randomized, blinded, placebo-controlled trial, the Generations Trial, to evaluate the clinical effects of Arzoxifene in a population of women with osteoporosis or low bone mass. Arzoxifene was associated with a 2.3% absolute reduction in the 3-year cumulative incidence of vertebral fractures and a 56% relative reduction in breast cancer. Like Tamoxifen and Raloxifene, there was a two- to threefold relative increase in thromboembolic events. The incidence of vertebral fractures was significantly reduced in the Arzoxifene group (2.6%) when compared to the placebo group (4.3%) (RR 0.61, 95% CI = 0.48–0.77, $p < 0.001$). Those in the Arzoxifene arm unfortunately had higher incidences of acute cholecystitis, osteonecrosis, lung metastases, chronic obstructive pulmonary disease (COPD), musculoskeletal complaints, and pneumonia (all $p < 0.03$) [37]. As a result, Arzoxifene development has since been discontinued.

Aromatase Inhibitors

Aromatase inhibitors (AI) have been considered an alternative agent for breast cancer prevention. These agents block estrogen synthesis as opposed to acting as tissue-specific estrogenic agonists or antagonists. They do this by inhibition of the aromatase enzyme which converts androgens to estrogens. They are not associated with an increased risk of endometrial cancer or thromboembolic events, as they do not have estrogenic agonistic properties. These agents are not indicated for use in premenopausal women and are contraindicated for use during pregnancy. The third-generation aromatase inhibitors approved for use and widely available include anastrozole, letrozole, and exemestane.

Exemestane

Exemestane is an oral steroidal aromatase inhibitor with mild androgenic activity. The NCIC Clinical Trials Group mammary Prevention.3 trial (NCIC CTG MAP.3) was an international, placebo-controlled, randomized, double-blinded trial to evaluate the use of exemestane as a breast cancer prevention drug in postmenopausal women. Exemestane was shown to decrease the incidence of invasive breast cancer by 65% and had a similar toxicity profile to that of Tamoxifen. Events such as hypertension, hot flashes, diarrhea, and musculoskeletal symptoms were significantly increased in the exemestane arm. Reportedly, there was no increase in "serious adverse events or end-organ toxic effects" attributable to exemestane although follow-up was fairly short [38, 39]. The standard dosage of exemestane is 25 mg daily for 5 years [2, 29].

Anastrozole

Anastrozole reversibly binds to the aromatase enzyme to block the conversion of peripheral androgens to estrogen by competitive inhibition. Anastrozole as a prevention agent was studied in the International Breast Cancer Intervention Study II (IBIS-II) trial which was an international, randomized, placebo-controlled, double-blinded study for prevention of breast cancer in postmenopausal women. The risk of developing cancer was reduced by 47% in the anastrozole group [40]. Women with atypical lesions (LCIS, atypical hyperplasia) made up 9% of the IBIS-II study population. A larger but not significant risk reduction was seen in patients with LCIS and atypical hyperplasia [40]. The toxicity profile of anastrozole is similar to that of exemestane: mainly musculoskeletal and vasomotor symptoms. The follow-up of the IBIS-II trial was 7 years compared to 5 years in the MAP.3, but both trials suggest aromatase inhibitors as superior prevention medications with a more favorable toxicity profile than either Tamoxifen or Raloxifene [38, 40].

Other Agents for Prevention

Given the undesirable toxic effects of the SERMs and AIs, the search for more natural better tolerated prevention agents remains the study of ongoing clinical trials. As previously mentioned, several of these novel agents are based on theoretical benefits of orphaned pharmaceuticals, holistic treatments, or medications currently in use for other conditions.

Based on the association identified previously between obesity, insulin resistance and breast cancer, novel uses for diabetic medications have been proposed. Recently, insulin has been implicated as a potential mediator and link between obesity and breast cancer through the signaling P13K and Ras-Raf signaling pathways. Metformin which is commonly used for diabetes treatment decreases hepatic glucose production and intestinal absorption of glucose while improving insulin sensitivity by increasing peripheral glucose uptake and utilization. Scientists hypothesize that metformin activates the AMP kinase pathway resulting in growth inhibition of epithelial cells and decreased mammalian target of rapamycin (mTOR) which in turn results in an overall decrease in mRNA translation inhibiting growth, proliferation, and differentiation of breast cancer cells [41–43].

Inhibiting the insulin-like growth factor 1 (IGF-1), also called somatomedin C, is another novel prevention hypothesis. IGF-1 is a protein in humans similar to insulin with potent mitogenic properties. IGF-1 is associated with proliferative and anti-apoptotic events after binding to the IGF-1R. It is also intimately linked with ERα which makes it an attractive target for prevention [44]. Pasireotide is a somatostatin receptor ligand that targets the mammary gland selectively. This results in inhibition IGF-1R activation, thus blocking the proliferative effects of IGF-1. It was additionally found to increase apoptosis in women with atypical hyperplasia [45, 46]. Further studies are currently underway.

Nonsteroidal anti-inflammatories (NSAIDS) are potent cyclooxygenase inhibitors and have been proposed for use as prevention for breast cancer based on the anti-angiogenesis properties of cyclooxygenase 2 (COX-2) inhibition. Celecoxib and meloxicam are selective inhibitors of COX-2 [47–49]. These medications have been implicated in adverse cardiac events and warrant consideration of their toxic effects prior to implementation as prevention for patients.

In 1998 the FDA approved Tamoxifen for use as a breast cancer reduction medication. This was followed by the FDA approval of Raloxifene for use as a breast cancer reduction medication in 2007. A recent meta-analysis of all studied agents showed aromatase inhibitors (anastrozole, exemestane) over Arzoxifene, Lasofoxifene, Raloxifene, Tamoxifen, and Tibolone to be significantly associated with a therapeutic effect and cancer reduction; however, it also notes that Arzoxifene, Lasofoxifene and Raloxifene have the best risk/benefit ratio [21]. Currently, Tamoxifen and Raloxifene are the only medications available in the United States with FDA approval for use in breast cancer prevention [2, 5, 29].

Health Benefits

In addition to breast cancer prevention benefits, these agents have been found to have other health benefits. Some studies have shown Tamoxifen to have significantly fewer gastrointestinal cancers [28]. In the NSABP P-1 study a reduction in hip, radius, and spine fractures was identified with Tamoxifen compared to placebo [3]. Raloxifene significantly reduces vertebral fractures and is even an approved treatment for osteoporosis [30, 31].

Risks of Prevention Medications

The landmark NSABP P-1 study identified elevated risks of endometrial cancer, stroke, pulmonary embolism (PE), and deep vein thrombosis (DVT) with use of Tamoxifen with the risk elevation predominantly in women over the age of 50 [3]. More hot flashes and vaginal discharge were also noted in the Tamoxifen group [3]. When the NSABP P-1 study was updated 8 years later, a slightly lower risk of PE and higher risk of endometrial cancer were reported although these differences were not found to be significant [27]. The IBIS-1 study similarly found higher rates of DVT and non-melanoma skin cancers in the first 10 years and noted a trend toward higher rates of endometrial cancer in the first 5 years in the Tamoxifen group.

Both Tamoxifen and Raloxifene increase the risk of venous thromboembolism between 4 and 7 events per 1000 women over 5 years, with events on Tamoxifen at the higher end of the reported range [2]. The risk of venous thromboembolism is higher in older patients and those with a family history of venous thromboembolism [2, 6]. Tamoxifen increases the risk of endometrial cancer by 4 more cases per 1000 women [2]. Current recommendation stresses the importance of timely workup of vaginal bleeding due to this elevated risk [29]. Vasomotor symptoms such as hot flashes are common adverse effects of both medications and may commonly affect adherence [2]. Tamoxifen is associated with a risk of cataracts, while Raloxifene is not [6].

While AIs have lower rates of thrombosis and endometrial cancer, they have higher rates of vasomotor symptoms and arthralgia [40, 50]. The MAP.3 trial did not observe any significant increased risk of major adverse events in its 3-year follow-up period [50]. Both MAP.3 and IBIS-II had increased rates of arthralgia and vasomotor symptoms with AIs vs placebo [40, 50]. Significantly more hypertension but not cardiac events were reported in IBIS-II [40]. One major barrier to the use of AIs is their influence on osteoporosis which limits their use in a substantial subset of the postmenopausal female population as 39% of postmenopausal women otherwise eligible for breast cancer prevention have documented bone loss [50].

Patient Selection and Determining Risk

Many risk models are available to determine breast cancer risk. Unfortunately each has a unique set of variables that are used to calculate risk and each has advantages and limitations. Understanding these models aids in determining prevention eligibility. Traditionally, the NSABP P-1 trial assessed risk by the Breast Cancer Risk Assessment Tool (BCRAT or Gail model). Patients were considered high risk and therefore eligible for prevention medications if they had a 5-year risk >1.7% (http://www.cancer.gov.bcrisktool/.com). More recently, clinicians have evaluated the Tyrer-Cuzick (IBIS) model (http://ems-trials.org/riskevaluator) to assess risk; however, clinicians lack similar randomized prospective data regarding the use of the Tyrer-Cuzick model projections and therefore agreed upon thresholds for prevention eligibility. Patients with heterogeneous or extremely dense breast tissue are noted to have an increased RR of 2–4 for breast cancer. Only recently though has breast density data been incorporated into the current Tyrer-Cuzick version.

Coopey and colleagues have reported the 10-year cancer risk for women with ADH, ALH, and severe ADH to be 17.3%, 20.7%, and 26.0%, respectively [11–13]. Recent data from the Mayo Clinic suggest the cumulative lifetime risk of breast cancer in patients with a history of atypia is nearly 30% at 25 years and certainly influenced by the number of foci of atypia present. King et al. explored the relationship between LCIS and future breast cancer risk and determined LCIS conferred approximately a 2% annual incidence of breast cancer [4]. With these data it is clear that patients with atypia or LCIS meet the thresholds for prevention medication eligibility especially as these medications are well documented to reduce the 10-year breast cancer risk for all atypia (p, 0.05) [51].

Clinical Guidelines

The American Society of Clinical Oncology (ASCO) released clinical practice guidelines for breast cancer prevention in 2013. These guidelines recommend prevention medications for women with an estimated 5-year breast cancer risk >1.66% or women diagnosed with LCIS [29]. They recommend Tamoxifen for premenopausal women over 35 years with elevated breast cancer risk and Raloxifene or exemestane for postmenopausal women who met the risk criteria [29]. They did not recommend the use of other selective estrogen receptor modulators (Lasofoxifene and Arzoxifene) or other aromatase inhibitors (anastrozole) outside of clinical trials [29]. The USPSTF recommends prevention medications for women with a 5 year breast cancer risk >3% acknowledging these women are more likely to have a favorable risk benefit profile with prevention medications. The USPSTF recommends either Tamoxifen or Raloxifene but does not comment on exemestane due to its lack of FDA approval for this indication [2].

Uptake of Prevention Medications

Overall uptake of breast cancer prevention medications is low. Meta-analyses demonstrate only 15% of eligible patients are offered prevention medications, and of those offered prevention, only 16% based on pooled estimates from multiple studies actually choose to take it [52, 53]. Positive predictors of uptake include older age, higher objective risk, and a low-risk/high-benefit ratio [52, 53]. Friedman et al. developed benefit/risk tables for the use of prevention medications in women 50 years and older [54]. These tables stratify women by risk, age, presence of a uterus, and even ethnicity. Clinicians can then use the tables to determine if the risk/benefit ratio is favorable. The USPSTF used these tables to conclude that women with an estimated 5-year breast cancer risk of 3% or greater had a favorable benefit risk ratio for use of Tamoxifen or Raloxifene [2]. Negative predictors of prevention medication uptake include fear of side effects, lack of survival advantage, and perception of Tamoxifen as a cancer drug [52, 53]. Overall, uptake has been shown to be higher among patients participating in a clinical trial than in a non-trial setting (25% vs 9%, $p = 0.001$) [53], and uptake does not appear to differ based on study agent [53]. Physician recommendations have a variable effect on uptake of breast cancer chemoprevention [52, 53].

A longitudinal study of the LCIS population found only 17% of the patients took a prevention medication which comparable to the pooled analyses assessing uptake in the overall eligible population [4, 53]. Some studies have shown a higher uptake in high-risk women with atypia as opposed to those considered high risk based on strong family history alone [55]. In a multi-institutional clinical study of high-risk women, the uptake was as high as 66% in women with AH or LCIS [55]. Exemestane has been shown to have a low uptake when presented as an option for prevention [50]. Figure 10.1 shows a suggested flowchart for selection of an appropriate prevention agent.

The question of which clinicians should prescribe these medications remains unanswered. While internists or family physicians, surgeons, or oncologists would be appropriate to do so, a study of general practitioners in the UK found that most were unfamiliar with the concept of breast cancer prevention medications and were reluctant to initiate therapy [56]. Further, clinicians working in the clinical genetics setting reported lack of perceived benefit and difficulty interpreting guidelines as perceived barriers to implementation of chemoprevention for breast cancer [56].

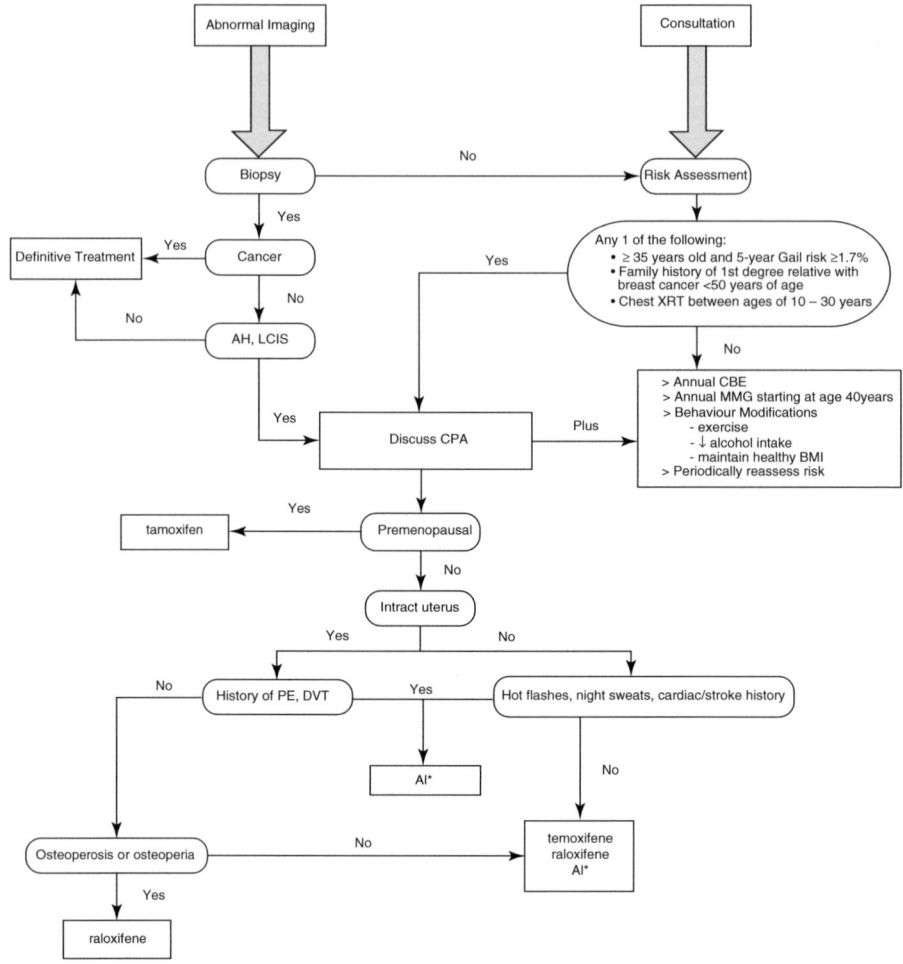

Fig. 10.1 Flow chart to determine risk and appropriateness for prevention medications. * – Off-label use; AH atypical hyperplasia, LCIS lobular carcinoma in-situ, IBIS International Breast Intervention Study, CPA chemoprevention agent, PE pulmonary embolus, DVT deep venous thrombosis, AI aromatase Inhibitor, CBE clinical breast exam, BMI body mass index, XRT radiation therapy, MMG mammography

Clearly, practicing clinicians need to be educated on the role, benefit, eligibility, and availability of prevention medications in addition to patients. This lack of knowledge likely hinders not only prescription of but also patient uptake if physicians lack confidence in their explanation of why prevention medications are important.

Adherence to Prevention Medications

Adherence to prevention medications is high in the short term but declines over 5 years [53]. In the IBIS-II trial, adherence at 6 months was 78% but only 14% at 5 years. King et al. [4] reported just under half of LCIS patients prescribed prevention medications completed 5 years of treatment with a median follow-up of 55 months, while Hermel et al. [55] noted fewer than 12% of patients completed 5 years of prevention medications [4, 55]. Lower adherence was associated with older age, smoking, depression, and allocation to Tamoxifen (vs Raloxifene or placebo) [53]. However, the NSABP P-1 trial documented an 84.3% adherence rate to Tamoxifen [57]. Negative predictors of adherence were smoking, gynecologic symptoms among moderate alcohol drinkers, baseline vasomotor symptoms in patients assigned to Tamoxifen, and adverse sexual symptoms among younger patients at 3 months [57]. The promotion of quality life measures and early management of symptoms may improve adherence [57].

Prevention medications for breast cancer are effective (Table 10.3). Clinicians must consider individual patient risks and benefits when counseling patients on recommendations. Low uptake and poor adherence despite the proven efficiency of prevention medications highlight a significant missed opportunity in the prevention of breast cancer. While the adverse effects associated with the medications may be a barrier to uptake and adherence, it is also important to consider the role of the healthcare provider in education of eligible patients.

Table 10.3 Randomized control trials assessing prevention medications for the prevention of breast cancer

Random controlled trials					
Trial	N	Arms/design	Follow-up mos. (median)	Population	Risk reduction; hazard ratio
NSABP P-1	13,388	TAM vs placebo	84	Pre or postmenopausal Gail >1.66	0.51
IBIS I	7152	TAM vs placebo	96	Pre or postmenopausal	0.75
STAR P-2	19,747	TAM vs Raloxifene	81	Postmenopausal	1.24 (TAM better)
NCIC-MAP.3	4560	Exemestane vs placebo	36	Postmenopausal	0.35
IBIS II	3964	Anastrozole vs placebo	60	Postmenopausal	0.47

TAM Tamoxifen, *NSABP P-1* National Surgical Adjuvant Breast and Bowel Project Breast Cancer Prevention Trial P1, *IBIS I* International Breast Intervention Study, *STAR P-2* National Surgical Adjuvant Breast and Bowel Project Study of Tamoxifen and Raloxifene P2, *MAP 3 NCIC-MAP.3* The National Institute of Canada Clinical Trials Group Mammary Prevention.3 trial, *IBIS II* The Second International Breast Cancer Intervention Study

References

1. Freedman AN, Graubard BI, Rao SR, McCaskill-Stevens W, Ballard-Barbash R, Gail MH. Estimates of the number of US women who could benefit from tamoxifen for breast cancer chemoprevention. J Natl Cancer Inst. 2003;95(7):526–32.
2. Moyer VA. Medications to decrease the risk for breast cancer in women: recommendations from the U.S. Preventive Services Task Force recommendation statement. Ann Intern Med. Practice Guideline Research Support, U.S. Gov't, P.H.S. 2013;159(10):698–708.
3. Fisher B, Costantino JP, Wickerham DL, Redmond CK, Kavanah M, Cronin WM, et al. Tamoxifen for prevention of breast cancer: report of the National Surgical Adjuvant Breast and Bowel Project P-1 Study. J Natl Cancer Inst. [Clinical Trial Multicenter Study Randomized Controlled Trial Research Support, U.S. Gov't, P.H.S.]. 1998;90(18):1371–88.
4. King TA, Pilewskie M, Muhsen S, Patil S, Mautner SK, Park A, et al. Lobular carcinoma in situ: a 29-year longitudinal experience evaluating clinicopathologic features and breast cancer risk. J Clin Oncol. [Evaluation Studies Research Support, N.I.H., Extramural Research Support, Non-U.S. Gov't]. 2015;33(33):3945–52.
5. Pruthi S, Heisey R, Bevers T. Personalized assessment and management of women at risk for breast cancer in North America. Womens Health (Lond). [Review]. 2015;11(2):213–23; quiz 23–4.
6. Vogel VG, Costantino JP, Wickerham DL, Cronin WM, Cecchini RS, Atkins JN, et al. Update of the National Surgical Adjuvant Breast and Bowel Project Study of Tamoxifen and Raloxifene (STAR) P-2 Trial: preventing breast cancer. Cancer Prev Res (Phila). [Comparative Study Multicenter Study Randomized Controlled Trial Research Support, N.I.H., Extramural Research Support, U.S. Gov't, P.H.S.]. 2010;3(6):696–706.
7. Statistics NCfH. Use of mammography among women aged 40 and over, by selected characteristics. Hyattsville: U.S.Government Printing Office; 2016. [cited 2017 October 1, 2017]; Available from: http://www.cdc.gov/nchs/hus/contents2016.htm#070
8. Neal L, Sandhu NP, Hieken TJ, Glazebrook KN, Mac Bride MB, Dilaveri CA, et al. Diagnosis and management of benign, atypical, and indeterminate breast lesions detected on core needle biopsy. Mayo Clin Proc. [Comparative Study Review]. 2014;89(4):536–47.
9. Walia S, Ma YL, Lu J, Lang JE, Press MF. Pathology and current management of borderline breast epithelial lesions. Am J Hematol Oncol. 2017;13(8):24–31.
10. Black MM, Barclay TH, Cutler SJ, Hankey BF, Asire AJ. Association of atypical characteristics of benign breast lesions with subsequent risk of breast cancer. Cancer. 1972;29(2):338–43.
11. Degnim AC, Visscher DW, Berman HK, Frost MH, Sellers TA, Vierkant RA, et al. Stratification of breast cancer risk in women with atypia: a Mayo cohort study. J Clin Oncol. [Research Support, N.I.H., Extramural Research Support, Non-U.S. Gov't Research Support, U.S. Gov't, Non-P.H.S. 2007;25(19):2671–7.
12. Hartmann LC, Degnim AC, Santen RJ, Dupont WD, Ghosh K. Atypical hyperplasia of the breast – risk assessment and management options. N Engl J Med. Research Support, N.I.H., Extramural Research Support, Non-U.S. Gov't. 2015;372(1):78–89.
13. Hartmann LC, Radisky DC, Frost MH, Santen RJ, Vierkant RA, Benetti LL, et al. Understanding the premalignant potential of atypical hyperplasia through its natural history: a longitudinal cohort study. Cancer Prev Res (Phila). [Research Support, N.I.H., Extramural Research Support, Non-U.S. Gov't]. 2014;7(2):211–7.
14. Hartmann LC, Sellers TA, Frost MH, Lingle WL, Degnim AC, Ghosh K, et al. Benign breast disease and the risk of breast cancer. N Engl J Med. 2005;353(3):229–37.
15. Menes TS, Kerlikowske K, Lange J, Jaffer S, Rosenberg R, Miglioretti DL. Subsequent breast cancer risk following diagnosis of atypical ductal hyperplasia on needle biopsy. JAMA Oncol. 2017;3(1):36–41.
16. Morrow M, Schnitt SJ, Norton L. Current management of lesions associated with an increased risk of breast cancer. Nat Rev Clin Oncol. 2015;12(4):227–38.

17. Page DL, Dupont WD, Rogers LW, Rados MS. Atypical hyperplastic lesions of the female breast – a long-term follow-up-study. Cancer. 1985;55(11):2698–708.
18. Page DL, Schuyler PA, Dupont WD, Jensen RA, Plummer WD, Simpson JF. Atypical lobular hyperplasia as a unilateral predictor of breast cancer risk: a retrospective cohort study. Lancet. 2003;361:125. 2003 Jun 7;361(9373):1994–1998.
19. Worsham MJ, Abrams J, Raju U, Kapke A, Lu M, Cheng JF, et al. Breast cancer incidence in a cohort of women with benign breast disease from a multiethnic, primary health care population. Breast J. 2007;13(2):115–21.
20. Maximov PY, Lee TM, Jordan VC. The discovery and development of selective estrogen receptor modulators (SERMs) for clinical practice. Curr Clin Pharmacol. [Comparative Study Research Support, N.I.H., Extramural Research Support, Non-U.S. Gov't Research Support, U.S. Gov't, Non-P.H.S. Review]. 2013;8(2):135–55.
21. Mocellin S, Pilati P, Briarava M, Nitti D. Breast cancer chemoprevention: a network ,meta-analysis of randomized controlled trials. J Natl Cancer Inst. [Meta-Analysis]. 2016;108(2):djv318.
22. Jordan VC, Robinson SP. Species-specific pharmacology of antiestrogens – role of metabolism. FASEB J. 1987;46(5):1870–4.
23. Wijayaratne AL, McDonnell DP. The human estrogen receptor-alpha is a ubiquitinated protein whose stability is affected differentially by agonists, antagonists, and selective estrogen receptor modulators. J Biol Chem. [Research Support, U.S. Gov't, P.H.S.]. 2001;276(38):35684–92.
24. Harper MJ, Walpole AL. A new derivative of triphenylethylene: effect on implantation and mode of action in rats. J Reprod Fertil. 1967;13(1):101–19.
25. Powles TJ, Hardy JR, Ashley SE, Farrington GM, Cosgrove D, Davey JB, et al. A pilot trial to evaluate the acute toxicity and feasibility of tamoxifen for prevention of breast-cancer. Br J Cancer. 1989;60(1):126–31.
26. Powles TJ, Ashley S, Tidy A, Smith IE, Dowsett M. Twenty-year follow-up of the Royal Marsden randomized, double-blinded tamoxifen breast cancer prevention trial. J Natl Cancer Inst. [Randomized Controlled Trial Research Support, Non-U.S. Gov't]. 2007;99(4):283–90.
27. Fisher B, Costantino JP, Wickerham DL, Cecchini RS, Cronin WM, Robidoux A, et al. Tamoxifen for the prevention of breast cancer: current status of the National Surgical Adjuvant Breast and Bowel Project P-1 study. J Natl Cancer Inst. [Randomized Controlled Trial Research Support, N.I.H., Extramural]. 2005;97(22):1652–62.
28. Cuzick J, Sestak I, Cawthorn S, Hamed H, Holli K, Howell A, et al. Tamoxifen for prevention of breast cancer: extended long-term follow-up of the IBIS-I breast cancer prevention trial. Lancet Oncol. [Multicenter Study Randomized Controlled Trial Research Support, Non-U.S. Gov't]. 2015;16(1):67–75.
29. Visvanathan K, Hurley P, Bantug E, Brown P, Col NF, Cuzick J, et al. Use of pharmacologic interventions for breast cancer risk reduction: American Society of Clinical Oncology clinical practice guideline. J Clin Oncol. [Review]. 2013;31(23):2942–62.
30. Cummings SR, Eckert S, Krueger KA, Grady D, Powles TJ, Cauley JA, et al. The effect of Raloxifene on risk of breast cancer in postmenopausal women: results from the MORE randomized trial. Multiple Outcomes of Raloxifene Evaluation. JAMA. [Clinical Trial Multicenter Study Randomized Controlled Trial Research Support, Non-U.S. Gov't]. 1999;281(23):2189–97.
31. Cauley JA, Norton L, Lippman ME, Eckert S, Krueger KA, Purdie DW, et al. Continued breast cancer risk reduction in postmenopausal women treated with Raloxifene: 4-year results from the MORE trial. Multiple outcomes of Raloxifene evaluation. Breast Cancer Res Treat. [Clinical Trial Multicenter Study Randomized Controlled Trial Research Support, Non-U.S. Gov't]. 2001;65(2):125–34.
32. Riggs BL, Hartmann LC. Selective estrogen-receptor modulators – mechanisms of action and application to clinical practice. N Engl J Med. [Research Support, Non-U.S. Gov't Research Support, U.S. Gov't, P.H.S. Review]. 2003;348(7):618–29.

33. Vogel VG. The NSABP Study of Tamoxifen and Raloxifene (STAR) trial. Expert Rev Anticancer Ther. [Review]. 2009;9(1):51–60.
34. Mirkin S, Pickar JH. Selective estrogen receptor modulators (SERMs): a review of clinical data. Maturitas. [Review]. 2015;80(I):52–7.
35. LaCroix AZ, Powles T, Osborne CK, Wolter K, Thompson JR, Thompson DD, et al. Breast cancer incidence in the randomized PEARL trial of Lasofoxifene in postmenopausal osteoporotic women. J Natl Cancer Inst. Randomized Controlled Trial Research Support, Non-U.S. Gov't. 2010;102(22):1706–15.
36. Suh N, Glasebrook AL, Palkowitz AD, Bryant HU, Burris LL, Starling JJ, et al. Arzoxifene, a new selective estrogen receptor modulator for chemoprevention of experimental breast cancer. Cancer Res. 2001;61(23):8412–5.
37. Cummings SR, McClung M, Reginster JY, Cox D, Mitlak B, Stock J, et al. Arzoxifene for prevention of fractures and invasive breast cancer in postmenopausal women. J Bone Miner Res. [Randomized Controlled Trial Research Support, Non-U.S. Gov't]. 2011;26(2):397–404.
38. Goss PE, Ingle JN, Ales-Martinez JE, Cheung AM, Chlebowski RT, Wactawski-Wende J, et al. Exemestane for breast-cancer prevention in postmenopausal women. N Engl J Med. [Multicenter Study Randomized Controlled Trial Research Support, Non-U.S. Gov't]. 2011;364(25):2381–91.
39. Goss PE, Ingle JN, Pritchard KI, Ellis MJ, Sledge GW, Budd GT, et al. Exemestane versus Anastrozole in postmenopausal women with early breast cancer: NCIC CTG MA.27 – a randomized controlled phase III trial. J Clin Oncol. [Clinical Trial, Phase III Comparative Study Historical Article Multicenter Study Randomized Controlled Trial Research Support, N.I.H., Extramural Research Support, Non-U.S. Gov't]. 2013;31(11):1398–404.
40. Cuzick J, Sestak I, Forbes JF, Dowsett M, Knox J, Cawthorn S, et al. Anastrozole for prevention of breast cancer in high-risk postmenopausal women (IBIS-II): an international, double-blind, randomised placebo-controlled trial. Lancet. [Multicenter Study Randomized Controlled Trial Research Support, Non-U.S. Gov't]. 2014;383(9922):1041–8.
41. Dowling RJO, Zakikhani M, Fantus IG, Pollak M, Sonenberg N. Metformin inhibits mammalian target of rapamycin-dependent translation initiation in breast cancer cells. Cancer Res. 2007;67(22):10804–12.
42. Goodwin PJ, Stambolic V. Obesity and insulin resistance in breast cancer – chemoprevention strategies with a focus on metformin. Breast. 2011;20:S31–S5.
43. Zakikhani M, Dowling R, Fantus IG, Sonenberg N, Pollak M. Metformin is an AMP kinase-dependent growth inhibitor for breast cancer cells. Cancer Res. 2006;66(21):10269–73.
44. Christopoulos PF, Msaouel P, Koutsilieris M. The role of the insulin-like growth factor-1 system in breast cancer. Mol Cancer. 2015;15:14.
45. Kleinberg DL, Axelrod D, Smith J, Singh B, Lesser M, Ameri P, et al. Breast cancer chemoprevention by IGF-I inhibition in women with atypical hyperplasia of the breast: A phase 1/2 proof of principle trial [abstract]. In: Proceedings of the 105th Annual Meeting of the American Association for Cancer Research. San Diego: Philadelphia (PA); 2014. AACR; Cancer Res 2014;74(19 Suppl): Abstract nr CT306. https://doi.org/10.1158/1538-7445.AM2014-CT306.
46. Smith J, Axelrod D, Singh B, Kleinberg D. Prevention of breast cancer: the case for studying inhibition of IGF-1 actions. Ann Oncol. 2011;22:i50–i2.
47. Harris RE, Beebe-Donk J, Alshafie GA. Reduction in the risk of human breast cancer by selective cyclooxygenase-2 (COX-2) inhibitors. BMC Cancer. [Research Support, N.I.H., Extramural Research Support, Non-U.S. Gov't]. 2006;6:27.
48. Masferrer JL, Leahy KM, Koki AT, Zweifel BS, Settle SL, Woerner BM, et al. Antiangiogenic and antitumor activities of cyclooxygenase-2 inhibitors. Cancer Res. 2000;60(5):1306–11.
49. Wang DZ, DuBois RN. Cyclooxygenase-2: a potential target in breast cancer. Semin Oncol. 2004;31(1):64–73.
50. Aktas B, Sorkin M, Pusztai L, Hofstatter EW. Uptake of exemestane chemoprevention in postmenopausal women at increased risk for breast cancer. Eur J Cancer Prev. 2016;25(1):3–8.
51. Coopey SB, Mazzola E, Buckley JM, Sharko J, Belli AK, Kim EMH, et al. The role of chemoprevention in modifying the risk of breast cancer in women with atypical breast lesions. Breast Cancer Res Treat. 2012;136(3):627–33.

52. Ropka ME, Keim J, Philbrick JT. Patient decisions about breast cancer chemoprevention: a systematic review and meta-analysis. J Clin Oncol. [Research Support, N.I.H., Extramural Review]. 2010;28(18):3090–5.
53. Smith SG, Sestak I, Forster A, Partridge A, Side L, Wolf MS, et al. Factors affecting uptake and adherence to breast cancer chemoprevention: a systematic review and meta-analysis. Ann Oncol. [Meta-Analysis Research Support, Non-U.S. Gov't Review]. 2016;27(4):575–90.
54. Freedman AN, Yu B, Gail MH, Costantino JP, Graubard BI, Vogel VG, et al. Benefit/risk assessment for breast cancer chemoprevention with raloxifene or tamoxifen for women age 50 years or older. J Clin Oncol. [Research Support, N.I.H., Extramural Research Support, N.I.H., Intramural Research Support, U.S. Gov't, P.H.S.]. 2011;29(17):2327–33.
55. Hermel DJ, Wood ME, Chun J, Rounds T, Sands M, Schwartz S, et al. Multi-institutional evaluation of women at high risk of developing breast cancer. Clin Breast Cancer. 2017;17(6):427–32.
56. Smith SG, Side L, Meisel SF, Horne R, Cuzick J, Wardle J. Clinician-reported barriers to implementing breast cancer chemoprevention in the UK: a qualitative investigation. Public Health Genomics. [Multicenter Study]. 2016;19(4):239–49.
57. Land SR, Walcott FL, Liu Q, Wickerham DL, Costantino JP, Ganz PA. Symptoms and QOL as predictors of chemoprevention adherence in NRG oncology/NSABP trial P-1. J Natl Cancer Inst. [Clinical Trial, Phase III Multicenter Study Randomized Controlled Trial Research Support, N.I.H., Extramural Research Support, Non-U.S. Gov't Research Support, U.S. Gov't, Non-P.H.S.]. 2016;108(4).

Prophylactic Mastectomy in Patients with Atypical Breast Lesions

11

Judy C. Boughey and Amy C. Degnim

Abbreviations

ADH	Atypical ductal hyperplasia
AH	Atypical hyperplasia
ALH	Atypical lobular hyperplasia
BPM	Bilateral prophylactic mastectomy
FEA	Flat epithelial atypia
LCIS	Lobular carcinoma in situ
TDLU	Terminal duct lobular unit

Introduction

Prophylactic mastectomy, removal of a "normal" breast without a cancer diagnosis, also known as risk-reducing mastectomy, decreases the risk of breast cancer development. Prophylactic mastectomy has been performed for decades, in women thought to be of elevated risk of breast cancer development. Initially the procedure most commonly performed for risk reduction was a subcutaneous mastectomy, and indications included personal or family history of breast cancer, multiple prior breast biopsies, challenging physical examination, mastodynia, and cancerphobia [1].

Risk Reduction with Bilateral Prophylactic Mastectomy

Studies of bilateral prophylactic mastectomy (BPM) in women with a family history of breast cancer have demonstrated that it decreases the relative risk of breast cancer development by 90–95% [1–5]. In a series from the Mayo Clinic of 214 women at high risk of breast cancer development, based on their family history, who underwent BPM, 3 developed cancer (1.4%) compared to the control group of these women's sisters, where 156 (38.7%) out of the 403 sisters developed breast cancer with 14.4 years of follow up, demonstrating a 90% risk reduction. In the 425 women at moderate risk of breast cancer development, 4 women developed cancer, compared to Gail model calculation which would have expected 37.4 women to develop breast cancer, reflecting an 89.5% risk reduction [1].

In a study of 483 BRCA 1 or BRCA 2 mutation carriers without a history of breast cancer, 105 underwent BPM, and 2 women (1.9%) developed breast cancer compared to 184 (48.7%) of the 378 who did not pursue BPM, resulting in a 90% risk reduction [3].

Risks and Benefits of BPM

Although BPM provides significant reduction of risk of breast cancer, removal of both breasts can be associated with complications related to the procedure and in the long term can be associated with significant negative psychosocial impact. A questionnaire of 572 women at a mean of 9.2 years after they underwent BPM reported that 70% were satisfied with the procedure, 11% were neutral, and 19% were dissatisfied. Importantly, 74% reported diminished emotional concern about breast cancer [6]. The most frequent adverse impact on psychosocial and social variables was satisfaction with appearance (36%), feelings of femininity (25%), sexual relationships (23%), and self-esteem (18%). At approximately 18.4 years follow up on 319 of these women, satisfaction remained high with 73% satisfied and 81% reporting they would make the same decision again [7]. Reconstruction and need for reoperations were associated with lower satisfaction with the decision to undergo BPM [8].

It is important for the patient to understand the difference between absolute risk reduction and relative risk reduction. BPM provides a relative risk reduction of 90–95% [1–5]. Therefore, for a woman at 70% risk of breast cancer development, it decreases the risk of breast cancer by 0.90×70, which is a 63% absolute risk reduction. However, for a woman who has a 25% risk of breast cancer development, the relative risk reduction is also 90%; but the absolute risk reduction is only 22.5%.

Thus, for women considering BPM, as with any surgical procedure, a full discussion of the pros and cons is imperative. BPM does not eliminate the potential to develop breast cancer, and cancer can still develop in residual tissue after a BPM [9]. Mastectomy is associated with potential surgical complications, both the general risks of a surgical procedure, such as venous thromboembolism, and anesthetic complications and also risks at the mastectomy site including bleeding, infection, skin flap necrosis, numbness, and chronic pain [10]. Mastectomy does result in permanent numbness of the chest wall, and even with advances in techniques, such as the use of nipple-sparing mastectomy, the nipple is still usually insensate. In many cases, breast reconstruction is performed, and this process can be started at the time of the mastectomy. In some cases, mastectomy and immediate implant reconstruction can be performed in a single step. However, usually reconstruction results in the need for further subsequent surgery, and reconstruction may fail. In a series of patients who underwent unilateral prophylactic mastectomy with reconstruction, 39% required at least one unplanned reoperation, and this was associated with lower satisfaction, lower likelihood of choosing prophylactic mastectomy again, and lower likelihood of choosing reconstruction again [8]. BPM is associated, as mentioned, with a potential negative impact on physical, emotional, and sexual well-being, and patients may regret their decision to pursue BPM. Advantages of BPM are significant decrease in risk of breast cancer, decrease in emotional concern regarding breast cancer risk, and no further need for breast imaging (no screening mammograms or screening MRIs). BPM offers a survival benefit for patients at the highest risk of breast cancer development who undergo the procedure at a young age. However, for women with a small increase in risk, there is no improvement in survival.

Indications for BPM

The Society of Surgical Oncology consensus statement from 2007 outlined the indications for BPM as; BRCA 1 or BRCA 2 mutations or other predisposition genes; strong family history of breast cancer; high-risk histology, including atypical ductal hyperplasia (ADH), atypical lobular hyperplasia (ALH), or lobular carcinoma in situ (LCIS) on biopsy, especially in women with significant family history; and rarely in cases for women with breasts that are difficult for surveillance, including extremely dense breasts, multiple prior biopsies, and strong concern for cancer risk [11].

On some occasions, it is appropriate to consider risk-reducing mastectomy for women with atypical breast lesions. However, due caution must be exercised with an understanding of which atypical breast lesions and which subsets of women with those atypical breast lesions have a breast cancer risk high enough to warrant considering this procedure. "Atypical breast lesions" is a catchall term that does not refer to a specific histologic diagnosis, and pathology details are critical when considering whether risk-reducing mastectomy may be appropriate. Prophylactic mastectomy should only be undertaken when a woman's long-term risk is high enough that the benefits of the surgery are judged to outweigh the risks. For this reason, more detailed understanding of risks associated with atypical breast lesions is necessary.

Atypical Hyperplasia

The classic atypical breast lesion is atypical hyperplasia (AH). There are two phenotypic variants of AH: atypical ductal hyperplasia (ADH) and atypical lobular hyperplasia (ALH). Both phenotypes are proliferative epithelial abnormalities involving the terminal duct lobular unit (TDLU) in breast tissue. In ADH, the proliferating epithelium demonstrates low-grade cytologic atypia combined with abnormal architectural structure (often a cribriform appearance with "punched out" spaces). The appearance is similar to ductal carcinoma in situ but measures <2 mm in size or involves less than two TDLUs. ALH is a proliferative process of the TDLU characterized by a proliferation of atypical small monomorphic epithelial cells lacking cohesion, where the process involves less than half of the acini within a TDLU [12]. In addition to these two lesions, other lesions that are sometimes considered atypical breast lesions include flat epithelial atypia (FEA), radial scar with atypia, and papilloma with atypia [13].

FEA is a columnar cell lesion with cytologic atypia and was defined more recently (2003) by World Health Organization (WHO) criteria [14]. Although initial descriptions of this lesion raised concern that women with FEA would have increased long-term risk, recent studies have shown that women with FEA do not have substantially increased breast cancer risk on the basis of this histologic finding alone [15–17]. ADH often occurs coincidentally with FEA (approximately 50% of cases) [18, 19]; in that situation those women have the long-term breast cancer risk that would be expected for a woman with ADH [17]. However, when FEA alone is present, the long-term breast cancer risk is considered to be increased approximately twofold, on a par with risk in women who have other benign proliferative breast lesions without atypia such as benign papilloma, florid ductal hyperplasia, sclerosing adenosis, or radial scar. It is also important to distinguish between lesions that have some form of atypia on percutaneous core needle biopsy, versus a final and definite diagnosis of AH. For lesions with cytologic atypia on core needle biopsy that do not meet criteria for AH (i.e., radial scar with atypia or papilloma with atypia), usually surgical excision is indicated to rule out the possibility of concurrent cancer and to determine if true AH is present or not. If findings meet criteria for ADH or ALH, then the AH present defines their future long-term breast cancer risk.

Long-Term Risk with Atypical Hyperplasia

In women who have a definite diagnosis of AH (ADH or ALH), there are multiple sources of data that corroborate the long-term increased risk of breast cancer in these women. The first report indicating increased breast cancer risk in women with AH came from the Nashville breast cohort in 1985. In that seminal report from doctors Dupont and Page, a four-fold increase was reported in breast cancer risk for women with atypical hyperplasia [20]. More recently, long-term breast cancer risk data have also been reported from the Nurse's Health Study [21, 22] and cohorts at the Mayo Clinic [23], the Partners Health group [24], and the Breast Cancer Surveillance Consortium (BCSC) [25]. The annual breast cancer risk associated with AH in these reports ranges from 0.6% per year [25] to approximately 2% per year [24], with the preponderance of data suggesting that risk in these women can be estimated at 1% per year. In the BCSC study, they reported only the risk of invasive cancer after ADH, whereas the Mayo Clinic and Partners studies reported a risk of both invasive cancer and ductal carcinoma in situ; this difference can explain in part the lower risk estimates reported from the BCSC study. Also, it is notable that standard breast cancer risk prediction models, such as the Gail model and the Tyrer-Cuzick/IBIS model, do not provide accurate risk prediction for women with AH [26, 27]. Therefore in women with AH, it is preferable to utilize the annual risk estimates above when estimating long-term breast cancer risk or else a risk model specifically designed and validated for women with AH. Estimating risk with annual absolute risk numbers also affords the ability to individualize long-term risk estimates based on a woman's age and expected longevity.

Early on, concern was raised that women who have both a family history of breast cancer and AH may have substantially increased risk compared to women with AH but no family history. However, that concern was raised based on a small subsample with large confidence intervals around the risk estimates [20]. Since then, data from the Mayo cohort and the Nurse's Health Study both show that in women with AH, a family history (in the absence of a known deleterious mutation) does not further significantly increase their breast cancer risk [22, 28]. Data from existing cohorts are also generally concordant that long-term breast cancer risk in women with AH is increased for both breasts, although there is an ipsilateral predominance [22, 24, 28]. Regarding possible differences in risk for ADH versus ALH, data across multiple cohort sources shows some variation, with some studies indicating higher risk in women with ALH [22] and some studies showing similar risk for both ADH and ALH [24, 28].

Risk Stratification Within Atypical Hyperplasia

It is important to remember that the absolute risks estimated in the preceding paragraph are based on large groups of women and that it may be possible to further discriminate risk among these women individually. One notable factor that appears to stratify risk significantly among women with AH is the number of foci of AH present within the benign biopsy specimen. This was first reported in the Mayo Clinic cohort [28, 29] and subsequently confirmed in the Nashville cohort [30]. Based on this stratification, women with a single focus of AH have estimated annual risk of 1%, women with two foci have estimated annual risk of 1.5%, and women with three or more foci have annual risk of approximately 2% [28–30]. In the Nurse's Health Study, a trend was observed for increased relative risk with increasing number of foci of AH, but the trend was not statistically significant overall. They further looked at the impact of number of foci of atypia in subsets of women with ADH versus ALH. In the subset analyses, they found higher risk in women with multiple foci of ALH but not in ADH, although these differences were not statistically significant either [22]. In the Mayo Clinic cohort, risk was higher for multiple foci of atypia in both ADH and ALH subsets. In the Nashville cohort, risk was increased for multiple foci of atypia in women with ADH or ALH, but the increase was statistically significant only in the subgroup with ADH [30].

This phenomenon of increased risk associated with larger volume of high-risk benign disease was also observed in a cohort of women with lobular carcinoma in situ (LCIS) at Memorial Sloan Kettering Cancer Center, where women with greater than half of the biopsy slides demonstrating LCIS had three-fold increase in risk, compared to women with less than half of their biopsy slides demonstrating LCIS [31]. When considering the number of foci of atypia, it is important to remember that most women with AH (~60%) have only a single focus, with a small minority having multiple foci [30]. Given that AH is a finding in only approximately 5–8% of all benign breast biopsies, only approximately 1–2% of all women with a benign breast biopsy will have multiple foci of AH. Therefore, although the number of foci of atypia appears to be a factor that stratifies risk in women with AH, this has not been corroborated in all studies, and it is a small minority of women who have multiple foci of atypia.

Bilateral Prophylactic Mastectomy in Women with Atypical Hyperplasia

For patients with AH, there are several clinical situations where prophylactic mastectomy may be reasonable. These include women with AH and extensive calcifications where excision of the whole area of calcifications would be disfiguring, women with multiple prior excisional biopsies for atypia and a new area of atypia identified, patients who develop new areas of atypia while on prevention therapy, patients with several sites of atypia who are unable to tolerate prevention therapy, and patients with atypia and extremely dense breast tissue or complex imaging that limits adequate surveillance imaging. Overall, these clinical situations are uncommon among women with AH, and the question is raised whether BPM may be appropriate for women with AH who do not fit the above scenarios.

Since a decision for prophylactic mastectomy would require a substantial increase in long-term breast cancer risk to justify the risk of the procedure, it is important to translate estimated annual risk into long-term or lifetime risk for an individual woman with AH. Generally, prophylactic mastectomy is considered justifiable if long-term/lifetime breast cancer risk is 50% or greater. Some women with AH may have long-term risk estimated in this range, although it is a minority of them, and they would be expected to have substantial risk reduction benefit from prevention therapy. For most women with AH, they are diagnosed in the sixth or seventh decade of life and have only a single focus of AH. With a life expectancy of 20–30 years, their lifetime risk is likely in the range of 20–30%, which falls short of a 50% lifetime risk. On the other hand, this degree of risk is not that different than the long-term risk associated with a PALB2 or CHEK2 mutation [32–34]. Furthermore, for a woman diagnosed with AH in her 40s, especially if she has multiple foci of atypia, her long-term risk likely does approach the 50% range. Therefore, in selected circumstances, it is reasonable to discuss risk reduction mastectomy in women with AH.

Decision-making about risk reduction mastectomy in women with AH is similar to decision-making in women at increased risk due to deleterious genetic mutations, in the sense that risks and benefits of the procedure must be weighed against the alternative approach of careful screening with a strategy of early detection. However, there is one important difference between the scenario of increased risk due to AH and increased risk due to a deleterious genetic mutation, which is the possibility of medical prevention therapy in women with AH. For women with AH, medical prevention therapy is proven to be highly effective. Prospective and retrospective data both confirm a substantial risk reduction benefit for prevention therapies in women with AH. In the NSABP P1 study of tamoxifen, a 70% reduction in breast cancer risk was observed in women with AH [35]. Similar risk reduction has been observed for anastrozole [36], raloxifene [37], and exemestane [38]. In the retrospective data of the Partners cohort, a similar 70% reduction in breast cancer risk was observed among women who took prevention therapy compared to those who did not [24].

In summary, final decision-making regarding prophylactic mastectomy depends on a woman's long-term absolute risk, her current age and anticipated residual risk, the risks of prevention medication versus risks of surgery, the degree of risk reduction anticipated from each approach, and the patient's preferences and values. Given the irrevocable nature of bilateral mastectomy, we would propose the following general risk-based recommendations regarding its use. For the minority of women with AH who have an estimated lifetime breast cancer risk of 50% or greater, prophylactic mastectomy should be discussed with them as an option, but a trial of prevention therapy should be strongly recommended before performing irrevocable surgery. For women with lifetime breast cancer risk of 25–50%, prevention therapy should be recommended. Prophylactic mastectomy may be considered in patients who are unable or unwilling to take prevention therapy and after thorough counseling. For women with lifetime risk of less than 25%, they should be advised against prophylactic mastectomy unless there are specific extenuating circumstances.

These guidelines provide a framework for discussion with women. However, there is no set risk above which BPM should be considered or below which BPM should be denied. Similarly, risk assessment provides good population-based estimations; however individual risk estimation is still limited. Thus, a careful evaluation of risk, life expectancy, and options for risk management together with shared decision-making taking into account patients' personal preferences are required when considering BPM for AH.

With improved risk prediction, potentially in the future we will be able to better discriminate risk among women with AH to help inform their risk management choices. Women with AH who have very high risk may benefit from BPM; however, chemoprevention and/or surveillance is favored over BPM for patients with AH.

References

1. Hartmann LC, Schaid DJ, Woods JE, Crotty TP, Myers JL, Arnold PG, Petty PM, Sellers TA, Johnson JL, McDonnell SK, Frost MH, Jenkins RB. Efficacy of bilateral prophylactic mastectomy in women with a family history of breast cancer. N Engl J Med. 1999;340:77–84.
2. Hartmann LC, Sellers TA, Schaid DJ, Frank TS, Soderberg CL, Sitta DL, Frost MH, Grant CS, Donohue JH, Woods JE, McDonnell SK, Vockley CW, Deffenbaugh A, Couch FJ, Jenkins RB. Efficacy of bilateral prophylactic mastectomy in BRCA1 and BRCA2 gene mutation carriers. J Natl Cancer Inst. 2001;93:1633–7.

3. Rebbeck TR, Friebel T, Lynch HT, Neuhausen SL, van t Veer L, Garber JE, Evans GR, Narod SA, Isaacs C, Matloff E, Daly MB, Olopade OI, Weber BL. Bilateral prophylactic mastectomy reduces breast cancer risk in BRCA1 and BRCA2 mutation carriers: the PROSE Study Group. J Clin Oncol. 2004;22:1055–62.
4. Rebbeck TR, Kauff ND, Domchek SM. Meta-analysis of risk reduction estimates associated with risk-reducing salpingo-oophorectomy in BRCA1 or BRCA2 mutation carriers. J Natl Cancer Inst. 2009;101:80–7.
5. Domchek SM, Friebel TM, Singer CF, Evans DG, Lynch HT, Isaacs C, Garber JE, Neuhausen SL, Matloff E, Eeles R, Pichert G, van't Veer L, Tung N, Weitzel JN, Couch FJ, Rubinstein WS, Ganz PA, Daly MB, Olopade OI, Tomlinson G, Schildkraut J, Blum JL, Rebbeck TR. Association of risk-reducing surgery in BRCA1 or BRCA2 mutation carriers with cancer risk and mortality. JAMA. 2010;304:967–75.
6. Frost MH, Schaid DJ, Sellers TA, Slezak JM, Arnold PG, Woods JE, Petty PM, Johnson JL, Sitta DL, McDonnell SK, Rummans TA, Jenkins RB, Sloan JA, Hartmann LC. Long-term satisfaction and psychological and social function following bilateral prophylactic mastectomy. JAMA. 2000;284:319–24.
7. Boughey JC, Hoskin TL, Heins CN, Hartmann LC, Frost MH. Long-term satisfaction and breast cancer outcomes after bilateral prophylactic mastectomy in women with a family history of breast cancer. Ann Surg Oncol. 2016;23:67.
8. Boughey JC, Hoskin TL, Hartmann LC, Johnson JL, Jacobson SR, Degnim AC, Frost MH. Impact of reconstruction and reoperation on long-term patient-reported satisfaction after contralateral prophylactic mastectomy. Ann Surg Oncol. 2015;22:401–8.
9. Mutter RW, Frost MH, Hoskin TL, Johnson JL, Hartmann LC, Boughey JC. Breast cancer after prophylactic mastectomy (bilateral or contralateral prophylactic mastectomy), a clinical entity: presentation, management, and outcomes. Breast Cancer Res Treat. 2015;153:183–90.
10. Hunt KK, Euhus DM, Boughey JC, Chagpar AB, Feldman SM, Hansen NM, Kulkarni SA, McCready DR, Mamounas EP, Wilke LG, Van Zee KJ, Morrow M. Society of Surgical Oncology Breast Disease Working Group statement on prophylactic (risk-reducing) mastectomy. Ann Surg Oncol. 2017;24:375–97.
11. Giuliano AE, Boolbol S, Degnim A, Kuerer H, Leitch AM, Morrow M. Society of Surgical Oncology: position statement on prophylactic mastectomy. Approved by the Society of Surgical Oncology Executive Council, March 2007. Ann Surg Oncol. 2007;14:2425–7.
12. Racz JM, Carter JM, Degnim AC. Lobular neoplasia and atypical ductal hyperplasia on core biopsy: current surgical management recommendations. Ann Surg Oncol. 2017;24:2848–54.
13. Racz JM, Carter JM, Degnim AC. Challenging atypical breast lesions including flat epithelial atypia, radial scar, and intraductal papilloma. Ann Surg Oncol. 2017;24:2842–7.
14. Tavassoli FA, Hoefler H, Rosai J, Holland R, Ellis IO. Intraductal proliferative lesions. In: Tavassoli FA, Devilee P, editors. World Health Organization classification of tumours: pathology and genetics of tumours of the breast and female genital organs. Lyon: IARC Press; 2003. p. 63–73.
15. Boulos FI, Dupont WD, Simpson JF, Schuyler PA, Sanders ME, Freudenthal ME, Page DL. Histologic associations and long-term cancer risk in columnar cell lesions of the breast: a retrospective cohort and a nested case-control study. Cancer. 2008;113:2415–21.
16. Aroner SA, Collins LC, Schnitt SJ, Connolly JL, Colditz GA, Tamimi RM. Columnar cell lesions and subsequent breast cancer risk: a nested case-control study. Breast Cancer Res. 2010;12:R61.
17. Said SM, Visscher DW, Nassar A, Frank RD, Vierkant RA, Frost MH, Ghosh K, Radisky DC, Hartmann LC, Degnim AC. Flat epithelial atypia and risk of breast cancer: a Mayo cohort study. Cancer. 2015;121:1548–55.
18. Peres A, Barranger E, Becette V, Boudinet A, Guinebretiere JM, Cherel P. Rates of upgrade to malignancy for 271 cases of flat epithelial atypia (FEA) diagnosed by breast core biopsy. Breast Cancer Res Treat. 2012;133:659–66.

19. Khoumais NA, Scaranelo AM, Moshonov H, Kulkarni SR, Miller N, McCready DR, Youngson BJ, Crystal P, Done SJ. Incidence of breast cancer in patients with pure flat epithelial atypia diagnosed at core-needle biopsy of the breast. Ann Surg Oncol. 2013;20:133–8.
20. Dupont WD, Page DL. Risk factors for breast cancer in women with proliferative breast disease. N Engl J Med. 1985;312:146–51.
21. London SJ, Connolly JL, Schnitt SJ, Colditz GA. A prospective study of benign breast disease and the risk of breast cancer. JAMA. 1992;267:941–4.
22. Collins LC, Aroner SA, Connolly JL, Colditz GA, Schnitt SJ, Tamimi RM. Breast cancer risk by extent and type of atypical hyperplasia: an update from the Nurses' Health Studies. Cancer. 2016;122:515–20.
23. Hartmann LC, Sellers TA, Frost MH, Lingle WL, Degnim AC, Ghosh K, Vierkant RA, Maloney SD, Pankratz VS, Hillman DW, Suman VJ, Johnson J, Blake C, Tlsty T, Vachon CM, Melton LJ 3rd, Visscher DW. Benign breast disease and the risk of breast cancer. N Engl J Med. 2005;353:229–37.
24. Coopey SB, Mazzola E, Buckley JM, Sharko J, Belli AK, Kim EM, Polubriaginof F, Parmigiani G, Garber JE, Smith BL, Gadd MA, Specht MC, Guidi AJ, Roche CA, Hughes KS. The role of chemoprevention in modifying the risk of breast cancer in women with atypical breast lesions. Breast Cancer Res Treat. 2012;136:627–33.
25. Menes TS, Kerlikowske K, Lange J, Jaffer S, Rosenberg R, Miglioretti DL. Subsequent breast cancer risk following diagnosis of atypical ductal hyperplasia on needle biopsy. JAMA Oncol. 2017;3:36–41.
26. Boughey JC, Hartmann LC, Anderson SS, Degnim AC, Vierkant RA, Reynolds CA, Frost MH, Pankratz VA. Evaluation of the Tyrer-Cuzick (International Breast Cancer Intervention Study) model for breast cancer risk prediction in women with atypical hyperplasia. J Clin Oncol. 2010;28:3591–6.
27. Pankratz VS, Hartmann LC, Degnim AC, Vierkant RA, Ghosh K, Vachon CM, Frost MH, Maloney SD, Reynolds C, Boughey JC. Assessment of the accuracy of the Gail model in women with atypical hyperplasia. J Clin Oncol. 2008;26:5374–9.
28. Hartmann LC, Radisky DC, Frost MH, Santen RJ, Vierkant RA, Benetti LL, Tarabishy Y, Ghosh K, Visscher DW, Degnim AC. Understanding the premalignant potential of atypical hyperplasia through its natural history: a longitudinal cohort study. Cancer Prev Res (Phila). 2014;7:211–7.
29. Degnim AC, Visscher DW, Berman HK, Frost MH, Sellers TA, Vierkant RA, Maloney SD, Pankratz VS, de Groen PC, Lingle WL, Ghosh K, Penheiter L, Tlsty T, Melton LJ 3rd, Reynolds CA, Hartmann LC. Stratification of breast cancer risk in women with atypia: a Mayo cohort study. J Clin Oncol. 2007;25:2671–7.
30. Degnim AC, Dupont WD, Radisky DC, Vierkant RA, Frank RD, Frost MH, Winham SJ, Sanders ME, Smith JR, Page DL, Hoskin TL, Vachon CM, Ghosh K, Hieken TJ, Denison LA, Carter JM, Hartmann LC, Visscher DW. Extent of atypical hyperplasia stratifies breast cancer risk in 2 independent cohorts of women. Cancer. 2016;122:2971–8.
31. King TA, Pilewskie M, Muhsen S, Patil S, Mautner SK, Park A, Oskar S, Guerini-Rocco E, Boafo C, Gooch JC, De Brot M, Reis-Filho JS, Morrogh M, Andrade VP, Sakr RA, Morrow M. Lobular carcinoma in situ: a 29-year longitudinal experience evaluating clinicopathologic features and breast cancer risk. J Clin Oncol. 2015;33:3945–52.
32. Antoniou AC, Casadei S, Heikkinen T, Barrowdale D, Pylkas K, Roberts J, Lee A, Subramanian D, De Leeneer K, Fostira F, Tomiak E, Neuhausen SL, Teo ZL, Khan S, Aittomaki K, Moilanen JS, Turnbull C, Seal S, Mannermaa A, Kallioniemi A, Lindeman GJ, Buys SS, Andrulis IL, Radice P, Tondini C, Manoukian S, Toland AE, Miron P, Weitzel JN, Domchek SM, Poppe B, Claes KB, Yannoukakos D, Concannon P, Bernstein JL, James PA, Easton DF, Goldgar DE, Hopper JL, Rahman N, Peterlongo P, Nevanlinna H, King MC, Couch FJ, Southey MC, Winqvist R, Foulkes WD, Tischkowitz M. Breast-cancer risk in families with mutations in PALB2. N Engl J Med. 2014;371:497–506.
33. Southey MC, Goldgar DE, Winqvist R, Pylkas K, Couch F, Tischkowitz M, Foulkes WD, Dennis J, Michailidou K, van Rensburg EJ, Heikkinen T, Nevanlinna H, Hopper JL, Dork T,

Claes KB, Reis-Filho J, Teo ZL, Radice P, Catucci I, Peterlongo P, Tsimiklis H, Odefrey FA, Dowty JG, Schmidt MK, Broeks A, Hogervorst FB, Verhoef S, Carpenter J, Clarke C, Scott RJ, Fasching PA, Haeberle L, Ekici AB, Beckmann MW, Peto J, Dos-Santos-Silva I, Fletcher O, Johnson N, Bolla MK, Sawyer EJ, Tomlinson I, Kerin MJ, Miller N, Marme F, Burwinkel B, Yang R, Guenel P, Truong T, Menegaux F, Sanchez M, Bojesen S, Nielsen SF, Flyger H, Benitez J, Zamora MP, Perez JI, Menendez P, Anton-Culver H, Neuhausen S, Ziogas A, Clarke CA, Brenner H, HArndt V, Stegmaier C, Brauch H, Bruning T, Ko YD, Muranen TA, Aittomaki K, Blomqvist C, Bogdanova NV, Antonenkova NN, Lindblom A, Margolin S, Mannermaa A, Kataja V, Kosma VM, Hartikainen JM, Spurdle AB, kConFab Investigators, Australian Ovarian Cancer Study Group, Wauters E, Smeets D, Beuselinck B, Floris G, Chang-Claude J, Rudolph A, Seibold P, Flesch-Janys D, Olson JE, Vachon C, Pankratz VS, McLean C, Haiman CA, Henderson BE, Schumacher F, Le Marchand L, Kristensen V, Alnaes GG, Zheng W, Hunter DJ, Lindstrom S, Hankinson SE, Kraft P, Andrulis I, Knight JA, Glendon G, Mulligan AM, Jukkola-Vuorinen A, Grip M, Kauppila S, Devilee P, Tollenaar RA, Seynaeve C, Hollestelle A, Garcia-Closas M, Figueroa J, Chanock SJ, Lissowska J, Czene K, Darabi H, Eriksson M, Eccles DM, Rafiq S, Tapper WJ, Gerty SM, Hooning MJ, Martens JW, Collee JM, Tilanus-Linthorst M, Hall P, Li J, Brand JS, Humphreys K, Cox A, Reed MW, Luccarini C, Baynes C, Dunning AM, Hamann U, Torres D, Ulmer HU, Rudiger T, Jakubowska A, Lubinski J, Jaworska K, Durda K, Slager S, Toland AE, Ambrosone CB, Yannoukakos D, Swerdlow A, Ashworth A, Orr N, Jones M, Gonzalez-Neira A, Pita G, Alonso MR, Alvarez N, Herrero D, Tessier DC, Vincent D, Bacot F, Simard J, Dumont M, Soucy P, Eeles R, Muir K, Wiklund F, Gronberg H, Schleutker J, Nordestgaard BG, Weischer M, Travis RC, Neal D, Conovan JL, Hamdy FC, Khaw KT, Stanford JL, Blot WJ, Thibodeau S, Schaid DJ, Kelley JL, Maier C, Kibel AS, Cybulski C, Cannon-Albright L, Butterbach K, Park J, Kaneva R, Batra J, Teixeira MR, Kote-Jarai Z, Olama AA, Benlloch S, Renner SP, Hartmann A, Hein A, Ruebner M, Lambrechts D, Van Nieuwenhuysen E, Vergote I, Lambretchs S, Doherty JA, Rossing MA, Nickels S, Eilber U, Wang-Gohrke S, Odunsi K, Sucheston-campbell LE, Friel G, Lurie G, Killeen JL, Wilkens LR, Goodman MT, Runnebaum I, Hillemanns PA, Pelttari LM, Butzow R, Modugno F, Edwards RP, Ness RB, Moysich KB, du Bois A, Heitz F, Harter P, Kommoss S, Karlan BY, Walsh C, Lester J, Jensen A, Kjaer SK, Hogdall E, Peissel B, Bonanni B, Bernard L, Goode EL, Fridley BL, Vierkant RA, Cunningham JM, Larson MC, Fogarty ZC, Kalli KR, Liang D, Lu KH, Hildebrandt MA, Wu X, Levine DA, Dao F, Bisogna M, Berchuck A, Iversen ES, Marks JR, Akushevich L, Cramer DW, Schildkraut J, Terry KL, Poole EM, Stampfer M, Tworoger SS, Bandera EV, Orlow I, Olson SH, Bjorge L, Salvesen HB, van Altena AM, Aben KK, Kiemeney LA, Massuger LF, Pejovic T, Bean Y, Brooks-Wilson A, Kelemen LE, Cook LS, Le ND, Gorski B, Gronwald J, Menkiszak J, Hogdall CK, Lundvall L, Nedergaard L, Engelholm SA, Dicks E, Tyrer J, Campabell I, McNeish I, Paul J, Siddiqui N, Glasspool R, Whittemore AS, Rothstein JH, Mcguire V, Sieh W, Cai H, Shu XO, Teten RT, Sutphen R, McLaughlin JR, Narod SA, Phelan CM, Monteiro AN, Fenstermacher D, Lin HY, Permuth JB, Sellers TA, Chen YA, Tsai YY, Chen Z, Gentry-Maharaj A, Gayther SA, Ramus SJ, Menon U, Wu A, Pearce CL, Van Den Berg D, Pike MC, Dansonka-Mieszkowska A, Plisiecka-Halasa J, Moes-Sosnowska J, Kupryjanczyk J, Pharoah PD, Song H, Winship I, Chenevix-Trench G, Giles GG, Tavtigian SV, Easton DV, Milne RL. PALB2, CHEK2 and ATM rare variants and cancer risk: data from COGS. J Med Genet. 2016;53:800–11.
34. Schmidt MK, Hogervorst F, van Hien R, Cornelissen S, Broeks A, Adank MA, Meijers H, Waisfisz Q, Hollestelle A, Schutte M, van den Ouweland A, Hooning M, Andrulis IL, Anton-Culver H, Antonenkova NN, Antoniou AC, Arndt V, Bermisheva M, Bogdanova NV, Bolla MK, Brauch H, Brenner H, Bruning T, Burwinkel B, Chang-Claude J, Chenevix-Trench G, Couch FJ, Cox A, Cross SS, Czene K, Dunning AM, Fasching PA, Figueroa J, Fletcher O, Flyger H, Galle E, Garcia-Closas M, Giles GG, Haeberle L, Hall P, Hillemanns P, Hopper JL, Kakubowska A, John EM, Jones M, Khusnutdinova E, Knight JA, Kosma VM, Kirstensen V, Lee A, Liindblom A, Lubinski J, Mannermaa A, Margolin S, Meindl A, Milne RL, Muranen TA, Newcomb PA, Offit K, Park-Simon TW, Peto J, Pharoah PD, Robson M, Rudolph A, Sawyer EJ, Schmutzler RK, Seynaeve C, Soens J, Southey MC, Spurdle AB, Surowy H,

Swerdlow A, Tollenaar RA, Tomlinson I, Trentham-Dietz A, Vachon C, Wang Q, Whittemore AS, Ziogas A, van der Kolk L, Vevanlinna H, Dork T, Bojesen S, Easton DF. Age- and tumor subtype-specific breast cancer risk estimates for CHEK2*1100delC carriers. J Clin Oncol. 2016;34:2750–60.
35. Fisher B, Costantino JP, Wickerham DL, Cecchini RS, Cronin WM, Robidoux A, Bevers TB, Kavanah MT, Atkins JN, Margolese RG, Runowicz CD, James JM, Ford LG, Wolmark N. Tamoxifen for the prevention of breast cancer: current status of the National Surgical Adjuvant Breast and Bowel Project P-1 study. J Natl Cancer Inst. 2005;97:1652–62.
36. Cuzick J, Sestak I, Forbes JF, Dowsett M, Knox J, Cawthorn S, Saunders C, Roche N, Mansel RE, von Minckwitz G, Bonanni B, Palva T, Howell A, IBIS-II Investigators. Anastrozole for prevention of breast cancer in high-risk postmenopausal women (IBIS-II): an international, double-blind, randomised placebo-controlled trial. Lancet. 2014;383:1041–8.
37. Vogel VG, Costantino JP, Wickerham DL, Cronin WM, Cecchini RS, Atkins JN, Bevers TB, Fehrenbacher L, Pajon ER, Wade JL 3rd, Robidoux A, Margolese RG, James J, Runowicz CD, Ganz PA, Reis SE, McCaskill-Stevens W, Ford LG, Jordan VC, Wolmark N, National Surgical Adjuvant Breast & Bowel Project. Update of the National Surgical Adjuvant Breast and Bowel Project Study of Tamoxifen and Raloxifene (STAR) P-2 trial: preventing breast cancer. Cancer Prev Res (Phila). 2010;3:696–706.
38. Goss PE, Ingle JN, Ales-Martinez JE, Cheung AM, Chlebowski RT, Wactawski-Wende J, McTiernan A, Robbins J, Johnson KC, Martin LW, Winquist E, Sarto GE, Garber JE, Fabian CJ, Pujol P, Maunsell E, Farmer P, Gelman KA, Tu D, Richardson H, NCIC CTG MAP.3 Study Investigators. Exemestane for breast-cancer prevention in postmenopausal women. N Engl J Med. 2011;364:2381–91.

The Nonsurgical Management of Ductal Carcinoma In Situ (DCIS)

12

Alastair M. Thompson

Natural History of DCIS

As described previously in Chap. 3, ductal carcinoma in situ (DCIS) is an intraductal epithelial proliferation with cellular atypia, not invading the basement membrane, and a non-obligate precursor of invasive breast cancer. DCIS has been recognized as prevalent in 8.9% of women in autopsy series of women who died of unrelated causes [1]. Literature describing the natural history of DCIS is rare and most reflects the prescreening era, where DCIS presented as symptomatic disease [2]. With the widespread adoption of breast screening, DCIS has increased from 1% to 2% of breast neoplasia to represent some 20% of screen detected lesions and 60,000 women diagnosed annually in the United States [3]. This has led to concerns regarding over diagnosis and potential overtreatment of DCIS [4], despite recent evidence that high rates of detection of DCIS through breast screening are associated with a reduction in the incidence of subsequent interval cancers [5]. Our contemporary understanding of the heterogeneous nature of DCIS has led some to propose that the word "carcinoma" should be stricken from the name altogether, in keeping with the change from the term lobular carcinoma in situ (LCIS) to lobular in situ neoplasia (LISN). A working group from the National Cancer Institute suggested that the word "cancer" to describe premalignant conditions such as DCIS should no longer be used, as this term almost mandates aggressive treatment to halt otherwise definite progression to a lethal disease process [6]. Advocates of the name change call upon studies linking patient anxiety and distress to overestimation of breast cancer risk [7, 8].

A recent series of women with DCIS diagnosed through the UK National Health Service (NHS) and the NHS breast screening program, followed 89 women with DCIS identified on core needle biopsy between 1998 and 2010 with a median

A. M. Thompson
Department of Breast Surgical Oncology, University of Texas MD Anderson Cancer Center, Houston, TX, USA
e-mail: AThompson1@mdanderson.org

follow-up of 5 years [9]. Invasive breast cancer developed in 29 (33%), with higher-grade DCIS developing invasive disease in a significantly higher proportion (48%) and more rapidly (median 38 months) than intermediate-grade (32% at median 60 months) or low-grade DCIS (18% at median 51 months). However, only one in seven of the women who died did so from breast cancer. Interestingly, subsequent invasive disease was significantly more common in DCIS where calcification was the predominant feature and, not unexpectedly, in younger women. Endocrine therapy did reduce the rate of subsequent invasive disease, consistent with clinical trial evidence following resection of DCIS in the NSABP B-24 [10] and UK DCIS trial [11], discussed further below. The authors concluded that surgical excision for high-grade DCIS should remain the treatment of choice, but for non-high-grade DCIS, the option of active surveillance within clinical trials should be considered [9].

Management of DCIS

The current management of DCIS largely mimics the treatment of invasive breast cancer with patient selection for surgery, for radiotherapy, choice of adjuvant endocrine therapy, and the potential for neoadjuvant therapy examined in therapeutic trials. Surgery remains the principle treatment for DCIS, with adjuvant radiation and endocrine therapy (for estrogen receptor (ER) positive DCIS) commonly used to prevent subsequent in situ or invasive events. NCCN guidelines [12] recommend lumpectomy (segmental or partial mastectomy) to achieve clear margins with irradiation as equivalent to mastectomy, with the decision between breast conservation and mastectomy for DCIS based on clinical, pathology, and patient factors. Improved locoregional control and event free survival can be achieved with the addition of adjuvant radiotherapy (in breast conservation) and endocrine therapies but come at the cost of additional morbidities.

Radiation Therapy

The Early Breast Cancer Trialists' Collaborative Group (EBCTCG) meta-analysis of randomized radiotherapy trials for DCIS demonstrated benefits for radiotherapy after breast conservation reducing the incidence of further invasive and DCIS events [13]. Risk stratification for 10-year ipsilateral breast events demonstrated a reduction in events for DCIS whether of size 1–20 mm or 20–50 mm or nuclear grades 1, 2 or, 3 [13]. Whole breast radiotherapy following breast conserving surgery reduced any local recurrence (DCIS and invasive breast cancer) from 28.1% to 12.9% and reduced the incidence of invasive disease recurrence from 11.0% to 5.0% at 10 years based on key trials such as the NSABP B17, NSABP B24 [14] and the United Kingdom/Australia New Zealand (UK/ANZ) [11] DCIS trials. While radiotherapy halves all types of in-breast recurrence, radiotherapy does not appear to alter long-term breast cancer-specific survival for those diagnosed purely with DCIS [12].

By contrast with treatment for invasive breast cancer, radiotherapy is only rarely used following mastectomy for DCIS [15].

While the extent of margin of clearance around DCIS has been hotly debated over the years, it is probable that at least a clear margin is required for the beneficial effects of breast radiotherapy to be realized. The dose and fractionation regimens for whole breast radiotherapy for DCIS after breast conservation mirror practices for invasive disease with a trend toward the use of hypo-fractionation and the potential added value of a boost to the tumor (DCIS) bed [16]. Whether less than whole breast irradiation to the DCIS resection bed, for example using intra-cavity radiotherapy techniques, is equivalent to external beam radiotherapy is currently unclear and should be practiced within the context of clinical studies [17]. The lower benefit of radiation therapy following BCT for DCIS in the elderly may also mirror invasive disease. Although avoidance of radiation is associated with increased risk for locoregional recurrence, omission of radiotherapy may appropriate for elderly patients with hormone receptor-positive disease on endocrine therapy, without impacting disease-free survival or overall survival [18, 19].

The selection of who receives breast radiotherapy after conservation surgery for DCIS appears to vary around the world. The tendency for high-grade DCIS to be associated with subsequent grade 3 invasive breast cancer, and the higher cumulative incidence of invasive disease [9], suggests that the biological behavior of DCIS is reflected in the histopathological appearances, as seen for DCIS recurrence following surgical resection [20]. Molecular triaging of DCIS to indicate a risk of future events has been developed with two tests available in the United States.

The Oncotype DCIS Score is a 12-gene assay, comprising proliferation, hormone receptor, and reference genes, that provides individualized 10-year risk of locoregional recurrence (of in situ and invasive disease) following treatment with breast-conserving surgery alone [21]. The DCIS Score was validated in two different patient populations as an independent predictor of recurrence risk beyond clinical and pathologic variables and may support the omission of radiation therapy in some patients with a low risk of recurrence [21, 22]. Critics believe that the rigid eligibility criteria for the landmark validation study, including 25 mm maximum size for low-/intermediate-grade DCIS, 10 mm for high-grade DCIS, and wide, 3 mm resection margins, historically high recurrence rates, and the timeframe when the patients were treated [21] limit the use of these results in current practice. However, subsequent validation in a more recent (1994–2003), geographically distinct series from Canada [22], together with clinical variables, may suggest a role for the DCIS Score in supporting decision-making for the use of radiotherapy following breast conservation.

In contrast to the distillation of data from invasive disease and redevelopment for DCIS that the Oncotype DCIS Score used, a more recently generated molecular test, the PreludeDx DCISionRT, has incorporated clinical variables with biomarkers ab initio. Clinical factors most impactful on subsequent further events (patient age, extent of lesion, margin status, palpability) together with discovery approaches to sets of biomarkers (hormone receptors, stress response genes, a cell cycle gene,

HER2 and Ki67) could allow prognostication and, unlike Oncotype DCIS, predict the benefits of breast radiotherapy. With multiple independent cross-validation studies in US and European series, the biological risk signature was most recently applied to the SweDCIS trial of breast conservation with or without radiotherapy conduced from 1987 to 1999 [23]. Using a cutoff score of ≤3 (low risk) versus >3 (elevated risk for further events), the biological risk signature predicted radiotherapy benefit for low risk (no benefit) and elevated risk (double the expected benefit for radiotherapy) in terms of subsequent invasive breast cancer [24].

While clinical application of these molecular-based scores for the management of DCIS is not widespread, they may inform clinicians and patients as to the likely benefits of adjuvant radiation therapy.

Endocrine Therapy

Following resection of ER-positive DCIS, the utilization of adjuvant endocrine therapy to prevent in-breast recurrence or invasive disease or prevent contralateral and distant breast events remains controversial. Indeed, not every DCIS is universally examined for ER status across the United States despite the NCCN guidelines recommending such testing [12]. Four large randomized clinical trials have addressed the relevance of adjuvant endocrine therapy for DCIS (Table 12.1).

In the NSABP B-24 trial for pre- and postmenopausal patients treated for DCIS by lumpectomy and adjuvant radiotherapy, tamoxifen reduced the risk of ipsilateral local recurrence by 30% and for contralateral breast cancer by 50% [25]. While the reduction in absolute risk at 5 years of any (invasive or noninvasive) breast cancer event was small (tamoxifen 8% vs placebo 13%), survival was not improved by the use of tamoxifen. The United Kingdom/Australia and New Zealand (UK/ANZ) trial examined the use of tamoxifen versus no adjuvant therapy following complete local excision of DCIS in the presence or absence of radiotherapy [11]. The trial demonstrated that, in the absence of radiotherapy, tamoxifen was associated with a 30% overall reduction in breast events through reduction in DCIS recurrence,

Table 12.1 Effects of endocrine therapy in DCIS trials

Trial	Endocrine therapy	Relative risk reduction to no endocrine therapy	Absolute reduction all events	Survival effect
NSABP B-24 [25]	Tamoxifen vs no endocrine therapy	Ipsilateral event 30%	5%	Not significant
		Contralateral event 50%		
UK/ANZ DCIS [11]	Tamoxifen vs no endocrine therapy	Overall reduction 30%	No benefit beyond radiotherapy	Not significant
NSABP B-35 [26]	Anastrozole vs tamoxifen	Not applicable	Anastrozole > tamoxifen, breast cancer-free interval	Not significant
IBIS II [27]	Anastrozole vs tamoxifen	Not applicable	Anastrozole = tamoxifen	Not significant

contralateral DCIS, and invasive disease events. Tamoxifen had no added benefit in patients who received radiotherapy and did not prevent ipsilateral invasive recurrence. Survival was not impacted by radiotherapy or tamoxifen in the UK/ANZ DCIS trial, with breast cancer accounting for only 20% of all deaths [11]. These two key trials suggest modest additional benefit of tamoxifen over a combination of breast conservation and breast radiotherapy to reduce local recurrence [11, 25].

More recently, two large randomized trials of the aromatase inhibitor anastrozole versus tamoxifen in postmenopausal women with DCIS have yielded conflicting data. In NSABP B-35 [26], which enrolled 3104 postmenopausal women who had undergone lumpectomy to clear margins and adjuvant radiation for DCIS, anastrozole treatment was associated with an improvement in breast cancer-free interval compared with tamoxifen (HR 0.73 [95% CI 0.56–0.96], p = 0.023), although disease-free survival was the same at 120 months (HR 0.89 [95% CI 0.75–1.07], p = 0.21) [26]. Among postmenopausal women under the age of 60 years (n = 1447), anastrozole demonstrated improvements in breast cancer-free interval HR 0.53 (95% CI 0.35–0.080) and disease-free survival HR 0.69 (95% CI 0.51–0.93), compared to tamoxifen [26]. In contrast, the International Breast Intervention Study (IBIS) II trial [27] of 2980 postmenopausal women who had undergone lumpectomy for DCIS to clear margins ± radiation failed to demonstrate an improvement with anastrozole compared to tamoxifen (HR 0.89 [95% CI 0.64–1.23], p = 0.49).

Overall, the potential for a reduction in contralateral and possibly local recurrence of DCIS with endocrine therapy should be balanced with the potential side effects of tamoxifen or anastrozole (Table 12.2) and impacts on quality of life. The side effects of tamoxifen and anastrozole are significantly different (Table 12.2) although the mortality within the trial was very similar with 33/1499 deaths

Table 12.2 Comparison of the side effects of anastrozole versus tamoxifen used as adjuvant therapy for DCIS in the IBIS II trial [27]

	Anastrozole number of patients (%)	Tamoxifen number of patients (%)	Odds ratio (95% confidence intervals)	Probability value
Musculoskeletal side effect				
Fractures	128 (8.5%)	99 (6.6%)	1.36 (1.03–1.81)	0.03
Arthralgia	832 (56.6%)	729 (48.3%)	1.41 (1.21–1.63)	<0.001
Joint stiffness	74 (5.0%)	35 (2.3%)	2.24 (1.46–3.47)	<0.001
Osteoporosis	97 (6.6%)	54 (3.6%)	1.91 (1.34–2.73)	<0.001
Cardiovascular side effect				
Deep venous thrombosis (no embolism)	7 (0.5%)	17 (1.1%)	0.42 (0.15–1.07)	0.05
Cerebrovascular accident	14 (0.9%)	3 (0.2%)	4.83 (1.34–26.27)	0.006
Hot flashes	818 (55.6%)	899 (59.6%)	0.85 (0.73–0.99)	0.03
Other side effect				
Non-breast cancer	60 (4.0%)	72 (4.8%)	0.85 (0.59–1.22)	0.4
Vaginal dryness	189 (12.8%)	159 (10.5%)	1.25 (1.00–1.58)	0.047
Hypercholesterolemia	43 (2.9%)	11 (0.7%)	4.11 (2.07–8.86)	<0.001

(one from breast cancer) in the anastrozole arm and 36/1489 (three from breast cancer) in the tamoxifen arm [27]. Furthermore, the issue of reduced adherence to endocrine therapy in the setting of DCIS – only 70% of women in the IBIS II [27] trial were still taking their endocrine agent at 5 years – if extrapolated to the wider community, would reduce the impact of adjuvant endocrine therapy for DCIS.

Neoadjuvant Therapy for DCIS

Neoadjuvant therapy has become a standard of care for downstaging invasive breast cancer and hence reducing the extent of surgery. However, the neoadjuvant approach for DCIS is less well developed. For ER-positive DCIS, targeting the estrogen receptor preoperatively has conceptual attractions, and the CALCB 40903 trial of 6 months of neoadjuvant letrozole tested the potential benefits of letrozole in this setting [28]. In 68 assessable patients, the MRI volume, but not the mammographic tumor diameter, significantly decreased with neoadjuvant endocrine therapy. For HER2-positive DCIS, a number of trials have used HER2-targeting agents including trastuzumab [29] or lapatinib [30] to test the feasibility of such approaches. Neoadjuvant therapy for DCIS may not be standard of care at the present time, but it is an important consideration when developing preoperative approaches and potential prevention strategies interrogating the biology of DCIS. At the present time, if there is a clinical need to defer conventional surgical intervention for DCIS, neoadjuvant endocrine therapy for ER-positive DCIS may provide a useful option.

Nonsurgical Management of DCIS

Approaches to managing DCIS have largely been derived from the treatment of invasive breast cancer, despite the probability that most women diagnosed with DCIS will not die from breast cancer [31]. Given the concerns regarding overtreatment of DCIS [4], the excellent long-term survival of women with DCIS [31, 32], and evidence from studies of the natural history of DCIS [9], opportunities for the nonsurgical management of DCIS have gained traction. While most agree that surgical excision for high-grade DCIS should remain the treatment of choice, for intermediate- and low-grade DCIS, the option of active surveillance has been proposed.

Active Surveillance

A small proportion of women in the United States (~1.5%) decline surgery and opt for surveillance with the potential addition of endocrine therapy if the DCIS is ER-positive. For low-grade DCIS, the 10-year disease-specific survival (DSS) was not significantly different between those undergoing surgical resection (DSS 98.8% in 8866 women) and those who did not have surgery (DSS 98.6% in 192 women) [32]. In support of nonsurgical management, prospective, population-based data suggests that segmental mastectomy or modified radical mastectomy (including for women with DCIS) may be associated with surprisingly high levels of chronic pain, disability, and psychological distress, often resistant to management, 4 and 9 months after breast surgery [33, 34]. These factors, along with the exceptional long-term survival for women with DCIS, have led some to question the need for surgery for all women with DCIS. In parallel, randomized trials of prostate cancer, thyroid neoplasia, and more recently small renal cancers (<2 cm) have employed active surveillance in place of more radical therapy. For prostate cancer, the Predict trial randomized 1643 men between active surveillance (based on Prostate-Specific Antigen (PSA) levels) and radical prostatectomy or radiotherapy. At a median follow-up of 10 years, survival in the active surveillance arm was not significantly different to conventional, radical therapy [35]. Similarly, a randomized trial of 1433 men, utilizing prostate biopsy with median follow-up of 4 years, identified active surveillance as a preferred strategy for men with low-risk prostate cancer [36]. Similar evidence emerging for other types of cancer suggests that active surveillance for selected patients may also be feasible in the setting of DCIS.

DCIS (like invasive breast cancer) exhibits a spectrum of phenotypic behaviors ranging from indolence through likely progression to invasive disease. Thus, for nonsurgical management of DCIS, targeting DCIS at low risk for progression as the focus for medical management alone is attractive. Internationally, there are three randomized and one single-arm trial aiming to determine the effect of nonsurgical management of low-risk DCIS. The Comparison of Operative to Monitoring and Endocrine Therapy (COMET) for low-risk DCIS trial [37] in the United States, the LOw-RISk DCIS (LORIS) trial [38] in the United Kingdom, and the management of LOw-gRaDe DCIS (LORD) trial [39] in mainland Europe are randomized studies comparing active surveillance to surgically based management. A fourth trial, the LOw-Risk DCIS with Endocrine Therapy Alone – TAmoxifen (LORETTA) trial, is a single-arm trial of no surgical intervention but tamoxifen treatment for ER-positive DCIS run through the Japan Clinical Oncology Group (JCOG 1505) [40]. The COMET and LORIS trials have already demonstrated the feasibility of randomizing patients between surgical and nonsurgical management. The US-based COMET trial, funded through the Patient Centered Outcomes Research Institute (PCORI) and run via the Alliance Co-operative Group, not only randomizes patients between guideline concordant care (surgery, with or without radiotherapy and/or endocrine therapy) and active surveillance (with the option of endocrine therapy) but also seeks to monitor outcomes in those not participating in the trial. Identification of subsequent invasive breast cancer is the primary outcome for both COMET and LORIS, although patient-reported outcomes, other breast outcomes, and health service impacts will also be studied and captured. There are subtle differences between the currently recruiting trials (COMET, LORIS, LORD, LORETTA) in terms of patient characteristics, imaging, and pathology features required for entry into the trial. There are also differences between the active surveillance arms, with mammographic surveillance every 6 months in COMET but every 12 months in LORIS and LORD, and the requirement for tamoxifen in LORETTA and option of endocrine therapy in COMET and LORIS but not LORD. The intent is for these trials to ultimately allow meta-analysis and thus to provide high-level guidance regarding the management options for DCIS.

Controversies for Nonsurgical Approaches

Understandable concern in the conservative management of clinically low-risk DCIS (active surveillance, endocrine therapy, observation alone) is the failure to identify the presence of invasive carcinoma at the time of diagnosis and the potential for progression of DCIS to invasive breast cancer. A meta-analysis examining 7350 cases of DCIS identified by core needle biopsy found invasive cancer at excision in 1736, thus underestimating 25.9% of cases [41]. More recent data from a national screening program with quality assurance measures in place for imaging and pathology suggest that the figure may still be around 20% [42]. Predictive variables associated with underestimating invasive disease include the presence of a palpable lesion, mammographic mass, the use of a smaller gauge biopsy device (14G vs 11G), and higher BIRADS categorization. Subsequent studies evaluating upgrade rates further identify seemingly cumulative risk factors [43] and have led to the creation of predictive nomograms [44, 45].

To evaluate the safety of observation in DCIS, a cohort of 296 patients who met some of the eligibility criteria for the LORIS trial were retrospectively identified at a single cancer center [46]. A majority of patients (82%) had intermediate-grade DCIS on core biopsy (likely to exclude them from the LORIS trial on central pathology review), though over half (62%) of the core biopsies in the study were performed with a vacuum-assisted 8-9G core needle. While this retrospective review did not mirror LORIS precisely, 20% of patients in this single center retrospective review were found to have invasive carcinoma on final pathology. Intermediate-grade DCIS was a statistically significant factor; 23% of intermediate-grade patients were upgraded based on final pathology compared to only 7% in low-grade DCIS, probably more reflective of the clinical trial underway. In a contemporary cohort of 307 patients diagnosed with DCIS by vacuum-assisted core biopsy, 81 met the eligibility criteria for the active randomized surveillance trials (COMET, LORIS, and LORD) [47]. Overall upgrade rate to invasive disease was 17% (53 of 307). However, upgrade rates in patients who met trial inclusion criteria were more reassuringly 6% for COMET, 7% for LORIS, and 10% for LORD, which is close to the 7% in low-grade DCIS previously suggested [46]. All upgraded cases were node negative, hormone receptor-positive (ER, PR), and HER2 non-amplified, indicating a traditionally favorable subset in terms of long-term survival. This provides strong reassurance that, using the current active surveillance trials criteria, any potential for missed, upgraded (invasive) lesions would likely not impact on patient survival.

Patient Reported Outcome Measures

A multitude of psychological, social, and physical stresses accompany the diagnosis and subsequent treatment of breast cancer. Anxiety, depression, fear of recurrence, pain, fatigue, body image issues, and sexual dysfunction have been found to affect quality of life and even long-term overall survival in patients with invasive breast cancer [48–50]. A recent meta-analysis of patient-reported outcomes identified these treatment-associated physical, mental, and sexual health issues also pertain to women with a diagnosis of DCIS [51]. Prospective randomized trials aiming to identify low-risk DCIS that can be safely managed with active surveillance may allow some women to safely avoid surgery and the associated physical and psychosocial morbidity [33, 34, 48–51].

Future Prospects

Treatment for DCIS, including surgery, radiation, and/or drug therapies, has largely followed evidence-based treatment guidelines utilized for invasive breast cancer. Radiotherapy and endocrine agents reduce locoregional events, without any apparent impact on survival. Trials are seeking to determine whether DCIS deemed low risk for progression may be managed without surgical intervention, relying on active surveillance with or without medical therapy to control breast neoplasia. Alternative strategies harnessing the immune system response using vaccination are currently being investigated [52, 53]. These could offer promising insights and novel treatment approaches to appropriately selected women. A key to determining how best to manage DCIS in the future is the global activity of randomized clinical trials and research activity now underway, though this will likely take some 5–10 years to produce clinically actionable data. In the future, not all women diagnosed with DCIS will require surgery; refining who those individuals are is a challenge of our times.

References

1. Welch HG, Black W. Using autopsy series to estimate the disease "reservoir" for ductal carcinoma in situ of the breast: how much more breast cancer can we find? Ann Intern Med. 1997;127:1023–8. https://doi.org/10.7326/0003-4819-127-11-199712010.
2. Erbas B, Provenzano E, Armes J, Gertig D. The natural history of ductal carcinoma in situ of the breast: a review. Breast Cancer Res Treat. 2005;97:135–44. https://doi.org/10.1007/s10549-005-9101-z.
3. Virnig BA, Tuttle TM, Shamliyan T, Kane RL. Ductal carcinoma in situ of the breast: a systematic review of incidence, treatment, and outcomes. JNCI J Natl Cancer Inst. 2010;102:170–8. https://doi.org/10.1093/jnci/djp482.
4. Independent UK Panel on Breast Cancer Screening. The benefits and harms of breast cancer screening: an independent review. Lancet. 2012;380:1778–86. https://doi.org/10.1016/S0140-6736(12)61611-0.
5. Duffy SW, Dibden A, Michalopoulos D, Offman J, Parmar D, Jenkins J, et al. Screen detection of ductal carcinoma in situ and subsequent incidence of invasive interval breast cancers: a retrospective population-based study. Lancet Oncol. 2016;17:109–14. https://doi.org/10.1016/S1470-2045(15)00446-5.
6. Esserman LJ, Thompson IM Jr, Reid B. Overdiagnosis and overtreatment in cancer: an opportunity for improvement. JAMA. 2013;310(8):797–8.
7. Partridge AH, Elmore JG, Saslow D, et al. Challenges in ductal carcinoma in situ risk communication and decision-making: report from an American Cancer Society and National Cancer Institute workshop. CA Cancer J Clin. 2012;62(3):203–10. https://doi.org/10.3322/caac.21140. Epub 2012 Apr 4.

8. Partridge A, Adloff K, Blood E, et al. Risk perceptions and psychosocial outcomes of women with ductal carcinoma in situ: longitudinal results from a cohort study. J Natl Cancer Inst. 2008;100(4):243–51. https://doi.org/10.1093/jnci/djn010. Epub 2008 Feb 12.
9. Maxwell AJ, Clements K, Hilton B, Dodwell DJ, Evans A, Kearins O, Pinder SE, Thomas J, Wallis MG, Thompson AM. Risk factors for the development of invasive cancer in unresected ductal carcinoma in situ. EJSO. 2018. https://doi.org/10.1016/j.ejso.2017.12.007.
10. Fisher B, Dignam J, Wolmark N, Wickerham DL, Fisher ER, Mamounas E, et al. Tamoxifen in treatment of intraductal breast cancer: National Surgical Adjuvant Breast and Bowel Project B-24 randomised controlled trial. Lancet. 1999;353:1993–2000.
11. Cuzick J, Sestak I, Pinder SE, et al. Effect of tamoxifen and radiotherapy in women with locally excised ductal carcinoma in situ: long-term results from the UK/ANZ DCIS trial. Lancet Oncol. 2011;12(1):21–9. https://doi.org/10.1016/S1470-2045(10)70266-7. Epub 2010 Dec 7.
12. National Comprehensive Cancer Network. Incorporated. https://www.nccn.org/patients/guidelines/stage_0_breast/. Accessed 10 Feb 2018.
13. Correa C, McGale P, Taylor C, et al. Overview of the randomized trials of radiotherapy in ductal carcinoma in situ of the breast. J Natl Cancer Inst Monogr. 2010;2010(41):162–77. https://doi.org/10.1093/jncimonographs/lgq039.
14. Wapnir IL, Dignam JJ, Fisher B, et al. Long-term outcomes of invasive ipsilateral breast tumor recurrences after lumpectomy in NSABP B-17 and B-24 randomized clinical trials for DCIS. J Natl Cancer Inst. 2011;103(6):478–88. https://doi.org/10.1093/jnci/djr027. Epub 2011 Mar 11.
15. Clements K, Dodwell D, Lawrence G, Ball G, Francis A, Pinder S, Sawyer E, Wallis M, Thompson AM, Sloane Project Steering Group. Radiotherapy after mastectomy for screen-detected ductal carcinoma in situ. Eur J Surg Oncol. 41(10):1406–10. 10/2015. e-Pub 8/2015. PMID: 26314790.
16. Romestaing P, Lehingue Y, Carrie C, et al. Role of a 10-Gy boost in the conservative treatment of early breast cancer: results of a randomized clinical trial in Lyon, France. J Clin Oncol. 1997;15(3):963–8.
17. Correa C, Harris EE, Leonardi MC, Smith BD, Taghian AG, Thompson AM, White J, Harris JR. Accelerated partial breast irradiation: executive summary for the update of an ASTRO evidence-based consensus statement. Pract Radiat Oncol. 2017;7(2):73–9. https://doi.org/10.1016/j.prro.2016.09.007. Epub 2016 Sep 17.
18. Kunkler IH, Williams LJ, Jack WJ, et al. Breast-conserving surgery with or without irradiation in women aged 65 years or older with early breast cancer (PRIME II): a randomised controlled trial. Lancet Oncol. 2015;16(3):266–73. https://doi.org/10.1016/S1470-2045(14)71221-5. Epub 2015 Jan 28.
19. Hughes KS, Schnaper LA, Bellon JR, et al. Lumpectomy plus tamoxifen with or without irradiation in women age 70 years or older with early breast cancer: long-term follow-up of CALGB 9343. J Clin Oncol. 2013;31(19):2382–7. https://doi.org/10.1200/JCO.2012.45.2615. Epub 2013 May 20.
20. Wallis MG, Clements K, Kearins O, Ball G, Macartney J, Lawrence GM. The effect of DCSI grade on rate, type and time to recurrence after 15 years of follow-up screen-detected DCIS. Br J Cancer. 2012;106:1611–7.
21. Solin LJ, Gray R, Baehner FL, et al. A multigene expression assay to predict local recurrence risk for ductal carcinoma in situ of the breast. J Natl Cancer Inst. 2013;105(10):701–10. https://doi.org/10.1093/jnci/djt067. Epub 2013 May 2.
22. Rakovitch E, Nofech-Mozes S, Hanna W, et al. A population-based validation study of the DCIS score predicting recurrence risk in individuals treated by breast-conserving surgery alone. Breast Cancer Res Treat. 2015;152(2):389–98. https://doi.org/10.1007/s10549-015-3464-6. Epub 2015 Jun 29.
23. Warberg F, Garmo H, Emdin S, et al. Effect of radiotherapy after breast-conserving surgery for ductal carcinoma in situ: 20 years follow-up in the randomized SweDCIS trial. J Clin Oncol. 2014;32:3613–8.

24. Warberg F, Garmo H, Folkvaljon Y, et al. A validation of DCIS biological risk profile in randomised study for radiation therapy with 20 year follow up (SweDCIS). In: San Antonio breast cancer symposium GS5-08, 2017 Dec 5–9; San Antonio, USA.
25. Fisher B, Land S, Mamounas E, et al. Prevention of invasive breast cancer in women with ductal carcinoma in situ: an update of the National Surgical Adjuvant Breast and Bowel Project experience. Semin Oncol. 2001;28(4):400–18.
26. Margolese RG, Cecchini RS, Julian TB, et al. Anastrozole versus tamoxifen in postmenopausal women with ductal carcinoma in situ undergoing lumpectomy plus radiotherapy (NSABP B-35): a randomised, double-blind, phase 3 clinical trial. Lancet. 2016;387(10021):849–56. https://doi.org/10.1016/S0140-6736(15)01168-X. Epub 2015 Dec 11.
27. Cuzick J, Sestak I, Forbes JF, et al. Anastrozole for prevention of breast cancer in high-risk postmenopausal women (IBIS-II): an international, double-blind, randomised placebo-controlled trial. Lancet. 2014;383(9922):1041–8. https://doi.org/10.1016/S0140-6736(13)62292-8. Epub 2013 Dec 12.
28. Hwang ES, Duong S, Bedrosian I, et al. Primary endocrine therapy for ER-positive ductal carcinoma in situ (DCIS) CALGB 40903 (Alliance). In: San Antonio breast cancer symposium GS5-05, 2017 Dec 5–9; San Antonio, USA.
29. Neoadjuvant Herceptin for Ductal Carcinoma In Situ of the Breast. ClinicalTrials.gov Identifier:NCT00496808.
30. Neoadjuvant Trial of Lapatinib for the Treatment of Women With DCIS Breast Cancer. ClinicalTrials.gov Identifier:NCT00555152.
31. Narod SA, Iqbal J, Giannakeas V, et al. Breast cancer mortality after a diagnosis of ductal carcinoma in situ. JAMA Oncol. 2015;1(7):888–96. https://doi.org/10.1001/jamaoncol.2015.2510.
32. Sagara Y, Mallory MA, Wong S, Aydogan F, Desantis S, Barry WT, et al. Survival benefit of breast surgery for low-grade ductal carcinoma in situ. JAMA Surg. 2015;150:739. https://doi.org/10.1001/jamasurg.2015.0876.
33. Bruce J, Thornton AJ, Scott NW, et al. Chronic preoperative pain and psychological robustness predict acute postoperative pain outcomes after surgery for breast cancer. Br J Cancer. 2012;107(6):937–46. https://doi.org/10.1038/bjc.2012.341. Epub 2012 Jul 31.
34. Bruce J, Thornton AJ, Powell R, et al. Psychological, surgical, and sociodemographic predictors of pain outcomes after breast cancer surgery: a population-based cohort study. Pain. 2014;155(2):232–43. https://doi.org/10.1016/j.pain.2013.09.028. Epub 2013 Oct 4.
35. Hamdy FC, Donovan JL, Lane JA, et al. 10-year outcomes after monitoring, surgery, or radiotherapy for localised prostate cancer. N Engl J Med. 2016;375:1415–24.
36. Leapman MS, Cowan JE, Nguyen HG, et al. Active surveillance in younger men with prostate cancer. J Clin Oncol. 2017;35:1898–904.
37. COMET. http://www.pcori.org/research-results/2016/comparison-operative-versus-medical-endocrine-therapy-low-risk-dcis-comet. Accessed 10 Feb 2018.
38. LORIS A phase III trial of surgery versus active monitoring for low risk ductal carcinoma in situ (DCIS). http://www.birmingham.ac.uk/research/activity/mds/trials/crctu/trials/loris/index.aspx Accessed 10 Feb 2018.
39. EORTC LORD. http://www.eortc.org/research-groups/breast-cancer-group/ongoing-and-future-projects/ Accessed 24 Feb 2017.
40. Kanbayashi C, Iwata H. Current approach ad future perspective for ductal carcinoma in situ of the breast. Jpn J Clin Oncol. 2017;47(8):671–7. https://doi.org/10.1093/jjco/hyx059.
41. Brennan ME, Turner RM, Ciatto S, et al. Ductal carcinoma in situ at core-needle biopsy: meta-analysis of underestimation and predictors of invasive breast cancer. Radiology. 2011;260(1):119–28. https://doi.org/10.1148/radiol.11102368. Epub 2011 Apr 14.
42. Nicholson S, Hanby A, Clements K, et al. Variations in the management of the axilla in screen-detected ductal carcinoma in situ: evidence from the UK NHS breast screening programme audit of screen detected DCIS. Eur J Surg Oncol. 2015;41(1):86–93. https://doi.org/10.1016/j.ejso.2014.09.003. Epub 2014 Oct 16.

43. Doebar SC, de Monye C, Stoop H, et al. Ductal carcinoma in situ diagnosed by breast needle biopsy: predictors of invasion in the excision specimen. Breast. 2016;27:15–21. https://doi.org/10.1016/j.breast.2016.02.014. Epub 2016 Mar 20.
44. Park HS, Kim HY, Park S, et al. A nomogram for predicting underestimation of invasiveness in ductal carcinoma in situ diagnosed by preoperative needle biopsy. Breast. 2013;22(5):869–73. https://doi.org/10.1016/j.breast.2013.03.009. Epub 2013 Apr 17.
45. Lee SK, Yang JH, Woo SY, et al. Nomogram for predicting invasion in patients with a preoperative diagnosis of ductal carcinoma in situ of the breast. Br J Surg. 2013;100(13):1756–63. https://doi.org/10.1002/bjs.9337.
46. Pilewskie M, Stempel M, Rosenfeld H, et al. Do LORIS trial eligibility criteria identify a ductal carcinoma in situ patient population at low risk of upgrade to invasive carcinoma? Ann Surg Oncol. 2016;23(11):3487–93. https://doi.org/10.1245/s10434-016-5268-2. Epub 2016 May 12.
47. Grimm LJ, Ryser MD, Partridge AH, Thompson AM, Thomas JS, Wesseling J, Hwang ES. Surgical upstaging rates for vacuum assisted biopsy proven DCIS: implications for active surveillance trials. Ann Surg Oncol. 24(12):3534–40. 11/2017. e-Pub 8/2017. PMID: 28795370.
48. Bower JE, Ganz PA, Desmond KA, et al. Fatigue in breast cancer survivors: occurrence, correlates, and impact on quality of life. J Clin Oncol. 2000;18(4):743–53.
49. Hawley ST, Janz NK, Griffith KA, et al. Recurrence risk perception and quality of life following treatment of breast cancer. Breast Cancer Res Treat. 2017;161(3):557–65. https://doi.org/10.1007/s10549-016-4082-7. Epub 2016 Dec 21.
50. Montazeri A. Health-related quality of life in breast cancer patients: a bibliographic review of the literature from 1974 to 2007. J Exp Clin Cancer Res. 2008;27:32. https://doi.org/10.1186/1756-9966-27-32.
51. King MT, Winters ZE, Olivotto IA, et al. Patient-reported outcomes in ductal carcinoma in situ: a systematic review. Eur J Cancer. 2017;71:95–108. https://doi.org/10.1016/j.ejca.2016.09.035. Epub 2016 Dec 15.
52. A HER-2/neu pulsed DC1 vaccine for patients With DCIS. ClinicalTrials.gov Identifier:NCT00107211.
53. A randomized trial of HER-2/neu pulsed DC1 vaccine for patients with DCIS. ClinicalTrials.gov Identifier:NCT02061332.

Surgical Treatment of Ductal Carcinoma In Situ

13

Meghan R. Flanagan and Kimberly J. Van Zee

Introduction

Historically, ductal carcinoma in situ (DCIS), or intraductal carcinoma, was a rare entity. With the advent of widespread routine screening mammography, the incidence has increased dramatically from 5.8 per 100,000 women in 1975 to 30.7 per 100,000 women in 2012 [1], such that it now comprises approximately 25% of all breast cancers diagnosed in the United States [2]. Standard treatment options include mastectomy, breast-conserving surgery (BCS), and BCS with adjuvant radiation therapy (RT) or endocrine therapy, or both. Local recurrence varies by treatment type, with meta-analyses finding 10-year rates of 2–3% with mastectomy, 13% after BCS+RT, and 28% after BCS alone [3, 4]. Approximately half of all local recurrences after BCS with or without RT are invasive, and there is a significantly increased risk of breast cancer mortality after experiencing an invasive recurrence [5, 6]. However, overall and disease-free survival following a diagnosis of DCIS are generally excellent with breast cancer-related mortality of 2–3% at over 10 years of follow-up regardless of treatment type [3, 4]. Thus, the overall goals of treatment are to prevent local recurrence and maintain high rates of disease-free survival while preserving quality of life.

Natural History

DCIS is the proliferation of transformed ductal epithelial cells contained within the basement membrane of the ducts of the breast. Autopsy studies have shown a prevalence of undiagnosed DCIS in about 9% of women [7], which is not unexpected given the long clinical course of breast cancer development and progression.

M. R. Flanagan · K. J. Van Zee (✉)
Breast Service, Department of Surgery, Memorial Sloan Kettering Cancer Center, New York, NY, USA
e-mail: flanagam@mskcc.org; vanzeek@mskcc.org

© Springer International Publishing AG, part of Springer Nature 2018
F. Amersi, K. Calhoun (eds.), *Atypical Breast Proliferative Lesions and Benign Breast Disease*, https://doi.org/10.1007/978-3-319-92657-5_13

Evidence that DCIS is a precursor to invasive cancer includes the coexistence of DCIS within an invasive carcinoma, the nearly identical genetic abnormalities in DCIS and invasive carcinoma, and the observation that even after treatment with complete surgical excision with or without RT, half of all local recurrences of DCIS are invasive. Furthermore, even after complete excision of DCIS, there is a higher risk of ipsilateral invasive cancer as compared to contralateral invasive cancer [3], and incomplete excision (i.e., positive margins) is associated with a doubling of invasive recurrence [5]. These observations provide further evidence that DCIS can progress to invasive cancer.

Although there are no prospective studies of the natural history of DCIS, there are three reports of "benign" excisional biopsy specimens that upon rereview decades later were found to contain DCIS. Rosen et al. and Sanders et al. both reported long-term outcomes of unrecognized and untreated low-grade DCIS lesions and found that 52% and 39% of the women, respectively, developed ipsilateral invasive cancer at an average of 10–15 years after excisional biopsy [8, 9]. Collins et al. found 13 cases of DCIS that were undiagnosed in excisional biopsy specimens, of which 6 (46%) were later diagnosed with ipsilateral invasive cancer an average of 9 years after the excisional biopsy [10]. The odds of developing invasive breast cancer among these women with missed DCIS was 13.5 (95% CI: 3.7–49.7). Because the DCIS was not recognized, there is no information on the margin status of the excisional biopsy specimen with respect to the DCIS. Therefore, it is possible that the unrecognized DCIS may have been completely excised in some of these patients, which suggests that the proportion of women with DCIS that would develop invasive cancer without excision may be higher.

A recent report of SEER data with a mean follow-up of 7.5 years found that over half (57%) of 146 women who did not undergo a surgical procedure for DCIS developed an ipsilateral invasive cancer [11]. Indirect evidence that DCIS progresses to invasive cancer comes from population-based studies correlating a rise in screening mammography and increased detection and treatment of DCIS and early invasive cancers with decreasing rates of invasive breast cancer and breast-cancer associated mortality [12]. This is consistent with the time course observed in prospective studies that show local recurrences of DCIS treated with BCS continuing even after more than a decade of follow-up [5, 6, 13, 14]. In a recent study of over five million women screened in the United Kingdom (UK) between 2003 and 2007, it was estimated that one invasive interval cancer was prevented with every three screen-detected cases of DCIS [15]. These findings contribute to the argument that DCIS can and does progress to invasive cancer and that detection and treatment reduce the rate of invasive breast cancer.

Mastectomy

Prior to the publication of randomized trials evaluating breast-conserving surgery for invasive breast carcinoma in the 1980s, standard treatment of all breast cancer, including DCIS, was mastectomy. Currently, it remains a surgical option for women with DCIS.

Table 13.1 Outcomes following mastectomy for ductal carcinoma in situ

Reference	Time period	Patients (N)	Median follow-up (years)	Local recurrence[a] N (%)	Invasive recurrence N (%)	Regional recurrence N (%)	Distant recurrence N (%)
Retrospective cohort studies							
Cutuli [16]	1985–1992	145	6.3	3 (2.0%)	3 (100%)	0	2 (1.4%)[b]
Carlson [17]	1991–2003	223	6.9	7 (3.1%)	6 (86%)	2 (0.9%)	2 (0.9%)[c]
Meijnen [18]	1986–2005	294	6.2	3 (0.9%)	2 (67%)	NR	1 (0.3%)[c]
Tunon de Lara [19]	1971–2001	342	9.8	7 (2.0%)	NR	NR	NR
Kelley [20]	1979–?	496	6.9	9 (2.0%)	9 (80%)	0	2 (0.4%)[c]
Owen [21]	1990–1999	637	12.0	12 (1.7%)	11 (92%)	2 (0.3%)	7 (1.1%)[c]
Meta-analyses							
Boyages [22]	1970–1990	1574	6.7	25 (1.4%)	19 (76%)	NR	NR
Stuart [4]	1940–2006	936	>10 years	22 (2.4%)	19 (86%)	NR	1.3%

NR, not reported
[a]Ipsilateral chest wall
[b]Not preceded by local recurrence
[c]Preceded by local recurrence

Several large retrospective studies have reported low rates of local (0.9–3.1%), regional (0.3–0.9%), and distant (0.3–1.4%) recurrence following mastectomy for DCIS, with median follow-up ranging from 6 to 12 years (Table 13.1) [16–21]. Local chest wall events are the most common first recurrence, and most are invasive (>80%). Studies have reported a mean time to disease recurrence of 3.3–5.6 years [17, 18, 20]. A few studies reported axillary management, which consisted of axillary lymph node dissection in approximately two-thirds of women. In a meta-analysis by Boyages et al. including 1574 patients who underwent mastectomy for DCIS, 25 (1.4%) were found to have a local recurrence with an average follow-up of 6.7 years [22]. Of the 25 recurrences, 76% were invasive. In an updated meta-analysis including studies published between 1974 and 2013 with at least 10-year follow-up, the local recurrence rate was 2.6% at 10 years, 86% of which were invasive. Breast cancer-specific mortality after mastectomy was 1.3% at 10 years [4].

Mastectomy is an effective treatment for DCIS with low rates of local recurrence and mortality. Current indications for the use of mastectomy in DCIS patients are the same as for invasive cancer and include multicentricity, the inability to completely resect all disease with clear margins while preserving a cosmetically acceptable appearance, and patient preference.

Breast-Conserving Surgery

Six randomized trials proved that mastectomy and breast-conserving treatment (BCT) resulted in equivalent outcomes for invasive breast carcinoma, leading to the widespread adoption of BCT for invasive cancer in the late 1980s and early 1990s [23–28]. This treatment approach was extended to DCIS without a randomized trial proving the equivalency of BCT and mastectomy in this patient population. There was a subset of patients in one of these trials, the National Surgical Adjuvant Breast and Bowel Project (NSABP) B-06, subsequently found to have pure DCIS instead of invasive cancer [29]. Central pathologic review of 2072 specimens found 78 patients with DCIS alone who were randomized to total mastectomy versus BCS with and without RT. At a mean follow-up of 4.7 years, there were seven ipsilateral breast tumor recurrence (IBTR) events (three DCIS, four invasive) in the BCS groups. Local breast recurrence occurred less frequently in patients treated with BCS+RT compared to those that underwent BCS alone (2/29 [7%] versus 5/22 [23%]). No local recurrence events were reported in the mastectomy group. Both the BCS+RT and mastectomy groups had one distant recurrence, with a breast-cancer related death in the mastectomy patient. The authors concluded that given the low rate of treatment failures in both groups, it was reasonable to consider BCT for DCIS patients.

Adjuvant Radiation After Breast-Conserving Surgery

Randomized Controlled Trials

In contrast to the lack of prospective trials comparing mastectomy and breast-conserving surgery outcomes for DCIS, there are four mature randomized controlled trials evaluating the benefit of adjuvant breast irradiation in unselected women with DCIS following surgical excision (Table 13.2). The majority of cases were screen-detected, ranging from 72% to 100%. In all trials, whole breast radiation was administered (generally 50 Gy in 2 Gy fractions), and a boost dose was not recommended (Table 13.2).

From 1985 to 1990, the NSABP B-17 trial randomized women with DCIS to either BCS alone ($n = 403$) or BCS+RT ($n = 410$) [5]. A negative margin was required, although 13% were subsequently found to have either positive or unknown margins. In the most recent update with a mean follow-up of 17.3 years, the 15-year cumulative incidence of IBTR in the BCS-alone arm was 35.1% compared to 20.0% in the BCS+RT arm. Overall, the addition of radiation resulted in a 52% relative reduction in the risk of invasive IBTR (HR 0.48, 95% CI: 0.33–0.69) and a 47% reduction in DCIS IBTR (HR 0.53, 95% CI: 0.35–0.80) but did not lead to a significant reduction in regional or distant recurrence. Radiation did not confer any overall mortality benefit (HR 1.08, 95% CI: 0.79–1.48) or breast cancer-specific mortality reduction (HR 1.44, 95% CI: 0.71–2.92) compared with BCS alone. Approximately half of the recurrences in each arm were invasive (56% BCS alone and 54% BCS+RT), and

Table 13.2 Outcomes of randomized controlled trials of women with ductal carcinoma in situ treated with breast-conserving surgery with or without adjuvant radiation

Reference	Time period	N	Median follow-up (years)	Radiation	Margin requirement	Local recurrence N (%)[a]		Type of IBTR	Breast-cancer specific mortality[a] N (%)		p-value
						BCS alone	BCS+RT		BCS alone	BCS+RT	
Randomized Controlled Trials											
NSABP B-17 [5]	1985–1990	813	17.25	WBRT (50 Gy); 9% received boost	No tumor on ink[b]	35%	18%	45% DCIS 55% invasive	3.1%	4.7%	NS
EORTC 10853 [6]	1986–1996	1010	15.8	WBRT (50 Gy); 5% received boost	No tumor on ink[c]	31%	18%	52% DCIS 48% invasive	5.0%	4.0%	NS
SweDCIS [14]	1987–1999	1046	17.5	WBRT (50 or 54 Gy)	Aim for macroscopic margin of ≥ 1 cm[d]	32%	20%	50% DCIS 50% invasive	4.2%	4.1%	NS
UK/ANZ[e] [13]	1990–1998	475	12.7	WBRT (50 Gy)	No tumor on ink[f]	25%	9%	51% DCIS 49% invasive	2.0%	1.5%	NS

(continued)

Table 13.2 (continued)

Reference	Time period	N	Median follow-up (years)	Radiation	Margin requirement	Local recurrence N (%)[a]		Type of IBTR	Breast-cancer specific mortality[a] N (%)		p-value
						BCS alone	BCS+RT		BCS alone	BCS+RT	
Meta-analysis											
EBCTCG [3]	1985–2000	3729	8.9			28%	13%	52% DCIS 48% invasive	3.7%	4.1%	NS

BCS breast conserving surgery, *RT* radiation therapy, *DCIS* ductal carcinoma in situ, *EORTC* European Organization for the Research and Treatment of Cancer, *EBCTCG* Early Breast Cancer Trialists' Collaborative Group, *NS* not significant, *NSABP* National Surgical Adjuvant Breast and Bowel Project, *UK/ANZ* United Kingdom, Australia, New Zealand, *WBRT* whole breast radiotherapy

[a]Local recurrence rates and distant disease/breast cancer mortality reported as: 15-year for NSABP B-17 and EORTC 10853, 20-year for SweDCIS, crude rates at 12.7 years for UK/ANZ, and 10-year for EBCTCG

[b]13% of margins involved or unknown

[c]16% of margins "not free", <1 mm, involved, or unknown

[d]11% positive, 9% unknown

[e]Patients in the UK/ANZ study underwent either a 2 × 2 randomization (n = 912), or chose randomization to one of the treatments (n = 782). Crude rates for local recurrence in this table are those patients who did not have tamoxifen treatment and were randomized to either BCS alone (n = 239) or BCS+RT (236). Crude rates for breast cancer specific mortality are based on those either randomized to or chose to have BCS alone (n = 544) or BCS+RT (n = 267).

[f]16% of margins were <1 mm, 15% of patients margin status was unknown

women with an invasive IBTR experienced a higher all-cause death rate (HR 1.75, 95% CI: 1.2–2.5) and breast cancer mortality (HR 7.1, 95% CI: 4.1–12.0).

The European Organization for Research and Treatment of Cancer (EORTC) 10853 trial randomized 1010 women between 1986 and 1996 with DCIS <5 cm, determined by either clinical measurement or extent of microcalcifications on mammogram, to BCS alone or BCS+RT [6]. The 15-year local recurrence rate was 31% among women who underwent BCS-alone compared to 18% in the BCS+RT group (HR 0.52, 95% CI: 0.40–0.68). The risk of local recurrence was highest during the first 5 years of follow-up (4.0% per year in BCS alone versus 2.0% per year in BCS+RT), decreasing to 2.0% and 1.2% over the next 5 years and then stabilizing at 1.3% and 0.6% per year after 10 years of follow-up. Of all local recurrences, 52% were invasive, which was associated with significantly worse overall (HR 5.1, 95% CI: 3.1–8.7) and breast cancer-specific survival (HR 17.7, 95% CI: 8.9–35.2) compared to those who did not experience a recurrence.

The Swedish DCIS (SweDCIS) trial was conducted from 1987 to 1999 [14]. In the most recent update with median follow-up of 17.5 years, there was a relative risk reduction for IBTR associated with receipt of RT of 37.5% at 20 years. There was a 67% reduction in DCIS IBTR and 13% reduction in invasive IBTR associated with adjuvant radiation. The largest risk reduction was seen in the first 10 years after diagnosis with an absolute risk reduction of 34.8% at 0–5 years, 9.8% at 5–10 years, and 0.7% at ≥10 years. Few DCIS recurrences occurred after the first decade. The hazard rate for invasive IBTR was higher in the BCS-alone arm compared to the BCS+RT arm in the first decade, but the hazard rates for invasive IBTR became similar after 12 years of follow-up. There was no significant effect of RT on overall or disease-specific survival. The 10-year breast cancer-specific death rate after a DCIS IBTR was nearly zero and was 20% after an invasive IBTR.

The United Kingdom, Australia, and New Zealand (UK/ANZ) DCIS trial accrued patients from 1990 to 1998, randomizing women in a 2 × 2 factorial design of RT, tamoxifen, or both following BCS [13]. Women could choose to participate in randomization for radiation or tamoxifen, or both. Among women who were randomized or chose not to take tamoxifen, 239 were randomized to BCS alone and 236 were randomized to BCS+RT. At a median follow-up of 12.7 years, there were 59 (24.7%) and 21 (8.9%) IBTR events in the BCS-alone and BCS+RT groups, respectively. DCIS constituted 49% of recurrences in the BCS-alone and 57% of recurrences in the BCS+RT group. There were no significant differences in overall or breast cancer-specific survival with the addition of adjuvant radiation.

The Early Breast Cancer Trialists' Collaborative Group (EBCTCG) performed an individual level meta-analysis of data from the 3729 women enrolled in these four randomized trials and reported 10-year outcomes [3]. In those women who underwent BCS alone, the 10-year cumulative rate of IBTR was 28%, as compared to 13% for BCS+RT. At 10 years after randomization, 48% of the local recurrences were invasive for both BCS alone and BCS+RT, and radiation halved the rates of both invasive and DCIS IBTR. Radiation reduced the rate of IBTR regardless of age, extent of resection, use of tamoxifen, method of detection (mammography versus clinical symptoms), margin status, multifocality, histologic or nuclear grade, comedonecrosis, architecture, or size. Adjuvant radiation resulted in a larger proportional reduction in IBTR for women ≥50 years compared to women <50 years (2p < 0.0004). For women <50 years, the 10-year absolute risk of IBTR was 29.1% for BCS alone versus 18.5% for BCS+RT, and for women ≥50 years, the risk was 27.8% for BCS alone versus 10.8% for BCS+RT. There was no difference in overall or breast cancer-specific mortality.

These four randomized controlled trials consistently show an approximate 50% reduction in IBTR with the addition of adjuvant radiation after BCS for DCIS with long-term follow-up of 13–17 years. Combining their data, the meta-analysis could identify no subset for which radiation did not approximately halve the risk of recurrence [3]. Furthermore, in the meta-analysis, approximately half of the ipsilateral recurrences were invasive, and radiation reduced the rate of invasive recurrence by half.

Prospective Trials of BCS Alone in Low-Risk DCIS

While radiation clearly reduces the risk of recurrence after BCS for DCIS, it can be associated with rare but potentially serious sequelae, such as cardiovascular disease and radiation-induced malignancy [30, 31]. Therefore, there has been an ongoing effort to identify subsets of women for whom radiation can be safely omitted.

The first prospective trial in the United States evaluating outcomes after BCS alone in low-risk DCIS patients included 143 patients with predominant grade 1 or 2 DCIS, size ≤2.5 cm on mammogram, excision with final microscopic margins ≥1 cm, and no tamoxifen use [32, 33]. The reported 10-year cumulative incidence of IBTR was 15.6% with a "substantial and ongoing" risk of local recurrence with longer follow-up. Of the IBTRs, 68% were DCIS and 32% were invasive, and there were no distant recurrences or deaths. Although this study demonstrated that there remained significant risk of recurrence, it also found that selecting women according to "low-risk" criteria resulted in similar recurrence rates with BCS alone as unselected women treated with BCS+RT in the randomized trials.

The second prospective study to evaluate recurrence risk in women with low-risk DCIS treated by BCS alone was the multi-institutional Eastern Cooperative Oncology Group (ECOG) 5194 trial [34]. This study included two cohorts of patients: cohort 1 included 561 patients with low- or intermediate-grade DCIS <2.5 cm; cohort 2 included 104 patients with high-grade DCIS ≤1 cm. Minimum negative margins were ≥3 mm, and a post-excision mammogram free of calcifications was required. The median lesion size for both groups was 0.7 cm, and tamoxifen was used by approximately 30% of patients. The 12-year IBTR rate was 14.4% in cohort 1 and 24.6% in cohort 2. Approximately half of recurrences were invasive in both cohorts (52% in cohort 1 versus 54% in cohort 2). The risks of developing an IBTR or an invasive IBTR increased without plateau over the 12 years of follow-up. Tumor size >1 cm was associated with a twofold increased risk of IBTR when compared to tumors ≤5 mm (HR 2.11, 95% CI: 1.23–3.62). Both cohorts had similar overall survival (84% cohort 1 versus 83% cohort 2). Both of these studies demonstrated that while there is a substantial risk of local recurrence even among women with low-risk DCIS, combinations of clinicopathologic factors can provide risk stratification for patients.

The third prospective study of low-risk DCIS is the Radiation Therapy Oncology Group (RTOG) trial of 9804 randomized women with "good-risk" DCIS that was mammographically detected, <2.5 cm, and was resected with surgical margins >3 mm to either RT or none following BCS [35]. Tamoxifen use was optional after 2001 and was taken by 62% of patients. The cumulative rate of local failure at 7 years was 6.7% in the BCS-alone arm compared to 0.9% in the BCS+RT arm, demonstrating that adjuvant RT substantially lessens the risk of recurrence even for low-risk DCIS. There were no significant differences in overall or disease-free survival.

Trends in Surgical Resection for DCIS

Several recent studies have evaluated national treatment trends for DCIS. In a study of 121,080 DCIS patients in the Surveillance, Epidemiology, and End Results (SEER) registry from 1991 to 2010, the most common treatment was BCS+RT (43.0%), followed by BCS alone (26.5%), unilateral mastectomy (23.8%), bilateral mastectomy (4.5%), and observation alone (2.3%) [36]. The proportion of patients undergoing BCS with radiation increased from 24.2% in 1991 to 46.8% in 2010, whereas there was a reduction in the rate of unilateral mastectomy (from 44.9% to 19.3%) and BCS alone (from 29.8% to 22.3%). In contrast, in a large single-institution study of 5865 patients at Moffitt Cancer Center treated from 1994 to 2007, mastectomy rates increased from 33% (1994–1998) to 44% (2004–2007) [37]. In a study of 212,936 women in the National Cancer Database (NCDB) treated between 1998 and 2011, mastectomy utilization decreased from 1998 to 2004, followed by an increase thereafter [38]. All three studies found mastectomy to be more common among younger women.

Studies specifically reviewing the utilization of contralateral prophylactic mastectomy (CPM) have consistently found increasing rates for all breast cancer, but particularly for DCIS. In a NCDB study evaluating CPM rates among women with unilateral breast cancer comparing the time periods of 1998–1999 with 2006–2007, women with in situ cancers more frequently underwent CPM compared to women with stage I, II, or III disease [39]. In a study using NCDB but focused specifically on CPM in DCIS, there was an increase from 12.7% in 1998 to 36.5% in 2011 [38]. Similarly, in a SEER study with 51,030 patients diagnosed with DCIS, the rate of CPM increased from 6.4% in 1998 to 18.4% in 2005 [40]. All of these studies found that CPM was associated with younger patient age, white race, and more recent year of diagnosis.

Factors Associated with Recurrence

Given the variability in local recurrence rates between different treatment options, and the excellent survival with all options, there is ongoing debate regarding optimal management for DCIS with concerns about both over- and undertreatment. It is important for an individual woman and her clinician to consider her priorities to choose the optimal treatment for her. Much work has been done to identify factors associated with recurrence, to help estimate risks, and to optimize individual treatment.

Treatment Period

The randomized controlled trials of radiation after BCS for DCIS had relatively high rates of local recurrence. Given that recurrence rates for invasive cancer have declined over time, Subhedar et al. examined recurrence rates of almost 3000 DCIS patients treated with BCS, with or without RT, over 30 years at a single institution to analyze temporal trends in DCIS recurrence [41]. A significant decrease in recurrence rates was observed (5-year IBTR rate: 13.6% for 1978–1998 versus 6.6% for 1999–2010 (HR 0.62, $p < 0.001$)). This decrease in risk remained significant (HR 0.75, $p = 0.02$) after controlling for clinicopathologic and treatment factors associated with IBTR or those that changed over time (age, family history, radiologic versus clinical presentation, nuclear grade, necrosis, number of excisions, margin status, receipt of radiation or endocrine therapy). Stratification by receipt of radiation revealed that the decrease in IBTR that remained after controlling for the nine clinicopathologic factors was limited to women not receiving RT (HR 0.62, $p = 0.003$). These data show that recurrence rates for DCIS have declined over time, with this decrease only partially due to increases in screen detection, negative margins, and use of radiation and endocrine therapies. The unexplained decrease in recurrence rates was driven by women who underwent BCS alone, suggesting that it is not due to improvements in radiotherapy but may be due to changes in radiologic detection and pathologic evaluation.

Age

Young age was first noted to be associated with a higher risk of IBTR for women with DCIS in 1999 [42]. This observation has subsequently been confirmed by several studies, including the four randomized trials discussed previously [5, 6, 13, 14]. However, in most analyses, age is categorized into two or three groups, without a full characterization of IBTR risk across the spectrum of age.

In a recent analysis of 2996 patients who underwent BCS for DCIS, IBTR was assessed by decade of age [43]. Among patients aged 20–92 years, the 10-year recurrence rate was significantly lower with increasing age, ranging from 27% for women <40 years to 7.5% for women ≥80 years. This inverse relationship between age and IBTR risk persisted after controlling for other clinical, pathological, and treatment factors, including radiation. The relationship between recurrence and age was particularly strong for invasive IBTR, with a sevenfold increased risk among women <40 years compared to women ≥80 years.

Younger age was also shown to be associated with increased mortality in a study of 108,196 women diagnosed with DCIS between 1988 and 2011 in the SEER database [11]. With a median follow-up of 7.5 years, investigators found that 20-year breast cancer-specific mortality was more than twofold (HR 2.58, 95% CI: 1.85–3.60) higher for women <35 years at diagnosis (7.8%) compared to older women (3.2%). The risk of dying of breast cancer was increased after an invasive IBTR (HR 18.1, 95% CI: 14.0–23.6).

In addition to young age being associated with a higher risk of recurrence, age is also associated with a differential benefit from radiation. In the meta-analysis of the four randomized trials of adjuvant radiation, there was a higher proportional risk reduction from RT for women ≥50 years compared to those <50 years (rate ratios: age <50 years 0.69, SE: 0.12; age ≥50 years 0.38, SE: 0.06, 2p = 0.0004) [3]. In the SweDCIS study specifically, where women were categorized by age <52, 52–60, and ≥61 years, the risk reduction associated with RT was not statistically significant in women <52 years (HR 0.69, 95% CI: 0.47–1.02). In particular, RT did not significantly reduce invasive recurrences in this youngest group, which had an absolute reduction in 10-year invasive IBTR of 3.9% (HR 0.86, 95% CI: 0.51–1.47) [14]. These findings should be incorporated when weighing treatment options, including surgical options as well as adjuvant radiation and endocrine therapies.

Method of Detection

Population screening with mammography has resulted in increased detection of DCIS, and several studies have suggested that mammographic detection is associated with lower local recurrence rates when compared to clinical detection. Using multivariable analysis of IBTR in 794 patients with a diagnosis of DCIS who had undergone BCS from 1990 to 2007 at the MD Anderson Cancer Center, Yi et al. found that initial presentation based on clinical exam was significantly associated with recurrence (HR 1.87, 95% CI: 1.03–3.37) [44]. On multivariable analysis of almost 3000 women who underwent BCS from 1978 to 2010 at Memorial Sloan Kettering Cancer Center, a clinical presentation consistently was associated with higher risk of IBTR in an adjusted analysis (HR 1.4, $p = 0.008$–0.03) [41, 43]. In a large population-based study in the Netherlands, women with screen-detected DCIS had a 25% lower risk of developing IBTR compared to those with a clinical presentation ($p = 0.02$) [45]. In analyses of EORTC 10853 and NSABP B-17, where 72% and 80%, respectively, of women were diagnosed with mammography, a diagnosis based on clinical symptoms was associated with a 1.3- to 1.5-fold increased risk of local recurrence [5, 6].

Margins

Of all the risk factors associated with recurrence, margin width is the only factor that is modifiable by the surgeon. With the exception of SweDCIS, the randomized trials of RT required microscopically negative surgical margins. Despite this requirement, 11–16% of patients were ultimately found to have involved or unknown margin status upon centralized pathologic review [3]. The meta-analysis showed that for both BCS alone and BCS+RT, there was a higher IBTR risk for women with positive margins [3]. However, these trials were not designed to evaluate the effect of margin width on IBTR, and specific negative margin widths were not reported.

In a study of 2996 DCIS patients treated with BCS over 30 years, Van Zee et al. found that for women who underwent BCS alone ($n = 1266$), the 10-year IBTR rate varied significantly by margin width with rates of 41% (positive), 27% (≤ 2 mm), 23% (>2–10 mm), and 16% (>10 mm) ($p = 0.0003$) [46]. However, among women who received radiation, there was no significant relationship. These findings remained true on multivariable analysis. This study suggests that wider negative margins may be important to reduce recurrence risk in women who do not undergo radiation but may not be necessary in those who undergo radiation.

In a study-level meta-analysis commissioned by a multidisciplinary consensus panel attempting to identify optimal margins for patients undergoing BCS+RT, positive margins were associated with a twofold risk of IBTR compared to negative margins [47]. They also found that more widely negative margins did not significantly decrease IBTR compared to 2 mm margins. Therefore, the group endorsed the use of 2 mm margins as the standard for an adequate margin in DCIS treated with BCS+RT [48]. No recommendation was made for women undergoing BCS alone.

Delays in Therapy

The four randomized trials clearly demonstrated a benefit for the use of radiation after BCS in patients with DCIS, but the optimal timing of this risk-reducing treatment was not evaluated. In a recent review, 1323 women treated with BCS+RT between 1980 and 2010 at a single institution were examined to compare local recurrence rates by timing of initial of adjuvant radiation (≤ 8 weeks, 8–12 weeks, and >12 weeks after surgery) [49]. With a median follow-up of 6.6 years and with 311 patients followed for ≥ 10 years, there were 126 (9.5%) IBTR events. On multivariate analysis, a delay in radiation >12 weeks was associated with a 1.9-fold increased risk of local recurrence compared to those who initiated treatment <8 weeks ($p = 0.014$). The authors suggest that the reason for an association between delay in radiation and IBTR is likely multifactorial, and although it may be related to time-dependent changes that affect the therapeutic effectiveness of radiation, others have also shown that delay in initiation of radiation may be associated with factors such as older age, ethnicity, being unmarried, and having increased comorbidities. Delay in initiation of adjuvant RT should be avoided if possible.

Pathologic and Histologic Characteristics

Nuclear Grade
Multiple studies have reported an increased risk of local recurrence associated with high-grade DCIS; however, these differences do not appear to be sustained with

longer follow-up. Among the four randomized controlled trials, the UK/ANZ trial found nuclear grade to be positively associated with risk of recurrence at a median of 4.3 years [50]. NSABP B-17 found that the initial differences noted at 5 years were no longer significant at 8-year follow-up [51, 52]. The EORTC 10853 and SweDCIS trials with median follow-up 15.8 and 17.5 years, respectively, found no difference in local recurrence based on nuclear grade [14, 53]. In a multi-institutional database of 268 women treated with BCT between 1967 and 1985, Solin et al. found a significantly higher risk of IBTR among women with high-grade DCIS at 5 years (7% high-grade versus 3% low-grade), but at 10 years, the relationship was reversed (13% high-grade versus 20% low-grade) [54]. Similarly, in a large retrospective study by Wallis et al. of 700 cases of DCIS identified from the National Health Service Screening Program, women with high-grade DCIS were not at increased risk of recurrence at a median follow-up of 15.3 years (low-grade, 14.7%; intermediate-grade, 16.1%; high-grade, 15.4%) [55]. However, median time to recurrence for high-grade lesions was 6.3 years compared to 10.9 years for low- and intermediate-grade lesions. These studies suggest that the higher rates of recurrence seen in the short-term studies of high-grade DCIS are due to earlier recurrence among high-grade lesions, but in the long term (i.e., 10–15 years), high-grade DCIS does not appear to have a higher recurrence rate.

Comedonecrosis

When consensus guidelines on the classification of DCIS were initially drafted, architectural features were divided into two main subtypes: comedo and non-comedo [56]. Non-comedo was further subdivided into cribriform, papillary, micropapillary, and solid. These subtypes are generally composed of cells with low-grade cytology and are frequently estrogen- and progesterone-receptor positive [57]. These features contrast with the comedo subtype, which demonstrates high nuclear grade cells, central necrosis, a lower rate of ER positivity, and higher rate of HER2 positivity [57–59]. The four randomized trials all demonstrated increased risk of IBTR in patients with comedonecrosis at short-term follow-up [50, 52, 53, 60]. However, in the long-term follow-up of results reported from the NSABP B-17 trial, there was no significant effect of comedonecrosis on recurrence among invasive IBTR events [5]. Solin et al. found the median interval to local recurrence was 3.1 years for high-grade lesions with comedo carcinoma versus 6.5 years for low-grade, non-comedo lesions [54]. Early differences in IBTR associated with comedo subtype and necrosis were no longer present at 10-year follow-up. The histopathologic diagnosis of comedonecrosis is inherently confounded with high grade and like high-grade lesions may be more associated with early, but not long-term, recurrence.

Decision-Making Tools

In an effort to aid patients and practitioners in the decision-making process for DCIS treatment, several tools have been created to estimate the risk of local recurrence and help guide treatment decisions, including the USC/Van Nuys Prognostic

Index [61, 62], the Memorial Sloan Kettering Cancer Center DCIS nomogram [63], and a 12-gene expression score, the Oncotype DX Breast DCIS Score [64].

University of Southern California (USC)/Van Nuys Prognostic Index (VNPI)

The USC/VNPI was developed to triage patients to optimal treatment: BCS alone, BCS+RT, or mastectomy [61]. Upon retrospective analysis of 425 patients, size of tumor, margin width, and pathologic classification were found to be predictive of IBTR [65]. After reports that young age was a risk factor for IBTR, the authors presented a revised version of the VNPI adding age as a fourth variable [62]. Recommendations for management are based on the 12-point scoring system: BCS alone for low risk (scores 4–6), BCS with adjuvant radiation for intermediate risk (scores 7–9), and mastectomy for high risk (scores 10–12). Attempts to externally validate the scoring system have been varied. In a retrospective review of 367 patients using the original USC/VNPI scoring system, de Mascarel et al. found that the local recurrence rate was significantly associated with the VNPI at a median follow-up of 5.9 years [66]. However, they found a relatively high rate of recurrence (9%) among the low-risk group compared to Silverstein's low-risk group (2%) [61]. Di Saverio et al. evaluated 259 patients treated with BCS with or without RT and at a mean follow-up of 10.8 years had 21 local recurrence events [67]. Of these local recurrences, there was a significant difference between the low- (4% recurrence), intermediate- (13%), and high-risk (25%) groups. However, in a study of 222 patients with mammographically detected DCIS in the United States, MacAusland et al. found a 5-year IBTR rate that did not distinguish between the three groups. They found no significant difference in freedom from IBTR between the low-risk (95%) and intermediate-risk (83%) groups ($p = 0.19$) [68]. Another study from the United Kingdom found that the USC/VNPI stratified 78% of patients into the intermediate-risk recurrence group and lacked discriminatory power to help guide management [69].

Memorial Sloan Kettering Cancer Center DCIS Nomogram (Fig. 13.1)

The Memorial Sloan Kettering Cancer Center DCIS nomogram was developed to provide individualized recurrence risk estimates for women treated with BCS for DCIS, using readily available clinicopathologic and treatment factors. It was created using data from 1868 DCIS patients treated with BCS between 1991 and 2006, of which 49% received radiation and 21% received adjuvant endocrine therapy [63]. There were 202 (10.8%) local recurrences, 80 (39.6%) of which were invasive. The influence on recurrence risk of age, family history, type of initial presentation (radiologic versus clinical), receipt of radiation, receipt of adjuvant endocrine therapy, nuclear grade (low versus intermediate/high), presence of necrosis, margins (negative versus positive/close), number of excisions (≤ 2 versus ≥ 3), and year of surgery is all integrated into the nomogram, which provides 5- and 10-year risk

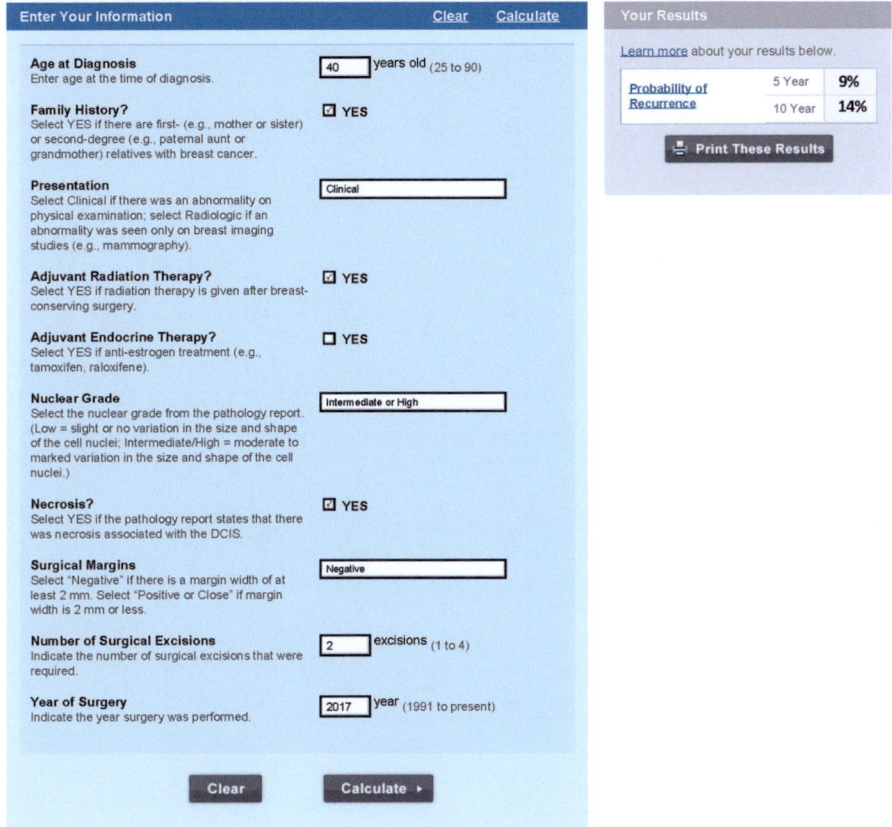

Fig. 13.1 MSKCC DCIS recurrence risk estimation nomogram

estimates of IBTR. It has been validated in at least five independent populations around the world with excellent calibration and correlation and good discrimination (Table 13.3) [44, 70–73]. The strengths of the nomogram are that it integrates numerous patient and disease characteristics that are readily available, provides recurrence risk estimates according to various adjuvant treatments, and has been externally validated in several different populations. Its individualized risk estimates are available free-of-charge online at www.nomograms.org.

Oncotype DX Breast DCIS Score

The Oncotype DX Breast DCIS Score was created using a 12-gene subset of a 21-gene assay used for invasive breast cancer and applied to data from 327 patients enrolled in ECOG 5194 [64]. Subsets with low, medium, and high scores had

Table 13.3 External validation of Memorial Sloan Kettering Cancer Center nomogram

Reference	Time period	N	Median follow-up (years)	Number of recurrences	10-year recurrence rate (%)	Concordance index or AUC	Correlation between 10-year predicted and observed (R)
Yi, 2012 MD Anderson Cancer Center [44]	1990–2007	794	7.1	62	10	0.63–0.65	NR
Sweldens, 2014 University Hospital Leuven, Belgium [70]	1973–2010	467	7.2	48	13	0.66	NR
Wang, 2014 National Cancer Center, Singapore [71]	1992–2011	716	5.8	42	7.4	0.67	NR
Collins, 2015 Harvard Pilgrim/Kaiser Permanente [72]	1990–2001	495	5.3	NR	13	0.68	0.95
Sedloev, 2016 Medical University Sofia, Bulgaria [73]	1998–2003	122	12.3	17	NR	0.92	0.91

AUC area under the receiver operating characteristic curve, NR not reported recurrence rates of 10.6%, 26.7%, and 25.9%, respectively. In a population-based study from Canada, similar results were found, with low-, medium-, and high-risk groups having 10-year IBTR rates of 12.7%, 33.0%, and 27.8%, respectively [74]. Invasive IBTR rates were 8%, 20.9%, and 15.5%, respectively. Thus, for overall and for invasive IBTR, a high score was associated with a lower risk than was an intermediate score. On multivariable analysis, the DCIS score remained significantly associated with IBTR (HR 1.68, 95% CI: 1.08–2.62). However, multifocality (HR 1.97, 95% CI: 1.27–3.02), tumor size >10 mm (HR 2.07, 95% CI: 1.15–3.82), and age <50 years (HR 1.75, 95% CI: 1.07–2.76) were all more predictive of IBTR. Therefore, women with age >50 and small DCIS size (<1 cm) but with a high DCIS score had a relatively low 10-year IBTR rate of 14.6%. In contrast, young women with a large area of DCIS (>2.5 cm) but with a low DCIS score had a high 10-year IBTR rate of 30.6% [75]. These data show that while the DCIS score does contribute to estimating the risk local recurrence, other clinical and pathologic variables are more predictive, indicating that the DCIS score should not be used in isolation and that clinicopathologic factors should also be included.

Management of the Axilla

The risk of nodal metastases in a woman with pure DCIS is very low [76]; however, a substantial proportion of women with DCIS found on core biopsy will be found to have invasive cancer on excision. A meta-analysis of 52 studies, including 7350 patients, reported that overall, 26% were found to have invasion at excision [77]. Variables that were significantly associated with higher risk of invasive cancer being found included the use of smaller core needle size, high-grade DCIS, lesion size >20 mm on imaging, Breast Imaging Reporting and Data System (BI-RADS) score of 4 or 5, mammographic mass, and palpability [77]. Currently, the American Society for Clinical Oncology and the National Comprehensive Cancer Network only recommend sentinel lymph node biopsy in the case of mastectomy or with excision in an anatomic location that could compromise the performance of a future sentinel lymph node procedure [78, 79]. Additional situations for which sentinel lymph node biopsy may be considered include when a mass lesion is seen on imaging and highly suggestive of invasive cancer, large areas of DCIS on imaging (≥5 cm) as these characteristics can suggest higher rates of upgrade to invasive cancer, and/or core needle biopsy pathology suspicious for invasive disease.

Conclusion

DCIS is an increasingly diagnosed early breast cancer with excellent survival, but with variable risk of local recurrence based on treatment type and various clinicopathologic factors. Approximately half of local recurrences are invasive, which portend a worse overall survival, thereby illustrating the importance of avoiding local recurrence. Radiation reduces the risk of any recurrence and invasive recurrence by half, in all identified subsets, but does not improve survival and is associated with rare but potentially serious side effects. Accurate and individualized risk estimates should be incorporated into a thorough discussion of the various treatment options, to help a woman weigh the risks and benefits of the various options so that she can make the best treatment decision for herself.

References

1. DeSantis C, Ma J, Bryan L, Jemal A. Breast cancer statistics, 2013. CA Cancer J Clin. 2014;64(1):52–62.
2. American Cancer Society. Cancer facts & figures 2017. Atlanta: American Cancer Society; 2017. p. 1–76.
3. Early Breast Cancer Trialists' Collaborative Group, Darby S, McGale P, Correa C, Taylor C, Arriagada R, et al. Effect of radiotherapy after breast-conserving surgery on 10-year recurrence and 15-year breast cancer death: meta-analysis of individual patient data for 10,801 women in 17 randomised trials. Lancet. 2011;378(9804):1707–16.
4. Stuart KE, Houssami N, Taylor R, Hayen A, Boyages J. Long-term outcomes of ductal carcinoma in situ of the breast: a systematic review, meta-analysis and meta-regression analysis. BMC Cancer. 2015;15(1):890.
5. Wapnir IL, Dignam JJ, Fisher B, Mamounas EP, Anderson SJ, Julian TB, et al. Long-term outcomes of invasive ipsilateral breast tumor recurrences after lumpectomy in NSABP B-17 and B-24 randomized clinical trials for DCIS. J Natl Cancer Inst. 2011;103(6):478–88.
6. Donker M, Litière S, Werutsky G, Julien J-P, Fentiman IS, Agresti R, et al. Breast-conserving treatment with or without radiotherapy in ductal carcinoma in situ: 15-year recurrence rates and outcome after a recurrence, from the EORTC 10853 randomized phase III trial. J Clin Oncol. 2013;31(32):4054–9.
7. Welch HG, Black WC. Using autopsy series to estimate the disease "reservoir" for ductal carcinoma in situ of the breast: how much more breast cancer can we find? Ann Intern Med. 1997;127(11):1023–8.
8. Rosen PP, Braun DW, Kinne DE. The clinical significance of pre-invasive breast carcinoma. Cancer. 1980;46(4 Suppl):919–25.
9. Sanders ME, Schuyler PA, Dupont WD, Page DL. The natural history of low-grade ductal carcinoma in situ of the breast in women treated by biopsy only revealed over 30 years of long-term follow-up. Cancer. 2005;103(12):2481–4.
10. Collins LC, Tamimi RM, Baer HJ, Connolly JL, Colditz GA, Schnitt SJ. Outcome of patients with ductal carcinoma in situ untreated after diagnostic biopsy. Cancer. 2005;103(9):1778–84.
11. Narod SA, Iqbal J, Giannakeas V, Sopik V, Sun P. Breast cancer mortality after a diagnosis of ductal carcinoma in situ. JAMA Oncol. 2015;1(7):888–96.
12. Cady B, Chung MA. Preventing invasive breast cancer. Cancer. 2011;117(14):3064–8.
13. Cuzick J, Sestak I, Pinder SE, Ellis IO, Forsyth S, Bundred NJ, et al. Effect of tamoxifen and radiotherapy in women with locally excised ductal carcinoma in situ: long-term results from the UK/ANZ DCIS trial. Lancet Oncol. 2011;12(1):21–9.
14. Wärnberg F, Garmo H, Emdin S, Hedberg V, Adwall L, Sandelin K, et al. Effect of radiotherapy after breast-conserving surgery for ductal carcinoma in situ: 20 years follow-up in the randomized SweDCIS trial. J Clin Oncol. 2014;32(32):3613–8.
15. Duffy SW, Dibden A, Michalopoulos D, Offman J, Parmar D, Jenkins J, et al. Screen detection of ductal carcinoma in situ and subsequent incidence of invasive interval breast cancers: a retrospective population-based study. Lancet Oncol. 2016;17(1):109–14.
16. Cutuli B, Cohen-Solal-Le-Nir C, de Lafontan B, Mignotte H, Fichet V, Fay R, et al. Ductal carcinoma in situ of the breast results of conservative and radical treatments in 716 patients. Eur J Cancer. 2001;37(18):2365–72.

17. Carlson GW, Page A, Johnson E, Nicholson K, Styblo TM, Wood WC. Local recurrence of ductal carcinoma in situ after skin-sparing mastectomy. J Am Coll Surg. 2007;204(5):1074–8. –discussion 1078–80.
18. Meijnen P, Oldenburg HSA, Peterse JL, Bartelink H, Rutgers EJT. Clinical outcome after selective treatment of patients diagnosed with ductal carcinoma in situ of the breast. Ann Surg Oncol. 2008;15(1):235–43.
19. Tunon-de-Lara C, André G, MacGrogan G, Dilhuydy J-M, Bussières J-E, Debled M, et al. Ductal carcinoma in situ of the breast: influence of age on diagnostic, therapeutic, and prognostic features. Retrospective study of 812 patients. Ann Surg Oncol. 2011;18(5):1372–9.
20. Kelley L, Silverstein M, Guerra L. Analyzing the risk of recurrence after mastectomy for DCIS: a new use for the USC/Van Nuys Prognostic Index. Ann Surg Oncol. 2011;18(2):459–62.
21. Owen D, Tyldesley S, Alexander C, Speers C, Truong P, Nichol A, et al. Outcomes in patients treated with mastectomy for ductal carcinoma in situ. Int J Radiat Oncol Biol Phys. 2013;85(3):e129–34.
22. Boyages J, Delaney G, Taylor R. Predictors of local recurrence after treatment of ductal carcinoma in situ: a meta-analysis. Cancer. 1999;85(3):616–28.
23. Arriagada R, Lê MG, Rochard F, Contesso G. Conservative treatment versus mastectomy in early breast cancer: patterns of failure with 15 years of follow-up data. J Clin Oncol. 1996;14(5):1558–64.
24. Van Dongen JA, Voogd AC, Fentiman IS, Legrand C, Sylvester RJ, Tong D, et al. Long-term results of a randomized trial comparing breast-conserving therapy with mastectomy: European Organization for Research and Treatment of Cancer 10801 trial. J Natl Cancer Inst. 2000;92(14):1143–50.
25. Fisher B, Anderson S, Bryant J, Margolese RG, Deutsch M, Fisher ER, et al. Twenty-year follow-up of a randomized trial comparing total mastectomy, lumpectomy, and lumpectomy plus irradiation for the treatment of invasive breast cancer. N Engl J Med. 2002;347(16):1233–41.
26. Veronesi U, Cascinelli N, Mariani L, Greco M, Saccozzi R, Luini A, et al. Twenty-year follow-up of a randomized study comparing breast-conserving surgery with radical mastectomy for early breast cancer. N Engl J Med. 2002;347(16):1227–32.
27. Poggi MM, Danforth DN, Sciuto LC, Smith SL, Steinberg SM, Liewehr DJ, et al. Eighteen-year results in the treatment of early breast carcinoma with mastectomy versus breast conservation therapy: the National Cancer Institute Randomized Trial. Cancer. 2003;98(4):697–702.
28. Blichert-Toft M, Nielsen M, During M, Moller S, Rank F, Overgaard M, et al. Long-term results of breast conserving surgery vs. mastectomy for early stage invasive breast cancer: 20-year follow-up of the Danish randomized DBCG-82TM protocol. Acta Oncol. 2008;47(4):672–81.
29. Fisher ER, Sass R, Fisher B, Wickerham L, Paik SM. Pathologic findings from the National Surgical Adjuvant Breast Project (protocol 6). I. Intraductal carcinoma (DCIS). Cancer. 1986;57(2):197–208.
30. Grantzau T, Mellemkjaer L, Overgaard J. Second primary cancers after adjuvant radiotherapy in early breast cancer patients: a national population based study under the Danish Breast Cancer Cooperative Group. Radiother Oncol. 2013;106(1):42–9.
31. Henson KE, McGale P, Taylor C, Darby SC. Radiation-related mortality from heart disease and lung cancer more than 20 years after radiotherapy for breast cancer. Br J Cancer. 2012;108(1):179–82.
32. Wong JS, Kaelin CM, Troyan SL, Gadd MA, Gelman R, Lester SC, et al. Prospective study of wide excision alone for ductal carcinoma in situ of the breast. J Clin Oncol. 2006;24(7):1031–6.
33. Wong JS, Chen Y-H, Gadd MA, Gelman R, Lester SC, Schnitt SJ, et al. Eight-year update of a prospective study of wide excision alone for small low- or intermediate-grade ductal carcinoma in situ (DCIS). Breast Cancer Res Treat. 2014;143(2):343–50.
34. Solin LJ, Gray R, Hughes LL, Wood WC, Lowen MA, Badve SS, et al. Surgical excision without radiation for ductal carcinoma in situ of the breast: 12-year results from the ECOG-ACRIN E5194 study. J Clin Oncol. 2015;33(33):3938–44.

35. McCormick B, Winter K, Hudis C, Kuerer HM, Rakovitch E, Smith BL, et al. RTOG 9804: a prospective randomized trial for good-risk ductal carcinoma in situ comparing radiotherapy with observation. J Clin Oncol. 2015;33(7):709–15.
36. Worni M, Akushevich I, Greenup R, Sarma D, Ryser MD, Myers ER, et al. Trends in treatment patterns and outcomes for ductal carcinoma in situ. J Natl Cancer Inst. 2015;107(12):djv263–10.
37. McGuire KP, Santillan AA, Kaur P, Meade T, Parbhoo J, Mathias M, et al. Are mastectomies on the rise? A 13-year trend analysis of the selection of mastectomy versus breast conservation therapy in 5865 patients. Ann Surg Oncol. 2009;16(10):2682–90.
38. Rutter CE, Park HS, Killelea BK, Evans SB. Growing use of mastectomy for ductal carcinoma-in situ of the breast among young women in the United States. Ann Surg Oncol. 2015;22(7):2378–86.
39. Yao K, Stewart AK, Winchester DJ, Winchester DP. Trends in contralateral prophylactic mastectomy for unilateral cancer: a report from the National Cancer Data Base, 1998–2007. Ann Surg Oncol. 2010;17(10):2554–62.
40. Tuttle TM, Jarosek S, Habermann EB, Arrington A, Abraham A, Morris TJ, et al. Increasing rates of contralateral prophylactic mastectomy among patients with ductal carcinoma in situ. J Clin Oncol. 2009;27(9):1362–7.
41. Subhedar P, Olcese C, Patil S, Morrow M, Van Zee KJ. Decreasing recurrence rates for ductal carcinoma in situ: analysis of 2996 women treated with breast-conserving surgery over 30 years. Ann Surg Oncol. 2015;22(10):3273–81.
42. Van Zee KJ, Liberman L, Samli B, Tran KN, McCormick B, Petrek JA, et al. Long term follow-up of women with ductal carcinoma in situ treated with breast-conserving surgery: the effect of age. Cancer. 1999;86(9):1757–67.
43. Cronin PA, Olcese C, Patil S, Morrow M, Van Zee KJ. Impact of age on risk of recurrence of ductal carcinoma in situ: outcomes of 2996 women treated with breast-conserving surgery over 30 years. Ann Surg Oncol. 2016;23(9):2816–24.
44. Yi M, Meric-Bernstam F, Kuerer HM, Mittendorf EA, Bedrosian I, Lucci A, et al. Evaluation of a breast cancer nomogram for predicting risk of ipsilateral breast tumor recurrences in patients with ductal carcinoma in situ after local excision. J Clin Oncol. 2012;30(6):600–7.
45. Elshof LE, Schaapveld M, Rutgers EJ, Schmidt MK, de Munck L, van Leeuwen FE, et al. The method of detection of ductal carcinoma in situ has no therapeutic implications: results of a population-based cohort study. Breast Cancer Res. 2017;19(26):1–10.
46. Van Zee KJ, Subhedar P, Olcese C, Patil S, Morrow M. Relationship between margin width and recurrence of ductal carcinoma in situ: analysis of 2996 women treated with breast-conserving surgery for 30 years. Ann Surg. 2015;262(4):623–31.
47. Marinovich ML, Azizi L, Macaskill P, Irwig L, Morrow M, Solin LJ, et al. The association of surgical margins and local recurrence in women with ductal carcinoma in situ treated with breast-conserving therapy: a meta-analysis. Ann Surg Oncol. 2016;23(12):3811–21.
48. Morrow M, Van Zee KJ, Solin LJ, Houssami N, Chavez-MacGregor M, Harris JR, et al. Society of Surgical Oncology-American Society for Radiation Oncology-American Society of Clinical Oncology Consensus guideline on margins for breast-conserving surgery with whole-breast irradiation in ductal carcinoma in situ. J Clin Oncol. 2016;30(33):4040–6.
49. Shurell E, Olcese C, Patil S, McCormick B, Van Zee KJ, Pilewskie ML. Delay in radiotherapy is associated with an increased risk of disease recurrence in women with ductal carcinoma in situ. Cancer. 2018;124(1):46–54.
50. Pinder SE, Duggan C, Ellis IO, Cuzick J, Forbes JF, Bishop H, et al. A new pathological system for grading DCIS with improved prediction of local recurrence: results from the UK/ANZ DCIS trial. Br J Cancer. 2010;103(1):94–100.
51. Fisher ER, Costantino J, Fisher B, Palekar AS, Redmond C, Mamounas E. Pathologic findings from the National Surgical Adjuvant Breast Project (NSABP) protocol B-17. Intraductal carcinoma (ductal carcinoma in situ). Cancer. 1995;75(6):1310–9.
52. Fisher ER, Dignam J, Tan-Chiu E, Costantino J, Fisher B, Paik S, et al. Pathologic findings from the National Surgical Adjuvant Breast Project (NSABP) eight-year update of protocol B-17: intraductal carcinoma. Cancer. 1999;86(3):429–38.

53. Bijker N, Peterse JL, Duchateau L, Julien JP, Fentiman IS, Duval C, et al. Risk factors for recurrence and metastasis after breast-conserving therapy for ductal carcinoma-in-situ: analysis of European Organization for Research and Treatment of Cancer Trial 10853. J Clin Oncol. 2001;19(8):2263–71.
54. Solin LJ, Kurtz J, Fourquet A, Amalric R, Recht A, Bornstein B, et al. Fifteen-year results of breast-conserving surgery and definitive breast irradiation for the treatment of ductal carcinoma in situ of the breast. J Clin Oncol. 1996;14(3):754–63.
55. Wallis MG, Clements K, Kearins O, Ball G, Macartney J, Lawrence GM. The effect of DCIS grade on rate, type and time to recurrence after 15 years of follow-up of screen-detected DCIS. Br J Cancer. 2012;106(10):1611–7.
56. The Consensus Conference Committee. Consensus conference on the classification of ductal carcinoma in situ. Cancer. 1997;80(9):1798–802.
57. Barnes NLP, Boland GP, Davenport A, Knox WF, Bundred NJ. Relationship between hormone receptor status and tumour size, grade and comedo necrosis in ductal carcinoma in situ. Br J Surg. 2005;92(4):429–34.
58. Barnes DM, Meyer JS, Gonzalez JG, Gullick WJ, Millis RR. Relationship between c-erbB-2 immunoreactivity and thymidine labelling index in breast carcinoma in situ. Breast Cancer Res Treat. 1991;18(1):11–7.
59. Poller DN, Silverstein MJ, Galea M, Locker AP, Elston CW, Blamey RW, et al. Ideas in pathology. Ductal carcinoma in situ of the breast: a proposal for a new simplified histological classification association between cellular proliferation and c-erbB-2 protein expression. Mod Pathol. 1994;7(2):257–62.
60. Ringberg A, Nordgren H, Thorstensson S, Idvall I, Garmo H, Granstrand B, et al. Histopathological risk factors for ipsilateral breast events after breast conserving treatment for ductal carcinoma in situ of the breast – results from the Swedish randomised trial. Eur J Cancer. 2007;43(2):291–8.
61. Silverstein MJ, Lagios MD, Craig PH, Waisman JR, Lewinsky BS, Colburn WJ, et al. A prognostic index for ductal carcinoma in situ of the breast. Cancer. 1996;77(11):2267–74.
62. Silverstein MJ. The University of Southern California/Van Nuys prognostic index for ductal carcinoma in situ of the breast. Am J Surg. 2003;186(4):337–43.
63. Rudloff U, Jacks LM, Goldberg JI, Wynveen CA, Brogi E, Patil S, et al. Nomogram for predicting the risk of local recurrence after breast-conserving surgery for ductal carcinoma in situ. J Clin Oncol. 2010;28(23):3762–9.
64. Solin LJ, Gray R, Baehner FL, Butler SM, Hughes LL, Yoshizawa C, et al. A multigene expression assay to predict local recurrence risk for ductal carcinoma in situ of the breast. J Natl Cancer Inst. 2013;105(10):701–10.
65. Silverstein MJ, Poller DN, Waisman JR, Colburn WJ, Barth A, Gierson ED, et al. Prognostic classification of breast ductal carcinoma in situ. Lancet. 1995;345:1154–7.
66. de Mascarel I, Bonichon F, MacGrogan G, de Lara CT, Avril A, Picot V, et al. Application of the Van Nuys prognostic index in a retrospective series of 367 ductal carcinomas in situ of the breast examined by serial macroscopic sectioning: practical considerations. Breast Cancer Res Treat. 2000;61(2):151–9.
67. Di Saverio S, Catena F, Santini D, Ansaloni L, Fogacci T, Mignani S, et al. 259 patients with DCIS of the breast applying USC/Van Nuys prognostic index: a retrospective review with long term follow up. Breast Cancer Res Treat. 2008;109(3):405–16.
68. MacAusland SG, Hepel JT, Chong FK, Galper SL, Gass JS, Ruthazer R, et al. An attempt to independently verify the utility of the Van Nuys Prognostic Index for ductal carcinoma in situ. Cancer. 2007;110(12):2648–53.
69. Boland GP, Chan KC, Knox WF, Roberts SA, Bundred NJ. Value of the Van Nuys Prognostic Index in prediction of recurrence of ductal carcinoma in situ after breast-conserving surgery. Br J Surg. 2003;90(4):426–32.
70. Sweldens C, Peeters S, van Limbergen E, Janssen H, Laenen A, Patil S, et al. Local relapse after breast-conserving therapy for ductal carcinoma in situ: a European single-center experience and external validation of the Memorial Sloan-Kettering Cancer Center DCIS nomogram. Cancer J. 2014;20(1):1–7.

71. Wang F, Li H, Tan PH, Chua ET, Yeo RMC, Lim FLWT, et al. Validation of a nomogram in the prediction of local recurrence risks after conserving surgery for Asian women with ductal carcinoma in situ of the breast. Clin Oncol. 2014;26(11):684–91.
72. Collins LC, Achacoso N, Haque R, Nekhlyudov L, Quesenberry CP, Schnitt SJ, et al. Risk prediction for local breast cancer recurrence among women with DCIS treated in a community practice: a nested, case-control study. Ann Surg Oncol. 2015;22(Suppl 3(S3)):S502–8.
73. Sedloev T, Vasileva M, Kundurzhiev T, Hadjieva T. Validation of the Memorial Sloan-Kettering Cancer Center nomogram in the prediction of local recurrence risks after conserving surgery for Bulgarian women with ductal carcinoma in situ of the breast. Barcelona; 2016. Available from: https://www.researchgate.net/publication/312232507_Validation_of_the_Memorial_Sloan-Kettering_Cancer_Center_nomogram_in_the_prediction_of_local_recurrence_risks_after_conserving_surgery_for_Bulgarian_women_with_DCIS_of_the_breast. Accessed 7 Nov 2017.
74. Rakovitch E, Nofech-Mozes S, Hanna W, Baehner FL, Saskin R, Butler SM, et al. A population-based validation study of the DCIS score predicting recurrence risk in individuals treated by breast-conserving surgery alone. Breast Cancer Res Treat. 2015;152(2):389–98.
75. Rakovitch E, Gray RJ, Baehner FL, Miller DP, Sutradhar R, Crager M, et al. Refined estimates of local recurrence risks and the impact of the DCIS score adjusting for clinico-pathological features: meta-analysis of E5194 and Ontario DCIS cohort studies. J Clin Oncol. 2017;35(Suppl 15): 528.
76. Leonard GD, Swain SM. Ductal carcinoma in situ, complexities and challenges. J Natl Cancer Inst. 2004;96(12):906–20.
77. Brennan ME, Turner RM, Ciatto S, Marinovich ML, French JR, Macaskill P, et al. Ductal carcinoma in situ at core-needle biopsy: meta-analysis of underestimation and predictors of invasive breast cancer. Radiology. 2011;260(1):119–28.
78. Lyman GH, Temin S, Edge SB, Newman LA, Turner RR, Weaver DL, et al. Sentinel lymph node biopsy for patients with early-stage breast cancer: American Society of Clinical Oncology clinical practice guideline update. J Clin Oncol. 2014;32(13):1365–83.
79. Gradishar WJ, Anderson BO, Balassanian R, Blair SL, Burstein HJ, Cyr A, et al. NCCN clinical practice guidelines in oncology: breast cancer, version 4.2017. 2nd ed. Journal of the National Comprehensive Cancer Network: 2018;16(3):310–20.

Index

A
Adjuvant radiation therapy, 45
American College of Radiology (ACR), 116
American Society of Clinical Oncology (ASCO), 138
Aromatase inhibitors (AI), 27, 96, 97, 134–137, 139, 140
Atypical ductal hyperplasia (ADH), 6, 129–130
    ALH, 79, 81, 85
    CNB, 82, 84–86
    DCIS, 79, 81
    definition, 79
    excisional biopsy, 83
    history, 80
    incidence, 82
    MRI, 81, 83
    ultrasound guided biopsy, 84
    upstaging rates, 84
Atypical hyperplasia (AH)
    ADH, 149 (*see also* Atypical ductal hyperplasia (ADH))
    ALH, 149 (*see also* Atypical lobular hyperplasia (ALH))
    breast cancer (*see* Breast cancer risk)
    FEA, 150
    long-term risk, 150, 151
    risk stratification, 151, 152
    in women, 152, 153
Atypical lobular hyperplasia (ALH), 6–7, 23, 24, 54, 79, 81, 85, 130

B
Benign breast lesions, 59
Bilateral prophylactic mastectomy (BPM), 149–153
    advantages, 148, 149
    atypical hyperplasia
        ADH, 149

        ALH, 149
        FEA, 150
        long-term risk, 150, 151
        risk stratification, 151, 152
        in women, 152, 153
    indications, 149
    risk reduction, 148
Bodian model, 106
Breast cancer risk, 103–110
    atypical hyperplasia
        chemoprevention, 110
        cumulative risk, 108, 109
        DCIS, 110
        extent of disease, 109
        family history, 109
        FEA, 111
        Gail model, 110
        invasive breast cancer, 107
        pateint age, 108–109
        types, 107, 108
        Tyrer-Cuzick model, 110
    LCIS, 104, 106
        Bodian model, 106
        chemoprevention, 105, 106
        cumulative risk, 104
        extent of disease, 105
        family history, 105
        ILC, 103
        patient age, 105
        pleomorphic LCIS, 106, 107
        Tyrer-Cuzick model, 106
Breast cancer surgery (BCS), 43
Breast-conserving surgery (BCS)
    low-risk DCIS, 178, 179
    randomized controlled trials, 174, 177, 178
    recurrence, 174
Breast Imaging-Reporting and Data System (BI-RADS) classification, 51
Breast-specific gamma imaging (BSGI), 125

C

Chemoprevention, 130, 131, 133–135, 139–141
    AI, 135
    AMP kinase pathway, 136
    anastrozole, 135, 136
    atypia, 129–130
    best risk/benefit ratio, 137
    clinical practice guidelines, 138
    diabetic medications, 136
    exemestane, 135
    health benefits, 137
    history, 130
    IGF-1, 136
    LCIS, 27–29
    metformin, 136
    NSAIDS, 136
    patient selection, 138
    prevention medications
        adherence, 141
        LCIS population, 139
        meta-analyses, 139
        non-trial setting, 139
        positive predictors of uptake, 139
        practicing clinicians, 140
        prevention agent selection, 139, 140
        risk of, 137–138
    Raloxifene, 132–134
    risk determination, 138
    SERM
        antiestrogen drugs, 130
        Arzoxifene, 134, 135
        ER, 131
        Lasofoxifene, 133, 134
        osteoporosis and fractures, 131
    Tamoxifen, 131, 132
Class lobular carcinoma in situ (CLIS), 90–92
Comparative genomic hybridization (CGH), 30–31, 40
Comparison of Operative to Monitoring and Endocrine Therapy (COMET), 165
Complex sclerosing lesion (CSL)
    atypical hyperplasia/breast carcinima, 57
    clinical symptoms, 56
    imaging characteristics, 56
    immunohistochemical stains, 56
    non-radial configuration, 55, 56
Contralateral prophylactic mastectomy (CPM), 179
Contrast-enhanced digital mammography (CEDM), 120, 121
Contrast-enhanced tomosynthesis (CET), 120, 121
Core needle biopsy (CNB), 66, 129
Cyclooxygenase 2 (COX-2) inhibition, 136

D

Deep vein thrombosis (DVT), 137
Digital breast tomosynthesis (DBT), 115, 119, 120
Distinguish from ductal carcinoma in situ (DCIS), 79
Ductal carcinoma in situ (DCIS), 42, 43, 174
    abnormal lesion/calcifications, 38
    amplification rates, 40
    BCS, 171
    benign breast disease, 40
    clinical outcome, 166
    clustered calcifications, 38
    comedonecrosis, 183
    endocrine therapy, 162–164
    ER expression, 41
    ER-negative comedo specimen, 39
    ER-positive specimens, 39
    field cancerization, 41
    future prospective, 167
    history, 38, 159, 160, 171, 172
    invasive carcinoma, 41
    K14, ARF6, and miR-10b, 39
    loss of 11q, 40
    management, 160
    margins, 181, 182
    mastectomy, 172, 173
    Memorial Sloan Kettering Cancer Center, 184–186
    method of detection, 181
    mortality, 44
    neoadjuvant therapy, 164
    non-genetic drivers, 40
    nonsurgical approaches, 166
    nonsurgical management, 164
    normal cells, 38
    nuclear grade, 38, 182, 183
    Oncotype DX Breast DCIS Score, 185, 187
    preoperative diagnosis, 41
    progressive changes, 39
    radiation therapy, 160–162
    recurrence
        accurate prediction, 43
        decision score, 43
        minimal-volume disease, 42
        molecular variables, 43
        patient outcomes, 42
        radiotherapy interaction, 43
        rate of, 42
        surgery and radiation, 42
    risk factors, 37
    surgical resection, 179
    survival benefit, 44, 45
    therapy, delay in, 182
    untreated results, 40
    USC/VNPI, 184

Index

E
Early Breast Cancer Trialists' Collaborative Group (EBCTCG), 160
Eastern Cooperative Oncology Group (ECOG), 42
E-cadherin staining, 91, 92
Endometrial cancer, 132
Estrogen receptor (ER), 23
    blockade, 130
    breast cancer cure, 130
    ERα, 131
    ERβ, 131
    normal uterine and bone tissue, 130
    Tamoxifen, 131

F
FEA, *see* Flat epithelial atypia
Fibroadenoma
    African-American women *vs.* Caucasians, 64
    diagnosis, 64
    imaging findings, 64–65
    incidence, 64
    management, 68
    non-palpable masses, 64
    normal-risk population, 68
    pathologic examination, 66–68
    physical examination, 64
    resection, 68
Fibroepithelial lesions, 64–74
    benign and malignant lesions, 63
    fibroadenoma
        African-American women *vs.* Caucasians, 64
        diagnosis, 64
        imaging findings, 64–65
        incidence, 64
        management, 68
        non-palpable masses, 64
        normal-risk population, 68
        pathologic examination, 66–68
        physical examination, 64
        resection, 68
    PASH
        imaging modalities, 69
        management, 70
        pathologic findings, 69, 70
        pre- and perimenopausal women, 68
        progesterone receptor expression, 69
        recurrences, 71
        slow-growing mass, 69
    phyllodes tumors
        clinical presentation, 71
        histology, 71
        imaging, 71
        malignant tumors, 71
        management, 73–74
        pathologic analysis, 72, 73
        population-based study, 71
        prognosis, 74
Fine-needle aspiration cytology (FNAC), 66
Flat epithelial atypia (FEA), 5, 111, 150
    definition, 57
    dilated acini and intraluminal calcifications, 58
    mammography, 58
    molecular evidence, 59
    pathologic evidence, 59
    reported upgrade rates, 58
    risk of, 59
    TBCRC 034 study, 58
    TDLUs, 58
Full-field digital mammogram (FFDM), 120

G
Gail model, 110

H
Hormonal receptors expression (HER), 93, 94
Hormone replacement therapy (HRT), 26

I
Inhibiting the insulin-like growth factor 1 (IGF-1), 136
Intermediate risk, 116
International Breast Cancer Intervention Study (IBIS-I) trial, 27, 132
International Breast Cancer Intervention Study II (IBIS-II) trial, 135
Intraductal papillomas
    ADH, 52, 53
    atypical papillomas, 54
    benign solitary papilloma, 54
    calcifications, 52, 53
    chemoprevention trials, 55
    classification, 52
    clinical decision-making, 54
    example, 54
    fibrovascular stalks, 52
    immunohistochemical stains, 52
    Mayo Clinic Surgical Index, 55
    meta-analysis, 52
    multiple papillomas, 54
    palpable mass, 52
    palpable papillomas, 54
    pathologic nipple discharge, 52
    Pathology Index, 55
    patient counseling challenging, 54
    radiologic-pathologic concordance, 53
    surgical excision, 53
    ultrasound, 52, 53

Invasive lobular carcinoma (ILC), 25, 103
  genomic similarities, 30, 31
  lobular histology, 30
  NSABP B-17 trial, 29

L
Lobular carcinoma in situ (LCIS), 23–26, 29–32, 90–93, 96–99
  bilateral mastectomy, 90
  bilateral risk of future carcinoma, 26
  biopsy, 22
  breast cancer risk, 103
  chemoprevention, 27–29
  contralateral breasts, 27
  evolution, 90
  excisional biopsy, 90
  HER, 93, 94
  histological analysis
    CLIS, 90–92
    florid, 93
    PLCIS, 92, 93
  incidence, 89
  initial surgery, 26
  ipsilateral breasts, 27
  ipsilateral carcinoma
    findings, 29
    ILC, 29–32
  ipsilateral vs. contralateral invasive breast cancer, 90
  LN
    clinical presentation, 25
    cytologic features, 23–25
    histologic findings, 23
    SEER database, 26
  malignant progression, 22
  management
    chemoprevention, 96, 97
    incidence, 98, 99
    pleomorphic LCIS, 98
    surgical intervention, 97, 98
    surveillance, 96
  pLCIS, 32
  risk factor and non-obligate precursor, 32
  upgrade rates, 94–96
  WHO, 89
Lobular neoplasia (LN)
  clinical presentation, 25
  cytologic features, 23–25
  histologic findings, 23
  SEER database, 26
LOw-RISk DCIS (LORIS) trial, 165, 178–179
LOw-Risk DCIS with Endocrine Therapy Alone– TAmoxifen (LORETTA) trial, 165

M
Magnetic resonance imaging (MRI), 38, 69, 72, 81, 83, 84, 96, 121–123, 125, 164
Mammogram, 38, 65, 177, 178
Mediator complex subunit 12 (MED12), 10
Memorial Sloan Kettering Cancer Center, 184–186
Molecular breast imaging (MBI), 125
Multiple Outcomes of Raloxifene Evaluation (MORE) trial, 133

N
National Surgical Adjuvant Breast and Bowel Project (NSABP) B-17 study, 27
NCIC Clinical Trials Group mammary Prevention.3 trial (NCIC CTG MAP.3), 135
Nonsteroidal anti-inflammatories (NSAIDS), 136

O
Oncotype DX Breast DCIS Score, 185, 187

P
PASH, see Pseudoangiomatous stromal hyperplasia (PASH)
Patient Centered Outcomes Research Institute (PCORI), 165
Per National Comprehensive Cancer Network (NCCN), 73
Phyllodes tumors (PT)
  clinical presentation, 71
  histology, 71
  imaging, 71
  malignant tumors, 71
  management, 73–74
  pathologic analysis, 72, 73
  population-based study, 71
  prognosis, 74
Pleomorphic lobular carcinoma in situ (PLCIS), 24, 32, 92, 93
"Popcorn"-like calcifications, 65
Positive predictive value (PPV), 124–125
Positron emission mammography (PEM), 125
Positron emission tomography (PET), 125
Postmenopausal Evaluation and Risk-Reduction with Lasofoxifene (PEARL) trial, 134
Progesterone receptor (PR) positive, 23

Index

Prophylactic mastectomy, *see* Bilateral prophylactic mastectomy (BPM)
Pseudoangiomatous stromal hyperplasia (PASH)
   imaging modalities, 69
   management, 70
   pathologic findings, 69, 70
   pre- and perimenopausal women, 68
   progesterone receptor expression, 69
   recurrences, 71
   slow-growing mass, 69
Pulmonary embolism (PE), 137

R

Radial scar
   architectural distortion, 55
   atypical hyperplasia/breast carcinima, 57
   biopsy specimen, 55
   BI-RADS classification, 56
   case-control study, 57
   clinical symptoms, 56
   concordance, 56
   imaging characteristics, 56
   obliterated ducts and acini, 55
   post-core biopsy mammogram, 56
   radiologic-pathologic concordance, 56
   risk of, 57
   vacuum-assisted device, 56
Risk lesions, 11
   ADH, 6
   ALH, 6
   clinical and histologic factors, 7
   clinical implications, 2
   DCIS, 3
   ER-negative neoplasia pathway, 4
   ER-positive neoplasia pathway, 4
   FEA, 5
   fibroepithelial lesions, 10
   gene expression profiling studies, 3
   genetic information, 3
   malignant potential, 1
   overall survival, 11, 12
   papillary lesions, 9
   precancerous lesions, 3
   radial scars, 8
   relative risks, 2

S

Screening mammography
   ACR, 116
   CEDM, 120, 121
   CET, 120, 121
   DBT, 119, 120
   sensitivity, 117
Selective estrogen receptor modulators (SERM)
   antiestrogen drugs, 130
   Arzoxifene, 134, 135
   ER, 131
   Lasofoxifene, 133, 134
   LCIS, 27
   osteoporosis and fractures, 131
Somatomedin C, 136
Study of Tamoxifen and Raloxifene (STAR) trial, 28, 133
Surveillance, Epidemiology, and End Results (SEER) database, 26, 44

T

Terminal duct lobular units (TLDUs), 80, 150
Translational Breast Cancer Research Consortium (TBCRC), 54
Tyrer-Cuzick model, 106, 110, 116, 138

U

Ultrasound, 52, 56, 64, 69, 72, 84, 123, 125
Unfolded lobules (ULs), 80
University of Southern California (USC)/Van Nuys Prognostic Index (VNPI), 184

V

Venous thromboembolism, 137, 148

W

World Health Organization (WHO) classification, 73, 89, 150

X

XRT, 44, 45, 140

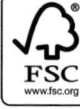

If you have any concerns about our products,
you can contact us on
ProductSafety@springernature.com

In case Publisher is established outside the EU,
the EU authorized representative is:
**Springer Nature Customer Service Center GmbH
Europaplatz 3, 69115 Heidelberg, Germany**

Printed by Libri Plureos GmbH
in Hamburg, Germany